"*Crisis and Contagion* supplies an intriguing addition to the growing critical literature on Covid-19. Assembling interviews and commentaries from a host of interdisciplinary thinkers, the volume examines how converging systemic factors have shaped the global coronavirus pandemic, engendering myriad forms of harm as well as new opportunities for resistance. The book's call for a 'revived and reimagined Left' to confront these challenges could not be more timely."

MARTHA LINCOLN, PhD, associate professor, Department of Anthropology, San Francisco State University, author of *Epidemic Politics in Contemporary Vietnam: Public Health and the State*

"The Covid-19 pandemic exposed how health inequities follow the fault lines of societal injustices. SARS-CoV-2 was the virus that wreaked havoc around the world, but the crisis of our times remains capitalism. In *Crisis and Contagion*, scholars, journalists, and activists call for an end to the neoliberal capitalist violence that wages war against life on earth. They remind us that our grief and rage can be marshalled for transformative action through social movements rooted in global solidarity. Indeed, collective resistance struggles that nurture just and caring societies are not only possible, but illuminate our way forward."

SAMIR SHAHEEN-HUSSAIN, MD, author of *Fighting for A Hand to Hold: Confronting Medical Colonialism against Indigenous Children in Canada*

"This expansive collection draws connections between capitalist and imperialist exploitation, inequality, environmental crisis, and the unequal impact of disease in an unjust and vulnerable world. From the late Mike Davis' humanity and intelligence, to Merlin Chowkwanyun's insight into history, race, and the power of the local, these interviews present astute thinkers from the broad political Left seeking to understand a global disease event—even as they lived it. *Crisis and Contagion* is essential reading for the historically conscious."

ESYLLT JONES, author of *Radical Medicine: The International Origins of Socialized Health Care in Canada*

"Covid-19 was not a one-off public health emergency, but a full-blown crisis triggered by internal contradictions within capitalism. In this provocative and often dazzling collection of interviews, the underlying link between the pandemic and capitalism is meticulously exposed, assiduously dissected, and scrupulously scrutinized."

VITTORIO BUFACCHI, Department of Philosophy, University College Cork, Ireland, author of *Everything Must Change: Philosophical Lessons from Lockdown*

CRISIS AND CONTAGION

CRISIS AND CONTAGION

Conversations on Capitalism and Covid-19

Edited by Ian McKay

Between the Lines
Toronto

Crisis and Contagion
© 2023 Ian McKay

First published in 2023 by
Between the Lines
401 Richmond Street West, Studio 281
Toronto, Ontario · M5V 3A8 · Canada
1-800-718-7201 · www.btlbooks.com

All rights reserved. No part of this publication may be photocopied, reproduced, stored in a retrieval system, or transmitted in any form or by any means, electronic, mechanical, recording, or otherwise, without the written permission of Between the Lines, or (for copying in Canada only) Access Copyright, 69 Yonge Street, Suite 1100, Toronto, ON M5E 1K3.

Every reasonable effort has been made to identify copyright holders. Between the Lines would be pleased to have any errors or omissions brought to its attention.

Library and Archives Canada Cataloguing in Publication
Title: Crisis and contagion : conversations on capitalism and Covid-19 / edited by Ian McKay. Other titles: Syndemic magazine
Names: McKay, Ian, 1953- editor.
Description: Essays previously published in Syndemic Magazine. | Includes index.
Identifiers: Canadiana (print) 20230491839 | Canadiana (ebook) 2023049188X | ISBN 9781771136396 (softcover) | ISBN 9781771136402 (EPUB)
Subjects: LCSH: COVID-19 Pandemic, 2020- —Economic aspects. | LCSH: COVID-19 Pandemic, 2020- —Social aspects. | LCSH: Capitalism—History—21st century. | LCSH: Economic history—21st century. | LCSH: Income distribution—History—21st century. | LCSH: Equality—History—21st century. | LCSH: Social conflict—History—21st century.
Classification: LCC HC59.3 .C75 2023 | DDC 330.9/052—dc23

Cover and text design by DEEVE

Printed in Canada

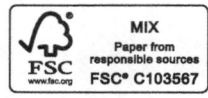 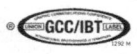

We acknowledge for their financial support of our publishing activities: the Government of Canada; the Canada Council for the Arts; and the Government of Ontario through the Ontario Arts Council, the Ontario Book Publishers Tax Credit program, and Ontario Creates.

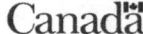 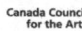 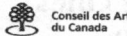 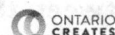 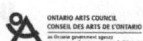 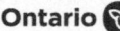

 For their financial support of this book we also thank the Future of Canada Project at McMaster University, administered by the Wilson Institute for Canadian History.

CONTENTS

Acknowledgements / ix

Introduction / 1

PART ONE
THE ORGANIC CRISIS OF NEOLIBERAL CAPITALISM

Nancy Fraser / 15

Mike Davis / 39

Mack Penner / 59

Andreas Malm / 83

Merrill Singer / 103

PART TWO
SACRIFICING THE SUBALTERNS

Nora Loreto / 123

Tithi Bhattacharya / 145

Chandrima Chakraborty / 161

Merlin Chowkwanyun / 173

Sanjay Nepal / 195

PART THREE
CHOPPY WATERS AHEAD

J. Michael Ryan / 213

Laura Spinney / 235

Naomi Klein / 247

Noam Chomsky / 263

Notes / 289

Index / 301

ACKNOWLEDGEMENTS

The pandemic has functioned as a prism—one that has compelled us to acknowledge its underlying causes and core contradictions—and our contributors, coming from distinctive intellectual and political locations, have all told us important new things about the persisting social system shaping our lives. We owe them our deepest thanks.

The funding for *Syndemic Magazine*, from which this book emerges, was provided by the Future of Canada Project at McMaster University, and much invaluable support was also extended by the university's Faculty of Humanities. I should also like to emphasize the collective work that made the project possible, with Samantha Clarke, Brandon Cordeiro, Ed Dunsworth, Eric MacPherson, Sarah Spike, and Sarah Whitwell all making invaluable contributions. Max Dagenais (then of the Wilson Institute) did much of the initial organizing for the series and Colin Czernada of the Faculty of Humanities was instrumental in guiding us through technical issues. Henry Giroux of McMaster cohosted and made possible our event with Noam Chomsky. Ann Herring and Susan Ferguson added their voices to the sessions with Merrill Singer and Tithi Bhattacharya, respectively. And none of it would have been possible without the IT savvy of my husband, Robert Vanderheyden.

INTRODUCTION

After more than three years, it still seems unbelievable: an entity so tiny its very existence was disputed until the 1930s—no bigger than 80–120 nanometres large (with a nanometre being a billionth of a metre)—brought much of the machinery of the capitalist world economy to a grinding halt, with millions urged to stay home, hospitals overwhelmed, and even in rich places like the US, the UK, and Europe, the loss of hundreds of thousands of people's lives. All because a contaminant had entered that world unannounced. One estimate contends that all the viruses that made Covid-19 such a life-altering and world-changing development could collectively fit into one Coke can.[1] One was asked to believe that invisible particles of the "coronavirus" (so named because its appearance under an electron microscope suggests a crown or perhaps a solar eclipse) were effecting visible, tangible differences, and that these particles could mutate, time and again, even though many authorities do not consider them to be alive at all. And one was expected "to reimagine activities that one once engaged in without a second's thought as ones that be fraught with invisible danger."[2] One encounter, perhaps, between one animal and another—likely a bat and a human being, with an intermediate species possibly in the mix—has led to convulsions throughout the world, Antarctica not excepted. Yet, on closer inspection, that a random ("stochastic") occurrence could have this impact on a world system tells us a lot about a system "markedly unprepared for its own blowback," whose rulers have for generations followed a playbook of facilitating its terraforming of the planet to serve the needs of profit-seekers.[3] Both that system's unexpected and acute weakness and its bizarre and irrational hold over our minds are unbelievable too.

In 2022, the Wilson Institute at McMaster University launched *Syndemic Magazine*, focused on the Covid-19 pandemic, to probe this unbelievable time.[4] It was a name we borrowed from Dr. Richard Horton of *The Lancet*, one of the world's most prestigious medical journals, who used it to suggest that the worldwide outbreak combined three elements: "the virus, the chronic conditions that make people more susceptible to it, and a situation of deepening poverty and inequality."[5] For medical anthropologist Merrill Singer, who invented the term in the 1990s (and discusses it here in chapter 5), the term describes various "disease-disease interactions caused, exacerbated, or intensified by adverse social conditions and environments."[6] For scholars interested in the wider social, cultural, and historical implications of Covid-19, and convinced they could only be grasped in a holistic and transnational context, the term, and the critical medical anthropology associated with it, opened a new vista onto our crisis-ridden world.

Over the six issues of *Syndemic*, from February to August, we attracted participants from around the world. The first issue examined neoliberalism and its implications for Covid-19 and contained essays from Mica Jorgenson on the environmental crisis and from Matt Sparke and Lucia Vitale on neoliberal capitalism as a "co-pathogenic driver" of Covid-19.[7] The second examined class, with essays from Ed Dunsworth, Nausheen Quayyum, Ranabir Sammadar, and Ethel Tungohan.[8] In April, *Syndemic* looked at "Gender and the Pandemic," with articles by Jennifer Wallace, Heather Howard-Bobiwash, Paige Castsellanos, Carolyn E. Sachs, and Ann R. Tickamyer.[9] The following month, *Syndemic* examined race and Covid-19, with contributions from Sarah Whitwell, Angela Mashford-Pringle, Sandria Green-Stewart, and Brandon Cordeiro.[10] In June, *Syndemic* looked at mass tourism, with contributions from Edward MacDonald, Karen Dubinsky, Luc Renauld, and Ligia Simba-Bolaños.[11] Finally, in summer 2022, we wrapped up this series of *Syndemic* with an issue focused on "Imagining and Remembering the Pandemic," with pieces from Brandon Cordeiro and Zachary Loeb.[12] Included in most issues were book reviews and summary "endnotes" by the editor. For anyone interested in the unfolding of Covid-19, *Syndemic* should be a valuable source of information and commentary.

This selection from *Syndemic* highlights another feature of the magazine: its interviews with leading authorities. Many of these interviews were public events and widely attended (virtually, on Zoom, since in-person gatherings were not possible during Covid-19). Some drew quite select crowds (with twenty participants or so); others found much larger audiences (with the most-attended session topping, as of November 2022, 130,000 viewers on YouTube).[13] Those interviewed ranged widely in gender, nationality, race/ethnicity, age (from twenty-somethings to ninety-somethings), and occupation (with activists, journalists, and freelance writers rubbing shoulders with professors and students). They also vary in their politics, with a good sampling of centrists and liberals jostling with those further to the left. Not all the interviews could be included in this collection, and readers are encouraged to explore the *Syndemic* site to find those that regretfully had to be left out for reasons of space.[14]

The fourteen interviews we have included can all be read independently but, to my eye, five themes tie them all together. The first is that neoliberal capitalism, whose intellectual history is distilled here by Mack Penner (chapter 3), has entered a period of profound crisis. For Nancy Fraser (chapter 1), this world system and civilization has been engulfed by a "perfect storm," potentially overshadowing those of the 1930s and 1970s. As a system, capitalism, although entailing by definition the market exchange of commodities with intrinsically different properties yet rendered equivalent through their translation into money values, could not persist were it fairly to pay for all the goods and services it acquires *gratis*. Through imperialism, western capitalists were able to seize vast lands, enslave large populations, and commandeer unending streams of natural resources from the colonized world, activities that bore more resemblance to looting and pillage than to the orderly exchange of equivalents. Through their command of public power, capitalists were also able to enshrine their property rights in law, and contrary to much of their talk, they have actually relied intensively upon the state (for such things as a stable money supply, publicly funded infrastructure, trained workforces, probusiness tariff policies, and a ready market, especially with respect to armaments). Capitalism also presupposes great reserves of energy, material inputs, and natural "sinks" for its waste, as well as a habitable planet, fertile fields, and resource-rich seas, all of which are regarded as "there for the taking and infinitely self-regenerating." And, of particular interest to feminists, a capitalist economy relies on the care work, disproportionately carried out by women, without which it would lack for workers capable of producing the commodities upon which it relies. For Fraser—and for Penner, Mike Davis, Andreas Malm, Noam Chomsky, and Naomi Klein (chapters 2, 4, 14, and 13, respectively), whose critique of the "shock doctrine" has been borne out by the strident reassertion of the politics of austerity in the wake of the pandemic[15]—these intricate arrangements, already riven with contradictions, have all become highly problematic, as Covid-19 has revealed so dramatically.

Some of these contradictions are similar to those driving earlier crises. By expropriating the surplus-value generated by workers over and above their costs of subsistence, and driven by the logic of competition to invest more and more in fixed capital, capital has a tendency to produce more goods than the producers it exploits can buy. One might imagine capitalists coming to the logical conclusion that they should, in their own collective interest, take a keen interest in righting this imbalance—that might be one reading of the Keynesian revolution in economics in the 1930s—but as Fraser, Malm, and Davis all remind us, such a "logical capitalism" is almost a contradiction in terms. For Chomsky, what we see in the 2020s is very much a continuation of capital's long-standing class conflict against workers and other producers. The drive to find cheaper and cheaper sources of labour and materials, even at the cost of destroying long-established industrial communities, derives in large part from the chaotically competitive nature of the system. While it might seem absurd to imagine a world in which industrial tasks are performed by robots, leaving the workers who once did that work in situations of desperate precarity and unable to purchase the very goods they used to produce, such automation might make perfect sense to an individual capitalist trying to beat competitors. And while it might also seem crazy to rob much of the Global South of its resources and drive many of its young people into desperate northward journeys, many now ending tragically in the Mediterranean or on the US border, it would not seem so to an individual investor with an eye on the bottom line and keen to obtain cheap inputs in the form of labour and materials. Especially since the 1970s, with the rise of neoliberalism and its misnamed "Free Trade Agreements," the entire planet has been targeted by a vast profit-making and transnational "megamachine," to use Fabian Scheidler's expression—a tightly integrated system geared to profit-making.[16] Some of the authors in this collection hope for more rational forms of our capitalist order, but it would be fair to say a skepticism of capitalism is a predominant motif within it.

The climate crisis, to broach the second unifying theme, is seen by many of the authors to be directly connected to the pandemic.

According to the "metabolic rift" thesis, capitalist property relations are disrupting flows "between humans and the rest of nature or within extra-human nature" (as Malm puts it). If some indications of that rift can be found in precapitalist times—deforestation in some areas was the flip side of the military might of the Roman Empire, for example—until the eighteenth century one could still realistically paint a general picture of humanity living within natural boundaries it could influence but not, finally, control. The coming of fossil capital—exploiting first coal, then oil and gas—qualitatively changed that pattern of living. By exploiting fossil fuels, capitalists could use "solar energy that had been preserved underground for millions of years," allowing "production to break through the limitations of wind, water, and muscle," in the words of ecological analyst Ian Angus.[17] The Second World War marked a second phase in the development of this rift, with the fabled "trente glorieuses" (c. 1945–1975) sending most metrics of planetary environmental upwards. With the advent of no-holds-barred capitalism under neoliberalism, those patterns intensified and the curves shot through the roof. By the 2020s, it has become apparent that such "natural" phenomena as hurricanes, forest fires, droughts, floods, and species extinctions are all connected to humankind's profit-driven project of planetary transformation in ways that place the continued existence of the species in danger. Yet, as Klein remarks, the only thing rising faster than our emissions of CO_2 is the output of words pledging to lower them.

Many of the authors in this collection would add "pandemics" to that list of calamities with the argument that global climate change, unchecked deforestation, and commercial agriculture, all accelerated by fossil capital, are disrupting the habitats of pathogen-carrying animals, who are then driven into new zones to survive. (Relatedly, some of those pathogens will breach the boundaries of the "gated communities" of pigs, chickens, and cows, factory farms that played a significant role in past pandemics—although, with the exception of mink farms in Europe, it seems they played a lesser role in this one.) First unaware of, and then indifferent to, the ecological consequences of its new capacities, humankind has been playing with fire. Covid-19 is, in large measure, the unhappy result—and it will be followed by many more "zoonoses" (i.e., diseases spreading from animals to humans).

Yet, of course, "humankind" implies some degree of common purpose and collective interest among human beings. In a capitalist society, such unifiers are undercut by contradictory purposes and irreconcilable interests—a third theme of this volume. The pandemic revealed how starkly class-divided human civilization has become. The initiatives of powerful human beings—cutting roads through jungles, opening mines, pumping cows full of antibiotics, raising interest rates, waging wars liable to kill millions if not billions—have consequences for those they rule over and actively disempower. Subaltern groups, the *classi subalterne*, "are always subject to the initiatives of the dominant group," even when they "rebel and rise up," even when they have seemingly triumphed. Because they lack political autonomy, are often made up of different races, and generally lack "initiative in the struggle," their history "is necessarily fragmented and episodic."[18] Class is the "underlying magnetic field of politics," and other subaltern identities—founded on religion, race, gender, nation, or region, none of which should be minimized—are often ways "in which class struggle comes to be organized at the level of civil society."[19] A defining characteristic of subalternity is "living in a world where the dominant scripts on offer have not been written by people like you," writes anthropologist Kate Crehan.[20] For Italian writer Antonio Gramsci, whose work we have been quoting, subalterns' understandings of reality tend to "common sense," a phrase that in English has a more positive connotation than it has in Italian. Gramsci means by it that subalterns are often unconscious of, or resistant to, ways of understanding their social world that go beyond a hodgepodge of superstitions, folkloristic beliefs, and "crudely . . . conservative sentiments."[21] As Davis suggests in this volume, and Pat Armstrong and André Picard revealed in their interviews with *Syndemic Magazine*,[22] some of the most sorely oppressed subalterns in 2020–23 were the senior citizens trapped in institutions (a.k.a. long-term-care facilities, old folks' homes, aged-care centres, *Pflegeheimen*, *maisons de retraite*, or *case di riposo*), a good many of them dying alone, some of thirst or starvation, lying in their own excrement, helpless and frightened. On the bright side, the corporations owning many of their institutions made handsome profits.

Such enormities of 2020–23 have seemingly generated no powerful movements to put an end to them. It is "common sense" that unelected plutocrats should be in charge of space travel and mass communication, that rivers should be turned to sludge and mountains levelled, that the poor and precarious must work so the system exploiting them can endure. And it is common sense that entrepreneurs have every right to squeeze profits from the bodies of the elderly (a process deemed not just legitimate but necessary, since neoliberalism provides us with a master key, a logic of rule, that should be extended to every sphere).

At the other end of the generational spectrum we find many questioning young people, already penalized by more than two years of school closures and physical distancing. They are re-entering a world of overburdened hospitals and disappearing social safety nets. Some of them are burdened with compromised immune systems. Their generation is forced to respond not just to the ongoing Covid-19 pandemic but to RSV, Strep A, and Long Covid—a crisis-ridden world whose transformation is a life-or-death proposition for them. Tithi Batthacharya (chapter 7) and Fraser underscore the role of the many women who are expected to do most of the work of care, much of it unpaid and unrecognized, without which our system could not socially reproduce itself. Such caregivers can also be numbered among the subalterns. Racialized minorities, often deliberately slotted into inferior positions in the profit-making megamachine, have uniquely suffered through the pandemic—as Chandrima Chakroborty (chapter 8) and Merlin Chowkwanyun (chapter 9) suggest—not because of any intrinsic biological deficiencies, but rather because they are called upon by the megamachine to perform particular subordinate functions rendering them directly exposed to the virus. Through much of the Global South, transnational tourism has left some poor but picturesque countries at the mercy of the fickle enthusiasms of those rich enough to visit them, as Sanjay Nepal (chapter 10) points out. Sexual minorities too have experienced their own version of Covid-19, as Nora Loreto (chapter 6) reminds us, as many of their centres of sociability and life-giving medications were disrupted (sometimes deliberately), and they were routinely if illogically scapegoated by spokespeople for the major monotheistic religions.

On the world scale, the metropoles of the Global North have helped themselves to the lion's share of vaccines, leaving vast numbers in the Global South unprotected, in an almost caricatural re-enactment of the harshest realities of nineteenth-century imperialism. Yet, as some of the authors suggest, and as an ever-growing mountain of evidence about global inequalities of wealth confirms, to some extent a levelling process is at work in the contemporary crisis, which, as Klein observes, threatens to turn the world as a whole into an environmental "sacrifice zone." Living in a "rich country" no longer means much for people routinely denied access to health care, living in deliberately deindustrialized communities without even modest guarantees of security—and, if they are undocumented workers, even those doing the "essential" work without which society could not function, all the while at the mercy of deportation regimes.

Gramsci offers us no magic formula for how all the subalterns cast in inferior positions by the master scripts of capitalism can be united. Yet, he does insist that we remember how *relational* classes are with respect to each other—there can be no aristocrats without serfs, no factory owners without workers.[23] Building on that insight, some reimagine the working class as a social force extending far beyond the workplace. While Gramsci never doubted that it was primarily up to wage workers to change society, partly because they alone are in a functional position to do so, they can only pull that off by interacting intelligently with those whose social interests could be related to their own. All such alliance-building among the unpropertied was bound to arouse fierce opposition from the propertied, suggesting as it did not just a more equitable division of wealth but, potentially, a rethinking of the very social system itself.

Today, the very conceptualization of class issues (to follow a suggestion by Bhattacharya) may be shifting: no longer centred strictly on workplace struggles (with those of Amazon workers deservedly prominent in 2020–23),[24] a new politics of class could address each of the major subaltern groups by reminding them of their common interest in the survival of the species. If such an alliance for people's struggle is ever to take shape, it will require new media, because as Loreto reveals, both corporate and the largely misnamed "social" media are allergic to approaches going beyond their individualistic practices and applied philosophies.

A fourth theme in this volume is the emerging conflict over the memory of Covid-19 and its future commemoration. In the conventional view, drilled home in countless editorials and think pieces, Covid-19 was a "once-in-a-lifetime" happening, paralleled only by the Great Influenza Epidemic of 1918–20 (popularly misnamed the "Spanish Flu"). Covid-19, it was said, was a serendipitous ("Black Swan") event. As Kate Winslet, playing the part of a scientist in *Contagion* (2011) puts it, "Somewhere in the world, the wrong pig met up with the wrong bat"[25]—or, perhaps in this case, the wrong pangolin, mink, ferret, snake, turtle, or white-tailed deer (the question of the intermediate species the virus might have travelled en route from bat to human is still unsettled).[26] This emphasis on Covid-19 as a peculiar and unanticipated "one-off" might be expected in societies whose leaders have long advised them that things are getting better and better thanks (naturally) to the perspicacity of those very same leaders. Certainly many citizens of rich countries had come to think that plagues were passé[27]—or at least that infectious diseases were henceforth to be confined to poor countries and poor people.

Others fit Covid-19 into patterns both primordial (humans have always contended with viruses, which have even shaped our DNA) and perennial (three or so times per century, such pandemics break out). Both lines of interpretation have their strengths. Still, those persuaded by the metabolic rift position suggest that by reassuringly minimizing the extent to which pandemics and neoliberal capitalism have expanded together, such conventional ways of approaching the pandemic are flawed. Granting the continuities in the human/virus relationship, these critical materialists urge us to see that we are now living in a time of its qualitative transformation.

In this line of interpretation, what's missing from many "historical" accounts of Covid-19 (with their relentless return to the Great Influenza Epidemic of 1918–20 as their primary historical reference point) is HIV/AIDS, sweeping the world since 1982 and thus far claiming far more lives than Covid-19. What are also missing are the many other outbreaks—MERS, Ebola, Zika, a succession of bird flus (each of them potentially entailing a far higher butcher's bill than Covid-19)—that have regularly erupted ever since the 1980s. As so many critics pointed out in 2020–23, one could fill a medium-sized library with reports, from the 1990s on, warning about coming epidemics. The locations of outbreaks—West Africa, Southeast Asia, and Latin America—align (as they have aligned since the 1920s) with areas of massive, highly exploitative capitalist colonization of hitherto lightly-touched zones. From this critical perspective, Covid-19 (alongside

HIV/AIDS) is a curtain-opener for an "Age of Pandemics," fuelled ("upstream") by the headlong conversion of the planet into an organic megamachine for the production of profits and ("downstream") disseminated by the unprecedented degrees of human interconnectivity that come with global capitalism, exemplified in the 2020s by the energy-guzzling container ship and the sensation-seeking tourist.

In the mainstream interpretation, Covid-19 can be deemed a "one-off," perhaps a judgment of God and a foreshadowing of Apocalypse or the result of a dastardly experiment by our (racialized) enemies (with China now filling a role once played by Russians and Islamists). In the critical materialist interpretation, by contrast, Covid-19 is better seen as an indication of the ongoing consequences of the species-threatening externalities of the capitalist mode of production. As the "first drafts of history" take shape—in the form of memoirs, polemics, opinion pieces, social science articles, and so on—the first interpretation, aligned with the individualist biases of our social and political order, will be privileged. And this "Whig Version of History" will likely prevail if there are no more mass pandemics, the climate emergency fades away, and enlightened leaders do develop a rational plan to close the metabolic rift and together devise a more stable future for humanity. If all these developments unfold, Covid-19 will be remembered, perhaps, as a minor bump in the road taking us to the ever-more-managed and profitable future imagined by *The Economist* and its countless disciples.

Unfortunately, such a liberal utopia, never very plausible to begin with in a capitalist world, is a mirage. More world-shaking pandemics are almost certain to follow this one. If humanity is lucky, if the diseases' basic reproductive rate (R_0) is in the ballpark of Covid-19 (i.e., hovering around three), the butcher's bill will be approximate to that of Covid-19 (perhaps a mere twenty million before it becomes endemic—which, we need to remember, still means it will destroy many lives, as does influenza every year). But if humanity is unlucky, that rate, and the case-fatality rate (CFR), could be far higher (as is the case with other zoonotic diseases, including some of the influenzas locally circulating in 2022). In that case, all bets for our species are off. If it is true that zoonotic spill overs affecting humanity are relatively rare, it is also true that, in this perverse game of Russian roulette, we are firing millions of shots every day. Only one or two need to hit the bullseye—and then, absorbed within the planetary megamachine, viruses released from their conventional habitats can once more engulf the world.

Will anyone remember Covid-19? Already in 2023, one senses a strong reluctance to dwell on it. The Great Influenza Epidemic of 1918–20, as Laura Spinney (chapter 12) notes, has gone almost uncommemorated (while there are tens of thousands of monuments to the First World War with which it coincided). The drive to "turn the page" and forget is strong. Schooled to imagine history as a narrative of Great Men Doing Great Things—that is, founding Great Countries and waging Great Wars—we will find it hard to put the events of this pandemic in any such narrative form. If there are heroes to be found in 2020–23, they were often militantly opposed to being considered heroes, and many of them were subalterns—women showing up as PSWs and risking their lives, nurses whose faces were scarred by wearing masks for endless hours in emergency wards, workers doing their jobs in manufacturing, underpaid clerks in grocery stores, gay men fighting for retrovirals in countries hostile to their very existence—who do not normally crowd the pages of our conventional history textbooks.

A fifth and final theme raised by these interviews relates to the pandemic's likely political impact. In the pandemic's first year, leftists hoped that the pandemic's harsh lessons for subalterns of all descriptions might result in their coming together in a united front capable of challenging a transparently self-destructive system. Instead, the radical right, some of it strongly reminiscent of classic fascism (and, in Sweden, Hungary, Italy, Ukraine, Brazil—and India, as Bhattacharya reminds us—drawing quite directly on fascist ideas and symbols) is on the march, attracting to its banners large numbers of discontented people. Added to this turbulence is a new Cold War in which, as before, liberals will find ways to reconcile their ostensible commitment to human rights with strategic and profitable alliances with regimes that routinely violate them.

Leftists, sometimes content to dismiss rightward-tending malcontents as racists, homophobes, xenophobes, sexists, and fanatics—all labels that in conspicuous cases seem quite fitting—are called upon to rethink their own strategies in such a time. They cannot "chide" their way to power, remarks Penner. Some, such as Malm, reflect on the limitations of a left that, over the past four decades and for understandable reasons, has dallied with a libertarian antistatism that is out-of-keeping with a world crisis unresolvable without some global (and scientifically reputable) authority to restrain capital's assault on the planet or, less modestly, to come up with a postcapitalist order founded on different principles. It may be, as Chomsky hints, that a better-managed capitalism is all that can be on the agenda for now, or, following Fraser and Bhattacharya, that a "feminism for the 99%" can achieve some substantial gains even within the system. Yet, if the crisis of that system grows ever deeper and its contradictions more species-threatening, perhaps a revived and reimagined left, reacquainting itself with class realities and the imperative of transforming the state, can once again imagine a different way of life for humanity. There is a lot—humanity itself—at stake.

PART ONE
THE ORGANIC CRISIS OF NEOLIBERAL CAPITALISM

PART ONE

THE ORGANIC CRISIS OF NEOLIBERAL CAPITALISM

AN INTERVIEW WITH

NANCY FRASER

29 OCTOBER 2021

Nancy Fraser has long been a leading progressive feminist thinker for our times and is a renowned figure for all who follow critical theory, socialist feminism, and the ideas of the transnational left. Her books have changed a generation's understanding of the complex past and contested future of global capitalism. Some of her earlier titles are *Justice Interruptus: Critical Reflections On The Post-Socialist Condition* (1997), which examines the impact of neoliberalism on the left; *Fortunes Of Feminism: From State-Managed Capitalism To Neoliberal Crisis* (2013), which charts a transition from redistribution to recognition in feminist thought; and *The Old Order Is Dying And The New Cannot Be Born* (2019), which examines the global ecological, economic, and social breakdown that has undermined any notion that neoliberal capitalism is beneficial for the majority. *Capitalism: A Conversation in Critical Theory* (2018) explores critical theory in a very conversational and accessible way through a conversation with Rahel Jaeggi on how best to conceive and transform the institutionalized social order that is contemporary capitalism.

FRASER: My topic is the "Covid Pandemic: A Perfect Storm of Capitalist Irrationality and Injustice."

We often hear that Covid-19 has lit up all the fault lines of our society, especially fault lines of gender and colour, of nation and class, and that is absolutely true. But I still believe we do not hear enough about the social system that generates those fault lines, even though it's the same social system, I will suggest, that brought us the virus in the first place, and that is blocking our efforts to deal with it.

So, my proposal in this talk is, in effect, to stop tiptoeing around and cut to the chase. What the pandemic really diagnoses, I claim, is the deep-seated dysfunctionality of capitalism. Truth be told, Covid is a "perfect storm" of capitalist irrationality and injustice.

More than anything in recent memory, certainly than anything in my lifetime, it discloses the system's multiple contradictions: ecological, political, social, and economic. All of these contradictions are baked into a social order that incentivizes a profit-hungry class of owners and investors to devour the essential conditions of their own existence, and what's worse, the essential conditions of *our* existence. It incentivizes them, in other words, to guzzle care work, to scarf up nature, to eviscerate public power, to wolf down the wealth of racialized populations, and to suck dry the energy and creativity of all working people.

Those things I just listed are, in my view, essential preconditions of production and accumulation, as well as of life on the planet. And that's precisely the rub. Capitalist society is structured in a way that begs the profit-makers to gobble them up in order to fatten their own share prices, even while it absolves them of any obligation to replenish what they take or to repair what they damage. So, the effect is not only to leave a trail of wreckage across the globe, but . . . also to periodically destabilize the whole jerry-built edifice of capitalist society. That's my diagnosis in a nutshell, and what I want to argue here is that Covid-19 offers a textbook demonstration of this proposition. The pandemic is a switch point where all of capitalism's contradictions converge— where the cannibalization of nature, care work, and political capacity, of peripheralized populations and working classes, merge together in a lethal binge.

Now, to see why, we need to revisit the concept of capitalism. Our received understandings focus too single-mindedly on the system's official economy. They identify the core injustice of capitalist society with the exploitation of free waged workers at the point of commodity production, and they designate the system's defining irrationality as its tendency to precipitate economic crises.

Now, these identifications are not so much wrong as incomplete. Capitalist societies do indeed generate class exploitation and economic crises as a function of their structural dynamics, but they also give rise to additional injustices and irrationalities that are equally structural and serious but that fail to appear on the radar screen of received understandings. These extra economic defects of capitalist society are deeply implicated, I'll try to show, in the present crisis. If we hope to interpret the latter correctly and figure out how to overcome it, we need to develop a new expanded conception of capitalism that foregrounds not just the system's economy but the relation of its economy to its noneconomic conditions of possibility.

So, let me just briefly mention four such noneconomic conditions for the possibility of a capitalist economy. The first is social reproduction, or as many now call it, care work. Included here are all the activities that create, socialize, nurture, sustain, and replenish the human beings who occupy positions in the economy. You can't have a capitalist economy without workers who produce commodities under the aegis of for-profit enterprises. And you can't have them without caregivers who reproduce human beings in settings external to the official economy. Care work includes gestation, birthing, nursing, feeding, bathing, socializing, educating, healing, protecting, solacing—in short, everything essential to sustaining beings (namely us) who are at once biological and social. Now, historically, much of this work has been unwaged and performed by women, often in households, but also in communities, neighbourhoods, and villages, in civil society associations, in public sector agencies, and increasingly, it must be said nowadays, in for-profit firms, including private schools and private nursing homes. But wherever it's done, social reproduction is an indispensable precondition for the production of commodities, for the making of profit, and for the accumulation of capital. Yet, capital goes to very great lengths to avoid paying for care work or, failing that, to pay as little as possible for it. And that is a setup for trouble because capitalist societies incentivize business to free ride on care work with no obligation to replenish it. They entrench a deep-seated tendency to social reproductive crisis as well as a gender order that subordinates women. So, that's number one.

Now, a second precondition for a capitalist economy is ecological. Just as a capitalist economy depends on care work, so too it presupposes the availability of energy to power production, of material substrates including so-called raw materials for labour to transform, and of sinks for absorbing waste. Capital relies, in short, on nature—in the sense, first, of specific substances inputted directly into production; and second, of general environmental conditions such as breathable air, potable water, fertile soil, relatively stable sea levels, and a habitable climate. But here again is the rub: by its very design, capitalist society incentivizes the owners to treat nature as a bottomless trove of noneconomic treasure—there for the taking and infinitely self-regenerating, not needing replenishment or repair. This too, we have finally realized, is a recipe for disaster. Capitalist societies institutionalize a structural tendency to ecological crisis as well as profound disparities in vulnerability to the ensuing fallout.

Now those disparities point to a third condition for the possibility of capitalist accumulation, namely wealth commandeered from subject populations. Almost always racialized, such populations are designated for expropriation as opposed to exploitation. Because they've been deprived of state protection and of actionable rights, their land and labour can be taken without remuneration and funnelled into the circuits of accumulation. Expropriation has often been seen as an early (superseded) feature of a system that piles up wealth by exploiting free workers in factories, but that's a mistake. Capitalist production would not be profitable without an ongoing stream of cheap inputs, including natural resources and unfree or dependent labour confiscated from populations who've been subjected through conquest, enslavement, unequal exchange, incarceration, or predatory debt and who are therefore unable to fight back. It's been said that "Behind Manchester stood Mississippi," meaning that slave labour supplied the cheap raw cotton that fed the iconic textile mills at the dawn of industrialization . . . The same is true today. "Behind Cupertino stands Kinshasa" (Cupertino, the headquarters of Apple; Kinshasa where coltan for iPhones and lithium for Tesla batteries are mined on the cheap, at times by enslaved Congolese children).

In truth, capitalist society is necessarily imperialist, continuously creating defenceless populations for expropriation. Its economy doesn't work if everyone is paid wages that cover their true reproduction costs. It doesn't work, in other words, without a global colour line dividing populations that are merely exploitable from those that are downright expropriable. By institutionalizing that division, capitalism also entrenches imperialism and racial oppression.

There is a fourth background condition for a capitalist economy, namely public power (paradigmatically, but not only, state power). Accumulation cannot proceed, after all, without legal systems that guarantee private property and contractual exchange nor without repressive forces that manage dissent, put down rebellions, and enforce the status hierarchies that enable corporations to expropriate racialized populations at home and abroad. Neither can the system function without public regulations and public goods (including infrastructure of various kinds) and a stable money supply. Indispensable for accumulation, these things cannot be provided through the market but only via the exercise of public power. Capital needs such power. But it is also primed to undermine it—by evading taxes, weakening regulations, offshoring operations, or capturing regulatory agencies. The result is a set of built-in tensions between the economic and the political and a deep-seated tendency to political crisis. On the one hand, capitalist societies tend to produce crises of governance in which the system destroys its own capacity to manage the problems it generates. On the other hand, it also tends periodically to precipitate crises of hegemony in which masses of people defect from politics as usual.

Now, in all four of these cases, capitalist societies, I've been suggesting, institute contradictory relations between economies and [their] noneconomic conditions of possibility. These relations become visible only when we understand capitalism broadly not as a mere economic system but as an institutionalized social order that also includes social reproduction, nature, wealth expropriated from racialized populations, and public power, all of which are essential to accumulation—and yet are depleted and destabilized by it. Viewed this way, capitalism harbours multiple crisis tendencies and structural injustices. Above and beyond its propensity to economic crisis, the system is primed to precipitate social, political, and ecological crises. Above and beyond economic exploitation, it entrenches gender and sexual subordination, racial imperial domination, environmental injustice, and denial of everyone's robust political freedoms. Largely invisible to received understandings, the full range of capitalist injustice and irrationality appears with blazing clarity when we assume the expanded view. That view, I want to suggest, provides the conceptual toolkit we need to parse the present crisis. The Covid-19 pandemic, as I noted before, is a switch point in my interpretation, where all of capitalism's injustices and irrationalities converge, where cannibalization of nature, care work, and the political capacity of peripheralized populations and working classes all merge together in a lethal binge.

Now, I want to take a closer look at Covid-19 and the present conjuncture. Let's consider first nature, which as I just suggested, is the site of the system's ecological contradiction. It was none other than capitalism's cannibalization of that vital support of its own existence and of ours that exposed humans to SARS-CoV-2 in the first place. Long harboured by bats in remote caves, the coronavirus that causes Covid-19 likely made the zoonotic leap to us in 2019 by way of some bridging species. But what brought the bats into contact with that intermediary and the latter into contact with us were the combined effects of global warming on the one hand and tropical deforestation on the other. Now, both of those processes are progeny of capital, driven by its hunger for profit. Together, deforestation and global warming eviscerated the habitats of innumerable species, triggering mass migrations, creating new proximities among previously distanced but now distressed organisms, and promoting novel transfers of pathogens among them. That dynamic has already precipitated a string of viral epidemics, each passed from bats or some other originating species to humans via some amplifying host. We have HIV/AIDS, Nipah, SARS, MERS, Ebola, and now of course Covid-19.

I hate to say it, but you already know it's true: more such pandemics will come. They are the nonaccidental by-products of a social order that puts nature at the mercy of capital [with its inherent incentive to] appropriate biophysical wealth as quickly and cheaply as possible, with no responsibility for repair or replenishment. Those dedicated to amassing profit decimate rainforests and bombard the atmosphere with greenhouse gases. Hell-bent on accumulation in every era but massively empowered by neoliberalism, they have let loose an escalating cascade of lethal plagues.

Now, Covid-19's effects on humans would be horrific under any conditions, but they have been incalculably worsened by another strand of the present crisis rooted in another structural contradiction of capitalist society that has also been sharpened . . . in the neoliberal era. It is, after all, not just nature that capital has cannibalized in this period but also public power. That too, as I suggested before, is an essential ingredient of its diet, avidly consumed in every phase of the system's development but devoured with special ferocity in the last forty years—and that's the catch. The political capacities that financialized capital has gorged on are precisely those we could have used to mitigate the pandemic—but no such luck. Well before the Covid-19 outbreak, most states bowed to the demands of the markets by slashing social spending, including in public health infrastructure and basic research. With a few exceptions, notably Cuba, they drew down stockpiles of life-saving equipment—PPE, ventilator, syringes, medicines test kits, and so on—they gutted diagnostic capacities, they shrank coordination and treatment capacities, closing public hospitals and ICU units. Having eviscerated the public infrastructure, moreover, our rulers devolved vital health care functions to profit-driven providers and insurers, to pharmaceuticals and manufacturers. Now these firms, which are constitutively uninterested in and unconstrained by the public interest, control the lion's share of the world's health-related resources, the labour forces and raw materials, the machinery and production facilities, the supply chains and intellectual property, the research institutions and personnel—all the things that together determine our fates, individual and collective. Committed to preserving their profit streams, they form a private force that blocks concerted public action on behalf of humanity. The effects are tragic but unsurprising: a social system that subjects matters of life-and-death to the law of value was structurally primed from the get-go to abandon untold millions to Covid-19. But that's not all.

The collapse of already weak public systems converged with another structural contradiction of capitalist society centred on social reproduction. Always a staple of capital's consumption, care work has been voraciously gobbled up by it in recent years. The same regime that divested from public health care infrastructure also weakened unions and drove down wages, compelling increased hours of paid work per household, including from primary caregivers. In other words, neo-liberalism offloaded care work onto families and communities at just the moment when it commandeered the social energies we needed to perform it. The effect was to turn capitalism's inherent tendency to destabilize social reproduction into an acute care crunch. Covid-19's advent has intensified this strand of crisis too, dumping major new care chores on families and communities, especially onto women, who still do the lion's share of unpaid care work. Under lockdown, as we know, childcare and schooling shifted into people's homes, leaving parents to take on that burden on top of others in confined domestic spaces ill-suited to those purposes. Many employed women ended up quitting their jobs to care for kids and other relatives, while many others were laid off by employers. Both groups face major losses in position and pay if and when they rejoin the workforce. A third group privileged to keep their jobs and work remotely from home (while also performing care work, including for housebound kids) have had to take multitasking to new heights of craziness. A fourth group, which includes both women and men, bears the honorific "essential workers" but is paid a pittance and treated as disposable—required to brave the threat of infection daily, along with the fear of bringing it home, in order to produce and distribute the stuff that enabled others to shelter in place.

Now in each of these cases, the work of social reproduction (now swollen by the pandemic) still falls largely to women, as it has in every phase of capitalism's history. But which women end up in which category depends on colour and class. So, let's turn now to them. A built-in feature of capitalist society, structural racism infuses every aspect of the current crisis. At the global level it colours the ecological strand, as capital quenches its thirst for cheap nature by seizing land energy and mineral wealth from racialized populations . . . deprived of political protection and actionable rights. Subjected variously to conquest, enslavement, genocide, dispossession by debt, and so on, these populations now bear an undue share of the global environmental load . . . Vulnerable to toxic dumping and so-called natural disasters, and to multiple lethal impacts of global warming, they now find themselves—no surprise—last in line for vaccination. At the national level, meanwhile, race infects the political and social reproductive strands of the crisis, as communities of colour are denied access to conditions that promote health, affordable high quality medical care, clean water, nutritious food, and safe working and living conditions.

So, it's no wonder their members were disproportionately infected and killed by Covid-19. The reasons are not mysterious: poverty and inferior health care; pre-existing medical conditions linked to stress, poor nutrition, exposure to toxins; overrepresentation in front line jobs that could not be performed remotely; lack of resources that would permit them to refuse unsafe work; lack of labour rights that would permit them to win protections; and inferior housing and living arrangements that don't allow for social distancing and that facilitate transmission and diminished access to the vaccine. Together these conditions have expanded the meaning of the slogan Black Lives

Matter, synergizing with its original reference to police violence and helping to fuel ongoing protests.

Colour, of course, is deeply entwined with class in the capitalist world system generally and in the present period particularly. In fact, the two overlapped considerably, as the category "essential worker" shows. If we leave aside medical professionals, that designation covers migrant farm workers, immigrant meatpacking and slaughterhouse workers, Amazon warehouse packers, UPS drivers, nursing home aides, hospital cleaners, supermarket stockers and cashiers, and those who deliver groceries and takeout meals. Especially dangerous in Covid-19 times, these jobs are mostly low-paid, nonunionized, precarious, bereft of benefits and labour protections, and subject to intrusive supervision and relentless speed-up. They are disproportionately filled by women and people of colour. Taken together, these jobs and those who perform them represent the face of the working class in financialized capitalism, no longer epitomized by the figure of the white male miner, factory operative, and construction worker. That class now consists paradigmatically of caregivers and low-wage service workers (paid less than the cost of its reproduction, when paid at all), [and] it is expropriated as well as exploited. Covid-19 has exposed that dirty secret as well. By juxtaposing the essential character of that class's work with capital's systematic undervaluation of it, the pandemic testifies to another major contradiction of capitalist society: the inability of markets in labour-power to accurately reckon the real worth of work.

In general then, Covid-19 is a perfect storm of capitalist irrationality and injustice. By ratcheting up the system's inherent defects to the breaking point, it shines a piercing beam on all the structural contradictions of our society. Dragging them out from the shadows and into the daylight, the pandemic reveals capital's inherent drive to cannibalize nature up to the very brink of planetary conflagration, to divert our capacities away from the truly essential work of social reproduction, to eviscerate public power to the point where it cannot solve the problems the system generates, to feed off the ever-decreasing wealth and health of racialized people, and to not only exploit but also expropriate the working class. We could not ask for a better lesson in social theory. But now comes the hard part: putting that lesson to work in political practice.

MCKAY: Thank you very much Dr. Fraser. I have a few questions I'd like to ask. The first one relates to your theme of crisis. You're really saying that there's a deep-seated tendency to ecological crisis at the very core of the capital system. This is in its DNA. There's a general crisis whose effects metastasize everywhere, shaking confidence in the established worldviews and ruling elites. I thought it was very pertinent that you used a quotation from Antonio Gramsci for one of your most recent books: "The old world is dying, and the new world cannot be born. In this interregnum, a great variety of morbid symptoms appear."[1] Well, few can doubt that we've passed through a world crisis in this pandemic, with manifold *fenomeni morbosi* (morbid phenomena).

But I wonder if there's a risk that crisis talk can, paradoxically, be both overwhelming and underwhelming—both suggesting something so vast that it seems beyond our power to control it (like global climate change) and yet, often, just a way to add juice to journalism (like the contemporary "crisis" afflicting the Montreal Canadiens, for example). In *Capitalism: A Conversation*, you yourself raised the question of the "Boy Who Cried Wolf." And you remark, there's a kind of absurdity in the posture of those who repeatedly announce the imminent collapse of capitalism and meanwhile everything carries on just as before. Are you suggesting, with your metaphor of "the perfect storm," something like Gramsci's organic crisis, a megacrisis combining a host of more particular ones? And could a hostile critic charge you yourself with "crying wolf"?

FRASER: Thank you, Ian, that's a very rich and beautifully formulated question. There are many different parts of it. Let me start with trying to distinguish the kind of loose crisis talk you refer to. (I don't know what's going on in Montreal—but I know that it's meant to be an example of the way people throw around this word.) Let's distinguish loose crisis talk from a critical-theoretical conception of crisis. And here, before we say too much about "crisis," we have to distinguish it from a crisis *tendency*.

In critical theory, and you find this in Marx and in subsequent critical theorists, the idea is that a social system can have built into it tensions or contradictions that incline it to precipitate crises under certain conditions (or absent other countervailing tendencies). The thing is that when these crises erupt (and they don't erupt that often, in my view), their roots lie in the social system itself—in the dynamics as triggered or facilitated by conjunctural developments.

The reason it's important to have this concept of "crisis" in critical theory is that we need it to distinguish between problems that are not deeply anchored in the social system and then can be fixed without a major overhaul of the social system, on the one side, and those that arise precisely as a result of the working out of the dynamics of the social system and might require a more radical fix. As I said in the talk, my view is that capitalism as a system has built into it at least four or five distinct tendencies to crises. That doesn't mean they're always in full flower, and it doesn't mean they always coincide.

Now we get to the part about organic crisis and so on. We should distinguish between a sectoral crisis and a general crisis. A sectoral crisis would be one in which, let's say, one of these crisis tendencies has been sort of rumbling along and piling up dysfunctionalities until there's a real apparent social blockage. You could say that, even though it didn't result in a full-scale collapse, the 2007–08 financial crisis was a sectoral crisis. It gave the appearance of being confined to the terrain of finance, and you might have expected, as I did, that a rational response would have included some major restructuring of how finance works. That didn't happen, and so I suspect there's still a ticking time bomb there, and we might not have heard the last of it. In any case, that's a sectoral crisis.

Now, what would happen, though, if all of the four crisis tendencies that I outlined here were to converge and burst into full flower at once? Then you would have a crisis of the whole social order. I think there have been some of these, but very few. This doesn't happen a lot. So, in other words, this Boy-Who-Cried-Wolf critique would apply if one were saying it's always happening, but I think we shouldn't be intimidated by that.

There's a great cartoon that appeared many years ago in the *New Yorker* that I've never forgotten in which some cows are standing around in a field. One cow comes running up to them and says, "Guys, I just found out where hamburger comes from." And the other one says to him, "Oh, you leftists and your conspiracy theories." So, in other words, let's not be intimidated by The Boy Who Cried Wolf—that is, talked into saying that capitalism doesn't tend to produce crises. It does. It's just that not too many of them have this spectacular form of a general crisis.

Maybe there have been three or four such crises in the history of capitalism. The last one was certainly in the 1920s and '30s. (There are those who would say that actually the whole period from the brink of the First World War to the end of the Second World War was one long general crisis of a whole social order.) My hunch (and there's no way you could know this for sure except *ex post facto*) is that we are living in a period now where the ecological crisis is converging with this crisis of public power, with the crisis of social reproduction, and with the crisis of livelihood and work. So, that doesn't mean capitalism is going to collapse tomorrow. This could fester for quite a long time, and there's no guarantee that it will be resolved at all or in a way that would be at all desirable.

There's one other distinction I would like to introduce and that's the distinction between a developmental crisis and an epochal crisis. A developmental crisis marks the sort of breakdown of one regime of capital accumulation, like liberal laissez-faire capitalism or social democratic New Deal capitalism. It marks the unravelling of a regime that managed for a while to keep the crisis at bay, that managed to finesse or soften the contradictions. When a regime unravels—here's where we get to the Gramsci language—there's an interregnum period, and that's when you get a lot of interesting political developments. All sorts of people begin to think outside the box. They're looking for something fundamentally different, for better or for worse (often for worse). In the past when such crises have happened, and they've been rare, they have been resolved not by the abolition of capitalism but by the reinvention of capitalism in a new form. So, with respect to liberal laissez-faire colonial capitalism, its crisis got solved through the creation of social democratic New Deal capitalism. The crisis of that regime in turn led to neoliberalism. It's the crisis of neoliberal capitalism that we are living in now. We can't know whether the outcome (if it's resolved at all) will be a new form of capitalism or a post- or noncapitalist alternative, meaning we don't know whether it's merely a developmental crisis in which capitalism develops a new form or whether it's a genuinely epochal crisis in which we get some brand new form of social organization.

Anyway, that's just a quick attempt to spell out some of the issues I think are packed into your very rich question. To end this answer, I should just reiterate that my hypothesis (which I can't fully substantiate) is that we are in a period of general crisis and, much as I don't want to be a crisis-monger, the global warming piece of it to me looks like a game-changer. I do feel something has to give and the politics of our moment, which may go on for some decades, are going to be extremely rocky as the dust settles and we figure out where the world is going to go.

MCKAY: I'm noticing that a lot of people are writing obits for neoliberalism. Unlikely suspects—the *Financial Times* of all things—are saying that radical changes to the social order . . . are now on the table.[2]

As a student of C. B. Macpherson, a political theorist of liberalism, I keep being struck by the links between its classical social reformist, corporate, and Keynesian forebearers and today's neoliberalism. To work with your metaphor of the perfect storm: after George Clooney (a.k.a. Captain Klein) goes down with the ship, having disregarded all the better-informed experts in his madcap voyage to Newfoundland's Grand Banks, can we really be sure that his successors will transform his hypercompetitive macho ways and limit their insatiable ego-driven drive to gobble up more and more stuff from nature? Or, to recall a metaphor from historian Adam Tooze, if neoliberalism has become a "bad brand," can we really be sure its manufacturers aren't just going to stick a new label on the tin? You argue in your book on *Capitalism*, "as a hegemonic project neoliberalism is finished, it may retain its capacity to dominate but it has lost its ability to persuade."[3] I really hope you're right, and yet I fear you're wrong. As Tooze went on to remark, "as a practice of government neoliberalism is a far harder beast to kill and if you think about neoliberalism as a structure of social interest, as a class project, it marches on unambiguously."[4]

So, Macpherson might say that what made today's neoliberals so persuasive to people (and maybe they're still persuasive) is that they repackaged age-old Lockean notions about property and the primacy of the individual and their possessions. These arguably toxic truisms persuade many of us still, in my view. So, are you really sure it's time to bid a dry-eyed adieu to the neoliberal age and its underlying individualistic assumptions?

FRASER: Well, that's a very challenging question. Just to clarify: I think that Tooze and I are in agreement. I think we're both saying that neoliberalism remains in force. The global financial architecture, the rules of the road of the world economy, are neoliberal. Nothing has changed. It remains in force. What I've been saying is that it doesn't command anywhere near the same level of mass support. I mean, there was a time when all sorts of working-class people in England and the United States thought their living conditions were problematic because there was too much government red tape and that the answer was to have more markets. I don't think anybody believes that now—or many fewer people believe that. The two pillars of hegemony for Gramsci are force and consent. Neoliberalism has force but doesn't have the same level of consent.

You see that in all of the resurgent forms of populism, especially on the right but in a few cases of populisms of the left. These are all, in one sense or another, protectionist. (Or at least that's how they campaign when they run for office—what they do when they get in power is another matter.) Populist strongmen represent the idea that "I'm going to work for you."

Now, it would help in this discussion if we try to say a little bit more about what neoliberalism is, because it's a word, as you say, that everybody uses and not everyone means the same thing by it. Every form of capitalism, whether we're talking about mercantile capitalism, liberal laissez-faire capitalism, social democratic capitalism, neoliberal—every form of historic capitalism has to, in some way or another, establish a relationship between the political and the economic, between production and social reproduction, between society and nature. These are sites of tension and contradiction, by definition, of any capitalist society. Each regime has a different way of finessing, massaging, and softening those contradictions.

Neoliberalism can be well understood by contrast to the previous period of social democratic capitalism. Social democratic capitalism relied on the Bretton Woods financial architecture to give states (especially wealthy states, of course, it must be said) a set of tools by which they could direct, steer, and manage their national economies through deficit spending, currency devaluation—all kinds of tools that allowed them to keep the social reproductive contradiction at bay, for example, by social spending, social insurance, all that kind of stuff. Neoliberalism took that away. We have a new relation between corporations and states now, and it was precipitated by the dismantling of the Bretton Woods capital controls, the dropping of the gold standard, and so on and so forth, which deprived states of this Keynesian toolkit. The exception of course is the US, because the dollar is world money. We can simply print more and more of it and can get away with murder, so to speak, in this realm as in others.

So, the previous regime, in a sense, empowered states to discipline capital for its own good. By contrast, the current regime allows markets and global investors to discipline states. Witness the gutting [in Greece] of the Syriza government's attempt to refuse austerity. So, states (with the exception of a very few) are weakened in their ability to manage the production/reproduction tension; they can't spend liberally to support schools health care, housing, et cetera for fear of having their bond ratings downgraded. Neoliberalism has also meant a huge change in the nature of labour markets. In this period, capital has recruited women en masse into labour markets and has changed the whole relation of production and reproduction as a result. In place of the old family wage (one salary can support a family), we now have the so-called two-earner family, which may sound gender-egalitarian and positive. In reality, it is a system for draining more and more hours of time from every household, with less and less remuneration. You've got people running around from one job to another, et cetera, and social reproduction is suffering. That's the condition the pandemic supervened on top of; it was already there.

With respect to the nature part, we've got all the new enclosures, privatization of water, knowledge, seeds, all kinds of things. Also, there's been a huge change in the character of environmental regulation. I rarely offer the US as a positive example of anything, but we did actually lead the way in the 1970s in establishing the Environmental Protection Agency. The jewel in its crown was the Superfund, tasked with cleaning up toxic waste dumps by taxing petrochemical and mining corporations. This was a far cry from today's profit-driven trading in emissions permits and carbon offsets using the market. This was using coercive state power: you dump the stuff, we take your money. That's a contrast to neoliberal environmental regulation, which is capital-friendly.

What I'm trying to suggest is that, if we think about what neoliberalism is from the standpoint of this enlarged view of capitalism, then we have to look at these fundamental four relations I identified and look at how they differ and how they quickly unravel—how very quickly they lead to unavoidable disaster. All sorts of things that shouldn't in a rational world exist, do exist. So, neoliberal capitalism at this point has no rational basis for continuing. That doesn't mean it won't continue in the future.

MCKAY: Thank you. I'd like to now switch to your very bracing, far-reaching, and controversial critique of what I would call the existing left, and I'd like to take up its three components in turn.

First, and most controversially perhaps, you present a sharp critique of actually existing feminism, at least in its predominant modes. Liberal feminists (along with many LGBTQ+ leaders) bought into what you explosively call "progressive neoliberalism." Lean-in-and-break-the-glass-ceiling corporate feminists offered charisma and excitement to what remained a highly oppressive system for the majority of the population. Progressives settled for diversity and inclusion—all of these buzzwords that come at us every day, on terms that consign most women to the same old oppression. Especially since the 1990s, you write, and I quote, "hegemonic currents of emancipatory movements became allied with neoliberal forces aiming to financialize the capitalist economy."[5] Do you detect signs of a postpandemic movement away from this very liberal and, of late, neoliberal form of feminism?

FRASER: I want to say that, first of all, there were always other feminisms. This is a critique of a hegemonic dominant current of feminism, one that has been elevated by the media to represent feminism per se, as if there were nothing else. But there have always been currents of Black feminism, of socialist and Marxist feminism, of Indigenous feminism, all kinds of feminism that wanted to represent a "feminism for the 99%."

Now, I think this whole question of hegemony that we were just talking about is relevant here too. 2016 was a watershed. Who was the candidate that Trump defeated? Hillary Clinton—the icon of liberal feminism. The person who wrote a book called *It Takes a Village* and gave behind-closed-door speeches to Wall Street for six-figure fees promising that she wasn't going to change any of the rules to regulate derivatives.

So, in other words, I think progressive neoliberalism was kind of exposed as a sham as all of these working-class people defected. Whether they went to Trump or Sanders made a great difference to me politically, but from this point of view, they were all rejecting progressive neoliberalism, and that meant that liberal feminism faced a kind of crisis as well.

Interestingly, it was around this time that, in the US, we began to see the election to Congress of a whole slew of Sanders-type female congresswomen, mostly women of colour, the so-called Squad. Now, they represent something else. They are certainly feminists, but they're not single-issue feminists. They are feminists who have a broader critique of the political economy. Some of them claim to be democratic socialists—I'm not 100 percent sure what exactly they mean when they use that phrase, nor am I sure that Bernie Sanders knows what he means when he uses that phrase—but there's something in the air.

It's probably the case in the Global South that there has long been what we can call (for shorthand) "feminism for the 99%" in a much more visible way, because in ex-colonial countries that have been ravaged by colonialism before and neoimperialism today, it's much harder to segregate some special class of things called women's issues from everything else that is destroying people's lives. So, I think there's a lot of feminism going on. We wrote a manifesto, *Feminism for the 99%*, in hopes of giving it a name, drawing the lines, saying we're at a fork in the road.[6] Liberal feminism is seemingly collapsing (OK, that might have been an exaggeration—but it's in trouble). Let's try something else.

So, I think in general that in a time of crisis like this—and now I'm talking about the hegemonic face of the crisis, not the structural face, but how people react—I think all the established political orientations begin to bleed support and there are opportunities for good alternatives to develop (as well as some of the very nasty alternatives that are unfortunately also developing).

MCKAY: That leads to the second group of leftists you're a bit critical of, conventional Marxists. Their purportedly mouldy models focus exclusively on capital/labour relations at the expense of all the hidden abodes you've documented so well, and without those hidden abodes capitalism couldn't exist. It seems Marxists characteristically ignore three big ways the system free-rides on those it deems outside itself. First of all, without the unpaid labour of mainly women, it could not function because their largely unremunerated work creates the very entities—workers—whose labour-power capitalism necessarily must exploit, not to speak of all the other caring functions you also enumerated. And without the supposedly free resources supplied by nonhuman nature, there would not, similarly, be any commodities upon which capitalism could profit. And without public power, what we misleadingly called "private enterprise" could neither come into being nor perpetuate itself. Now, I'm wondering—can the upshot of these three hard-hitting feminist and ecosocialist critiques still be called "Marxism"?

FRASER: I do call myself a Marxist. I'm not an orthodox Marxist. It's kind of awkward to start piling up adjectives: I'm a democratic socialist, feminist, antiracist, eco-something Marxist. Sometimes it's just easier to say, "Yes I'm a Marxist, but of a different kind."

I know this is going to sound absurdly presumptuous, so forgive me in advance—but Einstein didn't refute Newton. He resituated Newtonian physics in a broader frame within the field of objects of a certain size, not too small, not too big, et cetera. Newtonian physics works pretty damn well but there's a larger field, and so it's not the whole anymore. Something like that is what I've been trying to do with Marx. Not that I would compare myself to Einstein, but I think a lot of what Marx has to say about the official economy is right, it's just that the background conditions are presumed. He was very upfront about this in *Capital*, which presents an abstract idealized picture that assumes certain other things are in place that are not even talked about. So, I see myself as resituating the Marxian analysis of the capitalist economy, not refuting it.

MCKAY: Finally, I wanted to get to the tough words you have to say about anarchists and neoanarchists who have been so prominent in the post-1990s left through such movements as Altermondialisation, Occupy, and a host of identity-based leftisms. They fall short, you suggest, in three ways. First of all, although they preach a gospel of nondomination, in practice only a tiny minority people can devote their lives to demonstrations (and for a good many people demonstrating means the risk of deportation). Second, although they preach a radical democracy in practice, in the absence of clear structure, it's actually hard to tell how decisions are made. And third, although they preach challenging the foundations of capitalism, they deliver an unsustainable "constant meeting" guaranteed to burn people out rather than shake any of capitalism's foundations. Could we add to that list a fourth critique derived from the pandemic itself, which is that, contrary to the anarchist tradition, we have been taught in the harshest possible way that we need a global public power guided by science with the capacity to enforce measures necessary for the survival and flourishing of the species? So, what is your take on where the pandemic has left this powerful libertarian current of contemporary new leftism?

FRASER: Well, that's a very thoughtfully constructed question. I teach at the New School, where many of my students suddenly became anarchists at a certain point. It kind of drove me crazy, I have to say. We were a few blocks from Occupy, from Zuccotti Park. That whole movement had such enormous charisma. There was just this thing in the air that to be really radical, you couldn't have votes, you couldn't have spokespeople, you couldn't have leadership, you couldn't have a program, a set of demands, et cetera, et cetera.

There was (and maybe there still is) a certain crisis of organization on the left. And it's as if people think that because we don't want a Leninist party, therefore we don't want any party, therefore we don't want any sort of political structures. There's got to be something in-between, which I think we are still searching for. So, I agree with all of the points you raised about the failings of anarchism. I also agree very strongly with your last point that, again, if you wanted a textbook demonstration of why we need public powers, the pandemic is it. Maybe the most serious thing to say about anarchism is that it's too focused on the state. States can be very oppressive. But, if you simply focus on weakening states, what are you then going to have?

Is Exxon Mobil going to run things? Is Google going to run things? Facebook? So anyway, we have to target the corporations, the banks, the global financial institutions, as well as the repressive face of state power, and we have come up with new models for how public power is constituted and exercised. We on the left still need to think those issues through in a serious way.

Now, having said all of that, I know from my students that they believe that a lot of what I have just said to you, and what I've written on this subject, is much too simple-minded and doesn't take into account the great sophisticated new forms of anarchist theorizing that have gone on, which I confess I'm not deeply immersed in.

MCKAY: I'll just ask one more thing and then we should turn it over to our audience. The one thing I really appreciated about *Capitalism: A Conversation* was the way you went after moralizing finger-pointing—talking-down to rural and working-class people—often with the insinuation that they are culturally backward and stupid. I think you say that's a sure-fire way to generate resentment, not solidarity. So, if you dismiss people as a "basket of deplorables," lo and behold, they're apt to tune you out.

Many working people have been shaken loose from their accustomed ideological patterns and are desperate for some policy or person who can offer plausible-sounding alternatives to precarity and dispossession. But if leftists keep on talking to them in a condescending manner—as in, "We know the answers and you're too dumb and prejudiced and gullible to see them"—well, they are just undermining their own project. I think you point out the shallowness of that stance when you write, "[it] grossly exaggerates the extent to which the problems are inside people's head while missing the depth of the structural institutional forces that undergird them." And yet, I was taken by a comment from your sparring partner in *Capitalism: A Conversation*, when she suggests that, nonetheless, some social phenomena (one thinks of homophobia, sexism, racism) still need to be addressed. [7]

FRASER: A lot of progressive people, I think, overemphasize the interpersonal, the bad behaviour, the bad ideas, the bad language, et cetera (and I'm not trying to defend any of that bad stuff—it's bad). But if you try to build a politics on that, you become one of these Puritan scolds.

I just read a book I want to recommend. I think it's well-known because it's already been listed for many prizes, but Keeanga-Yamahtta Taylor's new book called *Race for Profit*, which is about housing. There is the most beautiful account of what the term "structural racism" or "institutional racism" ought to mean; there's a great political economy of real estate, of housing, of government programs, of the real estate industry, of developers, of appraisers, all of this in which race is at the centre. So, there are ways to address questions of race that don't first and foremost consist in calling out individuals.

Let me be clear because I don't want to be misunderstood. I don't care if people call out the David Dukes and the Richard Spencers. But there's a difference between that and people who might vote for Trump. I've called them opportunistic racists, not necessarily principled card-carrying racists. But they haven't gone to Ivy League colleges, they don't know that you're supposed to say BIPOC instead of Black or African American. We are too caught up on this level. I feel very strongly about it.

QUESTION FROM THE AUDIENCE: I work in finance and have done for many years, and one of the points about Covid-19 is that, when it started, there was a massive response from central banks, from governments. All of a sudden, the world was awash with cash. So, from my perspective, the real crisis starts now, as we start to reopen. What's the next step? Do we go back to how it was? Do we forge ahead with something new? What does that look like and who is going to influence that?

FRASER: Well, thank you for your question. A couple of thoughts about it. One is that the massive dumping or feeding of money into the system was another example of what we were talking about before—of non-neoliberal policy. All of a sudden, the idea of austerity disappeared and now we had a need for stimulus, for pump-priming, for income support, and so on. You would think again if we lived in a rational world that you wouldn't any longer be hearing from the "deficit hawks," but alas we have one in the United States Senate who is single-handedly blocking the passage of Biden's social spending bill on the grounds that it's too much debt to take on.

The other thing I want to say: I can tell you for the US that the picture you drew, of things getting better for everyone, is not the case. It's a two-thirds/one-third society. People who have good pension funds or 401Ks are doing well—of course the stock market is booming, they're not out spending lavishly on vacations and at restaurants and at the opera and so on and so forth—so yes, a lot of savings, and yes, a lot of appreciation. But for the two-thirds, for the working classes, it's been quite the opposite. My impression is that in many parts of the world this has been a disaster for livelihoods as well as for health.

Where are we going—back, forward? I don't think we're going back. It's hard to imagine how things could really stabilize as they are now because too much is out of the bag, so to speak, but that doesn't give us a clear picture of what might come next. If there's going to be a new form of capitalism, it's got to, in some sense or another, be green—and that's so hard to understand. Could four-fifths of the global capitalist class simply gang up on the fossil fuel energy sector and expropriate them and say you're out of business? But that's what they need to do.

MCKAY: Can I add something? On the one hand, I can see a kind of 1920s thing going on here, where we've gone through this enormous crisis. People want some kind of settlement of it. They want their sacrifices to be recognized and honoured. And, I think, there's an enormous exhaustion. I think people are just terribly tired of it all. For millions of people, there's also this terrible weight of bereavement and grief. So, it does remind me a little bit of the 1920s, with all of the immense dangers and possibilities of that decade.

On the other hand, there's been an interesting refusal of work going on where people are saying, "Well, we're just not going to do that job anymore. It's not worth it. Our lives are too important. Our time is too important." That's a really encouraging thing: a new willingness to resist. I would like to get your own prognostications. Can this be a new moment of resistance for working people?

FRASER: Yes, we've quoted Gramsci several times, so let's also bring in that other old chestnut we owe to him: "Pessimism of the intellect, optimism of the will."[8] I feel very energized. For me, this is a great time to be alive. I haven't felt that way since the 1960s.

People are defecting from the system. That's been really something. Black Lives Matter was the first mass national movement (and now even international movement) of militant antiracism in decades, so there are things going on. As I say, I think feminism is going through a kind of reckoning, and I see more visible alternatives to liberal feminism than I did. Ecopolitics is undergoing a huge, interesting change. It's no longer a single-issue movement. Now it's focused on questions like environmental racism or environmental justice and connected up with the defence of social reproduction and communities. So, there's a lot happening that has potential. The problem is, there's also antimask, antivax—a lot of insanity. There's a mass hysteria in the United States in some circles against the teaching of Critical Race Theory in elementary schools, which is another one of these insane fantasies that our right wing generates and our mainstream Republicans are happy to exploit. So, it's a mixed picture. But there are many good things in this picture and it's a great time to be alive and to fight for what you believe in.

AN INTERVIEW WITH
MIKE DAVIS
13 MAY 2021

California-based historian Mike Davis, who died of cancer on 25 October 2022, was one of the world's most important Marxist thinkers. He was the author of many works including *Prisoners of the American Dream* (1986), *City of Quartz* (1990), *Late Victorian Holocausts* (2001), *Planet of Slums* (2006), and *In Praise of Barbarians* (2007), *Old Gods, New Enigmas: Marx's Lost Theory* (2018).

More germane to our series are Mike's books on the global patterns of epidemic diseases, and here we have, in 2005, *The Monster at our Door*, which provides a disturbing analysis of the genesis of Avian Flu in the vast agrobusiness complex created by global neoliberalism. This book carried a message regarded as unduly alarmist by some critics: that unfettered capitalist accumulation was introducing humanity to an extended era of agrobusiness-accelerated diseases. In 2020, it was reissued with a new introduction under a revealing new name: *The Monster Enters*.

MCKAY: My first question. Along with others working in the Marxist tradition, for instance Bob Wallace, John Bellamy Foster, and Andreas Malm, you place special emphasis on the ways the present pandemic has been shaped by a corporate livestock revolution and Third World urbanization, elements of what many critical theorists have called the "metabolic rift." In essence, the metabolic rift [school] maintains that capitalist development, by despoiling the natural world, is undermining not only its own preconditions but menacing humanity's continued existence on the planet.

One theme raised by this emerging school is that the present pandemic and the general climate crisis are deeply interconnected, albeit in complicated ways. I was particularly struck by one passage in *The Monster at our Door* from 2005: "Contemporary influenza, like a postmodern novel, has no single narrative but rather disparate storylines racing one another to dictate a bloody conclusion."[1] What storylines strike you as particularly good ones to pursue as we come to grips with the legacy of this quite different disease called Covid-19?

DAVIS: Well, first of all, I wanted to acknowledge my debt to Rob Wallace and his brilliant book on *Big Farms, Big Flu*,[2] and also to Jim O'Connor, the great California Marxist economist, who really originated this idea of the metabolic rift. Before talking about the genesis and meaning of the current pandemic, I want to go back to something I discussed at length in the original 2005 version of my book. There's an incredible study that I quote by a large group of researchers and scientists.[3] What they show in extraordinary detail are the chief factors that influence the emergence, the spread, and also the pathogenicity of new diseases. Their account concerns West Africa. Now, traditionally, coastal West Africa, which is the most urban, fastest-urbanizing place on the planet, with the youngest population, derived its protein largely from fishing. There's a huge kind of artisan fishing industry in the Gulf of Guinea. But, in the 1980s, 1990s, huge factory fleets from Spain and Japan and northwest Europe rolled into the Gulf of Guinea, and they literally vacuumed up the fish stocks. Something like two-thirds of the fish protein was literally fished out, and this meant both the decline and destruction of parts of the native fishing industry, and also that fish prices rose in the cities—entailing an acute shortage of protein. At the very same time, multinational companies in Congo, Cameroon, Gabon, parts of Nigeria, were logging out hardwood forests on an industrial scale. To reduce their labour costs, they hired hunters basically to kill anything in sight. Some sixty to seventy wild animals, including primates, were put on the table in these logging camps. What happened then is that this "bush meat" (as it was called) also found an immediate market in the protein-deficient cities as a substitute for fish or, in some cases, for chicken. So, increasingly, bush meat found its way to the tables of people living in the slums of the large West African cities.

So you have, here, three different causalities: the ruthless mining-out of fish stocks in the Gulf of Guinea, the exploitation of tropical rainforests and the destruction of the barrier they provide between wild animal diseases and the viral reservoirs, and the growth (on an almost exponential scale) of informal and urban settlements lacking sanitation and potable water. So, these are the "perfect storm" conditions for the spread of Ebola, for HIV, and for God knows how many diseases in the future.

The primary actors in this are, of course, international corporations and governments financed by regressive taxes, who spend the minimum, if anything at all, on the provision of health infrastructure for these cities.

MCKAY: In that case, the storyline linking capitalist development to zoonotic diseases seems fairly straightforward. I'm not sure the storylines in Covid-19 have congealed yet to the point that we can be sure the "big farm creating disease" narrative is really the one that's going to be paramount. Some people then might say, "Well, doesn't that render the comparisons problematic, because maybe the genesis of this disease is quite different?" It might have had little to do with factory farming. How you would respond to somebody who says, "Well, this is a totally different script than the one of 'big farms caused big flu.'"

DAVIS: It would be easy enough to say, "Look, if there weren't the wet markets (the wild animal markets in China), you wouldn't have had a direct transmission belt between wild viral reservoirs and urban dwellers." Or you can take the Trump approach and see, behind this, a virus escape from a laboratory (a one-in-a-million event). But the truth is this: China, quite understandably given its agricultural reforms, is rapidly expanding the intrusion of agriculture into new areas, both in response to state policy but also simply as a survival strategy by poor villagers.

One thing we shouldn't forget is that Covid was anticipated to an extraordinary degree. After the outbreak of Avian Flu in 2003 in Southeast Asia, people knew a pandemic was coming. And they knew the virus would originate in contact between animals sold as food items and humans.

So, there was a major collaboration between a US-based NGO and the researchers at the Virology Institute in Wuhan. They were down for years exploring in the caves of Szechuan and discovered that bats (the most numerous mammals on the planet—some fifteen hundred species) were harbouring something like eight hundred different coronaviruses that might be capable of emergence and transmission. (Their program was abruptly ended by President Trump.) There are nineteen or twenty major reports from the US, Western Europe, the World Health Organization (WHO)—all detailing the likely progress of the pandemic.

The WHO, which was supposedly the frontline defence (and this was accepted, by treaty, by the 130 or more countries signatory to the WHO), became something of a hollow shell. Because countries didn't pay their contributions, the WHO became more and more dependent upon the United States and China (and also the Gates Foundation) for its financing. It had a structure where countries are given a veto over the public announcements and findings of the WHO.

If we might say that Ebola and HIV were "supply-driven" (by the destruction of natural barriers and the poverty driving people to bush food), in a sense Covid is "demand-driven." That is, the major factor is the absence of primary health care in so many parts of the world, as well as the states' failure (even in advanced countries with national health systems) to implement their own previous plans for pandemics. This has led to significant breakdowns of major global institutions, starting with the WHO.

If you look at the case of the European Union, its member countries are responsible for their own health care systems, but it has a pact that, in case of emergencies (whether those are earthquakes or tsunamis—but also pandemic disease), requires cooperation and mutual aid. Italy, which was the first major Western European country to be affected by the pandemic, invoked this statutory obligation. The response was immediate. France, Austria, other countries sealed their borders. In the end, the only two countries that quickly responded to the Italian emergency were China (which sent plane-loads of experts and supplies) and tiny little Cuba, which immediately sent doctors (Cuban doctors being on the front lines of every major epidemic).

Even if you can't tie coronavirus emergence directly to factory farms (in the way that you can with diseases carried by poultry or incubated in pigs), the fact is that a generation of understanding and planning was certainly discarded. And the pandemic was unleashed in a world in which there were, essentially, two immunological humanities.

MCKAY: What is amazing to people who read your work is how often the pandemic was not just anticipated but literally predicted. Right down to the end of 2019, people were developing scenarios at the official level of how an epidemic was going to work and how the state should respond. It's a major moment in which, notwithstanding all these predictions, the state has failed catastrophically.

Do you think we should steel ourselves for a future of pandemic after pandemic after pandemic? Some bleakly declared this our "starter pandemic." And, more concretely, then, what measures do you think states *should* take (apart from just gaming this out and running scenarios that nobody pays any attention to or commissioning all these reports you have mentioned that gather dust)?

DAVIS: The silver lining, of course, was that one part of the preparation was successful. And this is a direct result of the incredible revolution that's been occurring in bio-design and genetic design. The basis existed, the knowledge existed—and in some cases even the candidate vaccines existed—for the very rapid development of vaccines that specifically targeted Covid but also potentially further vaccines. In fact, it's quite within the realm of possibility that you could develop general or universal vaccines because what changes in these viruses as they mutate are mainly changes in the head of the surface protein. This is, inevitably, where variations will appear. They can't be stopped with the existing vaccines.

At the same time, if we put everything into vaccines, we'll miss the most important factor of all—which is the fact that so much of the world lives without primary health care. Even in the most advanced countries, particularly following the 2008 economic crisis, even in rich countries, public health and primary care have been totally eroded by job cuts and lack of finance. In the United States, for example, sixty thousand public health care workers' jobs were lost. They haven't been replaced. Similarly, look at Britain and the cutbacks that have eviscerated the National Health Service, and so on.

Now, one of the most important debates in the history of modern public health was the debate about social medicine. Essentially, there were two camps by the early twentieth century. On the one hand (with a genealogy that goes back to the father of pathology, Rudolf Virchow in Germany—Virchow had been at the barricades in 1848), we find one camp laying an emphasis on primary health care rather than specific cures for specific diseases. This also meant that, if you were going to provide adequate health care, you had to have major social change: raising wages, land reform, and so on.

And the place where the idea of social medicine gained its most important purchase was in South America. Particularly, take the case of Chile in 1939, when there was a brief Popular Front government. Its minister of public health was a young doctor who had written extensively about this idea of social medicine. His name was Salvador Allende. And the social medicine ideal was also embraced by social democrats in Western Europe and in the Soviet Union.

But, after the turn of the century, another school arose, from the US imperial experience in the Caribbean and the Philippines, which was essentially a *military* assault on a *specific* pathogen or that pathogen's major vectors, that is, the carriers of it. When I was a kid in the 1950s, I gobbled up all these books about Surgeon General [William Crawford] Gorgas and the heroic people who stopped yellow fever. This work was taken up by the Rockefeller Foundation. In the period between the two wars, the Rockefeller Foundation was the major financier and coordinator of these disease-specific campaigns.

A kind of last stand of the social medicine school was at a WHO summit in Alma Ata (in what's now Kazakhstan) in 1978–79. The Alma Ata Declaration declared that good health was a basic human right and more or less endorsed the social medicine position. But that has lost ground, of course, with the dismantling of the Soviet bloc and also with the growing power of Big Pharma, which endorses the view that hugely expensive government-subsidized vaccines are the only way to go. So, without discounting the importance of searching for new vaccines—particularly universal vaccines, which have come within our reach over the last five or ten years—I believe the fundamental questions in terms of world public health remain the questions posed by the social medicine movement.

MCKAY: I might just comment parenthetically that in Canada, why we have something progressive in our health system goes back in large measure to people who were inspired by the Soviet example in the 1920s and '30s and this quite revolutionary idea of "public health." But this leads me on to the next question. There seems to be a fundamental philosophical problem for neoliberals, who don't like the expansion of the welfare state and in many ways don't even like the idea of "the public" as an entity that has interests, a collectivity that should be cared for. This is a crisis for global neoliberalism and its way of thinking about the state and its way of thinking about humanity in general.

I sometimes think this might be the last nail in the coffin of neoliberalism as a plausible ideology, but then whenever I think that, I also reflect, "But consider how deeply this has sunk into the psyches of everybody who's been exposed to it in the last 40 years." Do you think we're hammering the last nail into neoliberalism's coffin, or is that premature?

DAVIS: Only if we have the hammer and are prepared to keep driving it in, relentlessly. There's neoliberalism and neoliberalism. And, in fact, most neoliberals—particularly as represented by New Labour [in Britain], the Democratic Party establishment here, and centrist regimes ([such as those of] German conservative parties)—don't discount the role of the state. They realize that different kinds of state-provided externalities are essential to a program of privatization and extending the contours for accumulation.

Capital itself will always find profitable opportunities in disasters, even those that it's brought about itself. Look at the United States. Amazon has emerged as this Leviathan over the bodies of hundreds of thousands of small business owners. The insurance companies are raking in the biggest profits in history in this country [the US]. Big Pharma has been given the profits for antivirals and vaccines that have been paid for by the American public with most of the research done in public universities. So, Covid, at least here in the United States, has been a bonanza for different sectors of capital, which look forward to an expansion of health care. And to coming pandemics! Important profit-points.

But what happened here is, of course, different in one way from anywhere else (except for Bolsonaro's Brazil). In this pattern, the state takes an active role in *disorganizing* the pandemic response. It becomes a major vector of the pandemic itself, which has yielded, of course, incalculable consequences.

It's not simply a partisan matter. If you look at states like New York and California, Democrats are completely culpable for massacres in senior homes and for the fate of low-wage workers, unprotected in essential industries. In Southern California, for instance, two-thirds of people who died from Covid are Latinos working in low-wage industries and living in congested housing. Likewise with farm workers. The United States and Brazil are examples of an almost fascist approach to disease.

It's my belief—not surprising—that the Republican Party has become the party of global death. It's been the major opposition to any kind of effective action about climate change. And it's now assured hundreds of thousands of unnecessary deaths—and more in the future. I tried to argue vigorously in the pages of *The Nation* that we shouldn't be worrying so much about a national inquiry into what happened on January sixth (when the far right invaded Congress), but more at the culpability of those responsible for allowing the pandemic, first of all, to get out of control, and then, secondly, attacking, disorganizing, demonizing necessary public health measures. This is murder. Most of the deaths, as pointed out by studies in *The Lancet* and even now by members of the Biden administration, were preventable and unnecessary.

Now, finally to the larger question. Can globalized neoliberalism—accumulation on a world scale through a division of labour that exports most productive jobs to relatively low-wage nations—continue without a serious infrastructure of global public health and control over the transmission of disease through air travel and trade?

I would say from the standpoint of a logical capitalism that this would be absolutely necessary. But we never actually deal with "logical capitalism." And the current chaos in the European Union, and all the initial disasters followed by second and third waves of the pandemic, and the fiasco of the vaccination campaign on the continent should raise some big questions about whether capital, independently organized or acting through the state, can really address emergencies—even while parts of it find in pandemics and plagues very new ways to engage in the neoliberal appropriation of wealth.

MCKAY: I'd like to go back to your idea of there being two distinct humanities, immunologically. One recalls Frederick Engels writing in Manchester in the 1840s about "social murder." He says that, even though mass deaths are happening without any one ⋰ . . individual explicitly murdering anybody, it is still kind of a social murder—it's a wilful abdication of responsibility for the lives of other people. In your book *Late Victorian Holocausts*, we see how the whole Indian economy was made subservient to the needs of the British Empire. So, while you had famines in India, you still had exports to Britain of the things the population needed. And that seems uncannily echoed today with India's experience with vaccines. A "vaccine powerhouse" essentially is really struggling to vaccinate its own people—and that's one reason the pandemic is getting out of control. Might Marxists celebrate 2020 as a moment in which class analysis and the critical analysis of empire came back squarely to centre stage—not only changing academic life but (more important) the progressive politics beyond the academy? Is that an overly optimistic analysis?

DAVIS: Perhaps. There's very little to celebrate in today's world.

MCKAY: But I do notice people are talking a lot more about class divisions.

DAVIS: True. But we have to translate that into real politics that has the ability to reach grassroots people, ordinary working people. Now India, apart from the great artificial famines of the 1870s and the 1890s, is where the majority of people killed by the 1918–20 flu lived. Some twenty to twenty-five million Indians died. And this is, again, an important case study for understanding the interactions between disease, capital, and, in this case, the imperial state. Because what happened in India is that the British torqued up, during the First World War, the requisition of grain and all kinds of other raw materials and supplies from India to support the Indian army, which was fighting the Ottoman Empire and on the Western Front. This coincided with a drought and widespread crop failure. So, when the H1N1 virus—the original one—disembarked from a ship in Bombay, millions of Indians were malnourished, already sick (there was also cholera). And they were absolutely decimated. And the British response was almost nothing—negligible, at the best.

Today in India, we see a model of growth that has produced a spectacular-looking twenty-first century, surrounded by immense belts of slums and misery. Most women in the Indian countryside, and in many cities, still have to defecate in the open. Potable water is often not available. So, India has subsumed within itself this division between immunological humanities. That is, on one side, there are people who live in societies like ours. (Remember, immunology determines so much of the pattern and the lethality of any pandemic.) We live in societies where it's the old and the poor, the people living in congested housing, immigrant populations, Native Americans, maybe about a quarter to a third of the population, who suffer from pre-existing conditions associated with enhanced mortality. On the other hand, in other places, like sub-Saharan Africa, the *majority* of people suffer from compromised immune systems, because of the lack of potable water, because of malnutrition, because of exposure to all kinds of toxic and environmental factors, and so on.

Now in India, we see these two worlds together: a newly-enlarged, fairly massive middle class, some of whom live in essentially American subdivisions within high-tech cities, but with the majority of the population lacking access to basic primary care, potable water, and so on. The "first" Indian humanity has been saved. The other's been neglected or condemned to pandemic. And, remember, if you allow RNA viruses free rein to spread in larger and larger populations, this increases the evolutionary space for these viruses to develop new and more deadly mutants. We've seen this happen before.

Here's where the fundamental break in human solidarity occurs. In India, the rich run to the clinics. The wealthy countries save each other. Pharmaceutical companies reap vast fortunes. But the larger part of humanity is totally left behind. Again, it's not only a matter of vaccines. It's the conditions that compromise immunity and healthy living conditions, which in many ways grow worse every year.

The UN has noted that, of its twenty-one key development goals, many of them have now been reversed, such as goals of reducing child poverty, and raising income, and better health, and education for women.

MCKAY: Even if you're a hard-nosed neoliberal, how could you possibly quarantine afflicted countries in a world that you have just globalized? We've been told for forty years that "the world is flat—we should level tariff barriers, encourage free movement of capital," et cetera. Well, how can a neoliberal then turn around and say, "We're going to quarantine India or Brazil?" Well, if you can't do that, then surely the next logical step is to say, "Well, we have to have some sort of global regime of public health that can force recalcitrant governments to do what the world requires."

DAVIS: Well, let me just repeat two earlier points. One is that it was the analysis of the social medicine tradition that health care is a human right and requires radical socioeconomic reforms, strong unions, the raising of incomes, agrarian reform. The other point is that there is no longer a pivot in the world, a kind of Archimedean point, for human solidarity and unity.

One thing the Cold War did was make every single inch of the earth valuable. If a small group of people, a tribal society say, decided they wanted to listen to Radio Moscow—well, the Americans were there a second later. The US side of the Cold War was forced to respond to the Soviet Union's anticolonialism and internationalism with its own vision of world progress. So, you had the Alliance for Progress and battling five-year plans across the planet. When the Cold War ended, any kind of real serious discourse about human development and progress as a whole was abandoned. And, of course, neoliberalism has dug that grave deeper and deeper.

Again, remember that even if suddenly vaccines were universally available everywhere, that would still leave the larger problem in place—which is that, a large portion of humanity is basically standing in front of the headlights of the next pandemic.

For Generation Z, the one that my younger children (who are still in high school) belong to, by every poll and measurement, some form of socialism wins out over capitalism any day of the week. This is an enormous development.

The emergence of this *new* new left has created a left-wing version of America First-ism. That was on full exhibit during the Democratic primary debates, when Bernie Sanders only marginally touched on international issues. Likewise, Elizabeth Warren. We suffer from a deficit of internationalism—which is why I can't help but be fond of the Argentine soccer fan currently inhabiting the biggest house in Rome. He [Pope Francis] is virtually the only world leader to stand up and insist on human solidarity, the unity of the human species, in almost every speech he makes.

MCKAY: In *Old Gods, New Enigmas*, you ask the question: To what extent does the informal proletariat—the most rapidly growing global class—possess historical agency? The old left hope was that the proletariat and trade unions, communist parties, to a point social democratic parties would be moving history forward. Since 1989 certainly, that's become far less plausible. Can there be ways this pandemic can mobilize people in other ways, maybe just by showing them the drastic costs of capitalism, unleashed?

DAVIS: Well, we've seen the new "vanguard of the proletariat" in action over the last year. I have, because of various ailments, spent an inordinate amount of time in hospitals and clinics over the last five years. At a big hospital, people are punching in the clock the same way people did into Ford factories or coal mines. But they're in some ways far more educated and conscious. And everything about the work that hospital workers of all kinds (and other people in essential services) do confronts them daily with the contradictions and failure of private medicine and a government directed against public welfare. It's no surprise, then, that the major union to support Bernie Sanders, and arguably the most militant union in the United States right now, is the National Union of Nurses.

I do believe that the pandemic around the world has radicalized health workers, with nurses often being in the vanguard. I think that's true for the National Health Service in Britain as well, and likely for other countries.

We shouldn't forget that a successful public health approach depends on popular mobilization, involvement from the grassroots level. So, for instance, Vietnam (considered middle-income but a poor country by our standards) has had an astonishing success in avoiding death on a large scale and containing the pandemic. One reason is that it has a medical elite with global stature because of its experiences fighting previous diseases like SARS and Avian Flu. But it also has a paramedical system reaching down to the village (paramedical workers and village nurses) and an aggressive approach to public health education. This doesn't exonerate the lack of democracy at the highest levels in that society, but it shows how absolutely important public participation is.

I recently blurbed a book by some Chinese new leftists based on interviews with people and experiences in Wuhan.[4] And, although the existence of a mass communist party that extends its tendrils down to every apartment building and so on played a crucial role in mobilization, much of what happened actually didn't occur through party channels. It occurred through popular organization, including swingeing critiques of the national cover-up by the government. They created these networks of popular self-help and resistance. And this really hasn't been measured or adequately reported in most accounts of the pandemic—the centrality of a popular role and the need for grassroots networks of public health medicine.

In fact, when you look at the whole issue of public health education, in the United States a hard-core 40 percent of the US population are also diehard pandemic denialists who regard a little reading in the *Bible* as far truer than any biology book. So, here, in supposedly one of most advanced scientific countries in the world, the degree of ignorance about basic science and the reign of religious superstition is, just simply, a staggering fact.

MCKAY: In some ways, that can be connected to neoliberalism's abandonment of any notion of responsibility to the people—in that rulers feel no responsibility to educate the people to whom they're supposedly answerable. So, in some ways, from this perspective, an uninformed populace is fine. Keep people fairly ignorant and superstitious, as long as they show up for work. What's the problem?

Maybe I'm being cynical, but I think there is a real way in which the neoliberal state entailed the abandonment of what Thomas Hobbes would have said was the primary responsibility of a government—which is to keep its people alive, basically, and protect them from each other. Why do we have a government? Upon what does its legitimacy rest? A long-standing argument would be: "Well, at least it keeps us alive." But these governments have not been doing that. Neoliberal governments almost universally have failed in that basic enterprise.

DAVIS: I agree with the interpretation that says we've entered a phase of apocalyptic capitalism, unable to prevent climate change, decarbonize the planet, provide universal public health. The global branded economy no longer creates jobs, which leads to an interesting Marxist paradox. The majority of the populations of Africa and Latin America toil in the informal economy. The formal economy hasn't created net jobs for years and years.

And, of course, waiting in the distance—how far we don't know, maybe much closer than we suspect—is the fact that nothing's been done to reduce the danger of nuclear war, particularly in some regional circumstances. In ensuring its own reproduction and survival, capitalism ensures a future of extinction for at least a large minority of the human race, particularly that part that's no longer requisite for its own reproduction.

Since the ending of the Cold War (and with that, any kind of universalist discourse), we kind of accept this in our daily lives. We kind of accept that millions of poor people are going to die. And it's becoming naturalized in the same way that homelessness has been in this country. My kids don't believe me when I tell them that, when I was a young adult, there was no homelessness in California. It's not a "natural" fact.

The triage of humanity is in place. That fact needs, I think, to guide and direct all of our thoughts and emotions and above all, our activism.

MCKAY: When you updated *The Monster At Our Door* of 2005 and you made it *The Monster Enters* in 2020, you wrote that you had to order in a copy of your own book because "unconsciously, I wanted it off my bookshelf in order to exorcise the anxiety involved in its writing."[5] That made me think of the extraordinarily terrible year this has been for people—of bereavement, of suffering, depression, mounting cases of "deaths of despair" through opioid addiction. Sometimes I wonder if we Marxists run the risk of adding our own little bit to an apocalyptic culture of despair, contributing to a sort of "collapsology" that some French writers critique, entailing almost an enjoyment of the idea of human collapse and the abandonment of humanism. Can we supplement our gloomy prognosis of all these enormous contradictions to generate something more inspiring for people? Surely a new global left will require a higher hope, a realistic hope, to aim for?

DAVIS: Well, I'm quite notorious on this point. I don't actually believe that hope is either a requirement of radical writing or a scientific concept. I think the obligation that I have, and others have, is to write as accurately and realistically as we can about the current crisis. People will fight because it is their way to realize their humanity, to defend their families and communities and class. People face the dark ages. And they offer resistance in return.

I'm very old school about this. And I suppose I'm very Brechtian about it, because Brecht's poems and writings in the late 1930s and the '40s had enormous influence on me when I was younger. We need to be ruthlessly honest about what we face and what our obligations are. I'm a socialist in the same way Billy Graham was a Baptist. I believe that it's the hope of the world, but we've lost an awful lot of ground, historically.

On a personal level, I'll contradict myself and say, I *am* hopeful. I have two kids still in high school. I have an older daughter in Belfast, where she was born. My kids are fierce fighters. They look ahead very, very clearly. They were active in the Black Lives Matter movement and so on. (My younger kids, by the way, are Mexican and their mother's Mexican). They go to an inner-city high school. It was amazing to me to see the kids in this high school. I'm not talking about rarities like my kids (growing up in a middle-class left-wing home with millions of books), but their friends, who were working-class Latino immigrants, Somalis, African Americans—just ordinary kids. The way they banded together and just erupted last spring and summer in the Black Lives Matter protest was astonishing to me. This is a generation of tigers and lions.

QUESTION FROM THE AUDIENCE: I like that you brought up the nurses and health care workers, but I can't help but think that, in Canada at least, it's illegal for nurses or other health care workers to go on strike. So, what advice or perspective would you have on organizing health care workers for more radical forms of labour protest?

DAVIS: Well, quite honestly, I (and most of the other people I know) have loads to learn from health care workers and their struggles. Now, labour movements in North America have always worked under legal disabilities, reactionary Supreme Courts, antistrike laws, states of emergency, and so on. And the traditional answer—not from the left, but even from such right-wing leadership as the American Federation of Labor, before the 1930s, was "No right to strike? Then Strike! Told not to go out in the streets and protest? Put your mask on, go out in the streets, and protest!" If strikes become impossible? Job actions of all kinds.

QUESTION FROM THE AUDIENCE: I have a spouse who works in health care. It's been an absolutely fascinating journey hearing about it. She said it's in many ways one of the most horrific diseases in terms of the comorbidities that were coming with it, so the people who were landing in hospital, they weren't just the 80-plusers, but people with hypertension, diabetes, and other comorbidities. Do you think that the general health of the *whole* nation (not just segments of the nation) will play a role not only in combating Covid but in the making of an optimal social policy?

DAVIS: Well, of course, epidemic disease always follows the contours of inequality and poverty. But, in this country, it was also driven by an administration that sabotaged every effort to protect people at the workplace.

Within the Department of Labor, we have the Occupational Health and Safety Administration (OSHA), which is supposed to protect workers at peril in various kinds of situations. There were hundreds of complaints filed with this agency by meatpacking workers, farm workers, other kinds of essential workers. And under Trump, OSHA refused to process any of these, refused to enact any fines or process grievances against any employers. In other words, it deliberately allowed the pandemic to spread through a largely minimum-wage workforce. A lot of people with existing comorbidities, as you say. The result was a slaughter—only surpassed by the massacre in nursing homes.

Last year, I issued a daily mailing of articles and comments on the pandemic, starting in March, taking stuff from scientific journals and sometimes my own editorials. The first thing I published was from a friend of mine who is the union rep for the nursing home employees in Kirkland, Washington, in a nursing home chain owned by one of the most notorious of these piratical companies. He pointed out—remember, this is the very beginning of take-off of the pandemic—that county health employees were shut out of the home from the very beginning. When they finally entered, nobody was asking questions about the staff in these homes. Nobody seemed to recognize, when people are so badly paid, that they often moonlight in a second job in another nursing home. He said: "So what's going to happen is, it's going to spread like wildfire through the entire system from coast to coast."

This disaster was entirely foreseen. He was absolutely right, down to the details. Basically, nothing happened. Again, regulation failed; there were no fines. About 40 percent of the people who died in the United States were [institutionalized] seniors, most of them because of the failure of state regulation. This is nothing but absolutely criminal. And, of course, it suggests the need for an entirely different system of taking care of the sick and elderly.

MCKAY: I think we need to retain that memory somehow, so that we don't just close the door on this pandemic and say, "Well, thank goodness, that's over! Back to Normal." The "normal" caused this problem.

DAVIS: I should mention a kind of personal experience here. My father was a member of the meat-cutters' union. He ended up losing his pension plan, and my mother went back to work as an aide in a nursing home. And I can't tell you how many nights she had to call my father to come to the nursing home to help her pick up an elderly patient who fell out of the bed, sometimes breaking bones, lying in their own urine and feces. Clean them, and put them back. The people who ran the nursing home refused to add more night shift workers. These people could have been in concentration camps.

So, this has been the case for a very long time. We have to get rid of the for-profit nursing home industry and replace it with something public, decent, and safe.

QUESTION FROM THE AUDIENCE: One thing you mentioned was how you were saying your kids don't believe you when you say there didn't used to be homeless people in California. So, I guess I'm just wondering if you think there's any main cause or factor that you attribute to the demise of labour and the welfare state that happened around the

1980s where we saw this privatization happen? I kind of wonder this because I feel like if there's no homelessness, why would people be driven to change the policies that were in place then?

DAVIS: Well, as old as I am, I've watched the evolution of homelessness and the ecology of homelessness through its different phases. In the beginning it was the shutting down of state mental hospitals and the idea that people would find jobs and shelter in their community. There would be this investment in community centres, and you would create a far more humane system. Well, institutions were shut down. People were forced out. But there wasn't the investment in either shelters or mental health facilities. And it wasn't too long before our jail systems became the major institutions for the mentally ill in the state.

Homelessness has changed over time. Right now, what is so striking is how many people are homeless, and homeless as family groups, including children, who don't fall into the categories of addiction, mental illness, or being dumped in the streets by the prison system. They're simply dehoused.

A few days ago, it was announced that California, for the first time in history, had lost population. This state has been in a continuous boom since I was born here in 1946, through my entire life. This is a historical watershed. And why is the population declining? Because huge numbers of working-class people, low-wage people, are fleeing the state. They can't afford shelter. And now, you're seeing this everywhere on the streets. It's just a screaming indictment, day-by-day, of the inhumanity of this system.

The housing crisis won't be resolved by the private sector, which builds mansions—it doesn't build affordable housing. You have to attack the system of private property. When I lived in London for years, I was always struck by the fact that, in the wealthiest neighbourhoods in Europe, you could still find council housing projects, brought by the victory of the Labour Government in 1945.

In my writing, I tried to stress that issues of gentrification and housing are insoluble unless you address the root cause of land inflation and speculation. We need to remove large parts of the city and to rescue it from land inflation. We need public housing. We need massive amounts of affordable housing that can't be built unless you control and stop the ever-rising prices of land.

Now my authority in all this is not Karl Marx, by the way. It's the most influential radical thinker of the late nineteenth century in the United States, Scotland, Ireland (I'm sure he had a big following in Canada as well): Henry George. He pointed out that the root causes of California's contradictions were land speculation and land profiteering. He proposed that, basically, you would tax away all gains in land value. People would own the real property—the house they built. The land, essentially, would be socialized.

One of the things that's kind of exciting right now is that questions, which formerly had been far beyond the horizon of even the most progressive politics, suddenly now have wide audiences. What Trotsky called "transitional demands"—ones that don't require the abolition of capitalism but are incompatible with traditional practices of profit-making—are finding an audience. And until you have the will, and have mobilized the support, to interfere in the land market and democratize urbanization, at least an important part of it, and also control sprawl, all attempts to prevent gentrification and the expulsion of people from cities will ultimately be unsuccessful.

AN INTERVIEW WITH

MACK PENNER

14 AUGUST 2022

Mack Penner is one of Canada's leading students of neoliberalism, and he is currently working on a major study of the Calgary School, a crucial nexus of right-wing thought in Canada from the 1980s, which played a role not only in steering many academics in a conservative direction but also helped propel Stephen Harper into the prime ministership. In addition to his stellar contributions to *Syndemic Magazine*, Penner has contributed to *Jacobin* and to numerous other projects.

MCKAY: Can you tell us what led you to the study of neoliberalism and why you think grasping it more rigorously is worthwhile?

PENNER: Before I began this work, roughly four years ago now, I was on at least three paths that led, in some way, to the study of neoliberalism broadly speaking. I was a historian of the left, a historian of twentieth-century Canada, and I was, and still am, a socialist. From each of these vantages, I was then interested in historical metanarratives, as it were, or in questions of how to think about the history of the twentieth century in terms of its characteristic *isms*.

So, for both intellectual and political reasons I am interested in the relations of capitalism, socialism, and liberalism, and it so happened that when I was in the early stages of conceptualizing my current project, the history of neoliberalism was being written up in ways that foregrounded these kinds of historiographical and philosophical questions. Within the last decade or so, there has been fascinating historical work published on the left-wing origins of neoliberalism, like Johanna Bockman's book, *Markets in the Name of Socialism*, which treats the relationship between socialism and neoclassical economics.[1] There's been work on neoliberalism and empire, like Quinn Slobodian's book, *Globalists*.[2] Amy Offner, a historian somewhat skeptical of the term "neoliberalism," has written brilliantly in *Sorting out the Mixed Economy* about how what we call neoliberalism is historicized best as an adaptive kind of capitalism rather than an abrupt political-economic rupture.[3] There's also great work on neoliberalism and democracy, like political theorist Wendy Brown's *Undoing the Demos*.[4] This is the sort of literature I've been engaged with, and I've found reading it immensely productive in terms of my interest in the historical dynamics of *isms*.

This rich historiography leaves the historian of neoliberalism with so many interesting questions and issues with which to work. And yet, the abundant international literature on neoliberalism has not (yet) had much apparent influence on Canadian historians. There is some great journalism, from people like Linda McQuaig and Donald Gutstein, that emerged more or less contemporaneously with the advance of neoliberalism in Canada and some academic political science that takes up certain themes of historical neoliberalism in Canadian contexts, but professional historians have had very little to say about these things.

I thought that studying neoliberalism from what I'd call a Canadian-transnational perspective was not simply a way to plug Canada into an existing narrative, but [a way] to explore the interplay between local contexts and the conditions of global neoliberalism. I very quickly became aware, for example, of how little the existing historiography on neoliberalism had to say about settler colonialism—and how difficult it was to ignore the presence of settler concerns among the Canadian proponents of neoliberalism.

Generally, then, grasping neoliberalism more rigorously is valuable in the first instance simply because it can be done, but more importantly, it is worthwhile for the way it enables thinking about the world we live in (and the world we would like to live in instead). Especially to the extent that my socialism is of the Marxian sort, and I am thus inclined to think of history in terms of broad structural antagonisms, I would insist that "neoliberalism" is a hugely important category for grasping the historical dynamics of our time.

MCKAY: The literature on neoliberalism is now enormous, and some, such as historian Daniel Rodgers, believe the term itself has reached its "best-before" date.[5] Many who might be considered promoters of the paradigm in free-market think tanks and business schools routinely roll their eyes when they heard hear the word, which in their view has become little more than a pejorative term for all the things about capitalism a given writer happened to dislike. "One often hears," remark theorists Damien Cahill and Maritjn Konings, "that it is a somewhat lazy way for left-wing critics to group together any number of heterogeneous things to which they happen to be opposed. Imprecision would seem to characterise its use, sometimes even among those for whom the concept is central to their analysis, and its overuse is seen to have resulted in loss of analytical value." [6]

Others query the coherence of the term, given the radically disparate policies self-proclaimed neoliberals have advanced over the past eighty years, often stitching together ad hoc responses to particular challenges together in ways that only seem coherent. Some, coming at neoliberalism from a more orthodox political economy perspective, see it as, essentially, an epiphenomenon of underlying capitalist social relations, sometimes with the suggestion that neoliberal ideas were just so much window dressing for defences of capitalism going back decades, if not centuries. For them, neoliberalism is the superstructure, capitalism the base.

The history of neoliberalism as an organized tendency certainly confirms the drive by its principal figures to preserve capitalist market relations and the possessive-individualist assumptions bolstering them, and in ways that would not have seemed unfamiliar to many Victorian capitalists. The reliance on figures like F. A. Hayek on Herbert Spencer, important when considering the genealogy of "spontaneous order" about which you have written, underscores this theme of capitalist continuity. And the American antistatism that had so warmly embraced Spencer in the nineteenth century turned with equal enthusiasm to the emigrant Austrians in the twentieth, in both cases reducing holistic and complicated theories to straightforward "up-with-business" arguments in favour of the unfettered rights of private property.[7] It is telling that, even today, rightists like Brazil's Bolsonaro profess their commitment to social liberalism, without, one suspects, much immersion in the arcana of neoliberal economics.

Yet, from a slightly different perspective, one might point out with respect to all major ideological formations that they change over time and that treating them as just so much window dressing unrealistically minimizes their real-world impact. Ideologies are an "objective and operative reality," highly significant to how historical processes are both shaped and experienced.[8]

Moreover, while neoliberalism undoubtedly draws upon, indeed reifies, the age-old precepts of liberal possessive individualism, within it those assumptions were qualitatively radicalized. In this more historicist approach to neoliberalism, it *first* emerged as a relatively small tendency among extreme rightists and liberals in the 1930s alarmed by the emergence of mass democracy and labour movements; *then* became a far more powerful ideological current with the coming of the Cold War in the 1940s, developing an impressive complex of academic and business institutions; *next* it crossed over the membrane of the state in the 1970s in far-reaching experiments in Latin America, the United States, and Britain, which succeeded in humbling and even destroying left and labour movements; *then* attained a new global stature in the 1990s as a doctrine of financialization, as such institutions as the World Bank, the International Monetary Fund, and even the United Nations adopted neoliberal precepts and practices, effectively empowering market forces over states; and *finally* has, in our own time, become a hegemonic logic of rule, to the point that, in many ostensibly public institutions, one still has to speak the language of neoliberalism if one wants to participate in decision-making. Yet, throughout all these changes, the notion that "true freedom resides in the market" was upheld.[9] We are dealing, in one formulation, with "an always mutating project of state-facilitated market rule, propelled not least by its own limitations, contradictions, and reactionary tendencies," which in a complicated, heterogeneous world, will never be found in "pure, uncut, or unmediated form."[10]

Simplifying heroically, one might see this as a debate between "fundamentalists" insisting on the perduring realities of capitalism and "neo-Marxists" who see those realities as interpreted and reshaped within ideological frameworks which, once they became hegemonic, attain a real-world significance: they have come to be almost compulsory, establishing categories that seem unquestionable (until the moment, that is, that they enter into crisis). How do you navigate this debate?

PENNER: In the first place, I tend to be of two minds about the "neoliberalism debates" that you refer to and in which the likes of Rodgers,

Cahill, and Konings are participants. On the one hand, it seems to me that those who employ neoliberalism as conceptual apparatus are under more pressure to defend and define themselves than are the employers of just about any other *isms* as analytical categories. In my weaker moments, this irks me.

At times, these debates boil down to mere politics. For sure, as you suggest, critics on the right who associate neoliberalism with a left-wing critique of capitalism will sometimes dismiss the term as if it were a mere pejorative, with conveniently shifting referents. Indeed, the term is sometimes used this way on the left. But the debate in this form is tiresome insofar as it poses the trading of insults as if it were substantive analysis.

More importantly, there are aspects of the neoliberalism debates that I find invigorating and generative. I routinely find myself learning a great deal from those who are, in some ways at least, wary of overusing the concept of neoliberalism. Take, for example, the historian Amy Offner whom I have mentioned already. In *Sorting out the Mixed Economy*, which focuses especially on the United States and Colombia in the middle part of the twentieth century, Offner describes how, when capitalist economies in the Americas encountered economic and political crisis in the 1970s and '80s, those crises were managed in part with existing policy tools inherited from the mixed-economies of the postwar era. Offner's book concludes with a rousing suggestion: "We might recognize that when we take issue with neoliberalism, we are often struggling with much more enduring features of capitalism, and take aim accordingly."[11]

It would be possible to read this as a suggestion that, indeed, neoliberalism is minimally important, a distraction from the real historical force of capitalism. But I much prefer an alternative takeaway: neoliberalism must be understood historically. It is folly to attempt to understand neoliberalism as if the period from the 1970s to the present had unfolded in exquisite historical isolation according to logics and principles all its own. As Offner points out, this view tends to feature in the self-perceptions of many right-wing intellectuals— and in the ostensibly critical accounts of certain leftists who have been over-inclined towards accepting narratives of intellectual and political heroism on the part of neoliberal true believers.[12] In these tales of heroism, the great crises of the 1970s, including the demise of the

Bretton Woods system, the oil shock, and stagflation, spelled the end of the era of postwar capitalism. The postwar arrangement had ceased to function. Neoliberal ideas just happened to be lying around—here I'm paraphrasing Milton Friedman—and thanks to the valiant action of neoliberal politicians, intellectuals, and businesspeople, a sort of neoliberal revolution, or historical break, took place.

The reality is far messier. Here, the work of historical sociologist Greta Krippner offers some clear guidance. Krippner has shown in the case of the United States that neoliberalism was the result of an ad hoc process where, over a period of years, policymakers worked out solutions to the most acute crises they faced. Moreover, the solutions they went with were more like band-aids that stopped the bleeding than they were like surgical operations that addressed root causes. In short, at the outset, neoliberalism was about assigning responsibility for distributional outcomes to the market in order to shift the blame away from government.[13] That is, neoliberalism is at least as much a history of frightened policymakers as it is one of principled ideologues.

This being the case, I tend to be quite comfortable with using "neoliberal capitalism" as a synonym for "neoliberalism." Clearly neoliberalism implies the preservation of capitalist market relations, as you say. And yet, if I can manifest a certain kind of interlocutor, it could be said that the construction "neoliberal capitalism" does privilege the latter half of the compound; "neoliberal" modifies "capitalism." So, to this interlocutor, I must be a vulgar fundamentalist to whom ideology is a mere epiphenomenon!

But I'd like to hope not. There tends to be a problem in these debates, I think, where emphases are treated like exclusions and accents are deemed oversights. Why should a history of partial continuity in the history of capitalism, like the one we get from Offner, be treated as if it implied a disregard for the significance of neoliberalism as an ideological project? It is indeed a history of partial continuity, and surely we can trace some of that partiality to the fact that, as you put it, neoliberalism "qualitatively radicalized" some pre-existing tenets in the liberal tradition. Why, reverting again to asking rhetorical questions, should a materialist approach to the history of neoliberalism foreclose upon our ability to appreciate the "objective and operative reality" of ideology, especially in common sense or hegemonic forms? As the French theorist Grégoire Chamayou has put it, supposedly spontaneous market order "holds together only thanks to demiurges who somehow patch it up permanently and who defend it tooth and nail against the new enemies it makes for itself every day."[14] If capitalist market relations can only endure thanks to "tooth-and-nail" defences, it would seem clear that those defences, which we could just call ideology, are of huge historical significance. The "neoliberal" modification of "capitalism" matters a great deal.

MCKAY: So, going back to flogging my tentative five-part periodization—briefly, neoliberalism as a fringe rightist ideology in Europe morphing into a transatlantic research and political program in the Cold War and then in the 1970s into a state practice in both the Global South (Latin America) and the Global North (in the United States and the United Kingdom, especially), which in the 1990s morphs once again into a world-reshaping praxis of capitalist globalization and the encasement of market relations from democracy, before, after 2008–10, slipping into a phase of serious crisis calling out for repeated and massive state bail-outs—would you agree that, as is the case with the coronavirus, it's very important to make clear what variant and period of neoliberalism one is addressing? I find it telling, for instance, that in one narrative about neoliberalism (Michael Roberts), it arises out of the crisis of profitability in the 1970s but after 1997 is undone by the realities of the "long depression"; whereas for Quinn Slobodian, neoliberalism's foundational moment is the coming of the WTO in 1995 with its profound acceleration of accumulation on a world scale. In short: in the works of these two leading scholars, there is scarcely any overlap in their conceptions of the "Age of Neoliberalism."

PENNER: I agree with your periodization, but I would want to stress the permeability of the boundaries at each step. This point is connected, also, to the "historicity" of neoliberalism. The headline dynamics in any given phase do not necessarily extinguish pre-existing trends, just as the arrival of a new headline dynamic need not imply its prior nonexistence. To take just one example from within the periodization, consider the issue of state bail-outs and their centrality in the period after 2008. As the American Federal Reserve stepped into its role as "global lender of last resort" by pumping liquidity into the trembling international financial system after the collapse of Lehman Brothers, we could be forgiven for seeing novelty. The scale of the Fed's intervention, as Adam Tooze has made very clear, was stunning.[15] It's appropriate to stress crisis and state intervention after 2008. But it is also true, as Perry Anderson has argued in a review of Tooze's work, that the Fed's crisis fighting tools in the crash of 2008 and afterwards were far from unprecedented. Anderson writes that "virtually all of the daring innovations with which Tooze credits the US authorities for stopping the crisis of 2008—and more—had been pioneered by their Japanese counterparts, most of them well beforehand, starting in the nineties, and in wider and ampler measure, without resort to chest-thumping." This is true of quantitative easing, or QE, whereby the Fed created systemic liquidity by massive purchasing of bonds and an accordant expansion of its own balance sheet, but it is also true of less-famous measures that featured in the Fed's heroic crisis-fighting efforts.[16] Crisis, like the Asian financial crisis of 1997, featured in the neoliberal period before 2008, and so did massive state-led crisis intervention.

In short, periodizations are important and they are helpful, but they depend on where we're looking. We should not expect them to be perfect heuristics. On the importance of clarity about our reference points, then, I agree; I would just add that our clarity should be as expansive as possible with regard to time, space, metrics, and so on.

MCKAY: At the same time, at least from my perspective, I'm repeatedly struck by what one might call neoliberalism's "aggressive unoriginality" (I'm borrowing the phrase from Lars Lih, writing in a totally different context).[17] That is, when we read Hayek in the mid-twentieth century on the dire threat of the "fetish of democracy," duly echoed by the likes of Alan Greenspan in this century when he salutes the workings of the global market as far superior to those made by elected politicians, I am drawn to the very similar sentiments of such Victorian liberals as John Stuart Mill and Herbert Spencer, to the point that I'd be tempted to call many "folk neoliberals" today Spencerians, not just in their "let-the-weak-go-to-the-wall" ethics, but in their unwavering conviction that a better future awaits us, made possible through the wonders of the "spontaneous order" a global marketplace somehow makes possible.

PENNER: Yes, it is a point made too rarely that when we are dealing with neoliberalism we are still, in very large measure, dealing with liberalism. This is yet again a place where we should be attentive to continuity and rupture simultaneously. The crisis of liberalism in the 1930s, which prompted the initial efforts of the neoliberal intellectuals at the Lippmann Colloquium in 1938 and later, in the 1940s, at the Mont Pèlerin Society, was to my mind a moment of (substantial) adjustment more than a total restart. The point was to rearticulate a form of liberalism that was up to the historical moment. In my own work on the neoliberal political scientist Tom Flanagan, a Calgary Schooler, while I would say for sure that Hayek is the strongest intellectual influence, John Locke, for example, is also alluded to frequently. Neoliberals are happy to enlist the tenets of an older tradition as it suits them.

MCKAY: If we can consider neoliberalism since the 1970s as "an always mutating project of state-facilitated market rule," and since the 1990s as a globally applied philosophy of encasing markets to protect them from democratic pressures and safeguarding the elaborate transnational networks of capitalist accumulation,[18] what are this framework's strengths? I imagine *The Economist* would tell us that neoliberalism and the competitive world economy has lifted millions out of poverty around the world; many shoppers at Wal Mart and Costco would implicitly second the motion that this revolution in political and economic thought has paid off in the form of cheaper articles of consumption; Ayn Rand's many devotees would tell us that it has liberated creative, self-starting individuals from the repressive dead weight of state bureaucracies. I am struck by how broadly and enthusiastically "market rule" is hailed as a liberating force, even by people who would seem to have every reason to be skeptical of it—and also by how reluctant many Marxists are to undertake realistic examinations of the acceptance of this core neoliberal principle, this ideological formation's capacity to shape common sense and political expectations. This "governing rationality," to use Wendy Brown's term, entails everyday people internalizing notions of competitiveness, branding, property accumulation as a key to self-worth, and so on, so that "economics becomes the model of everything," not excepting democracy.[19]

One objection one might make to the "base-and-superstructure" dismissal of neoliberalism as a mere epiphenomenon of capitalism is that its precepts, endlessly circulated in mass and social media and duly repeated by our governors, have a real purchase on people's daily lives and thoughts. Can we reconcile this perception of neoliberalism as a strong hegemonic force with one that presents it as just so many ad hoc responses calculated to safeguard the particular interests of certain powerful classes? Does minimizing neoliberalism's philosophical and political coherence, emphasizing its "ad hocery," so to speak, run the risk of rendering us blind to its hold on millions of people?

PENNER: I would concede each of those points that you make on behalf of neoliberalism, its apostles, and its allies. Yes, while exact figures vary in accordance with the metrics used, global poverty has been reduced a great deal from the 1980s, although any number that I could spit out here would have to be qualified in all sorts of ways. Suffice to say, hundreds of millions of people, at least, have escaped extreme poverty. The stunning growth of the Chinese economy in the last three or four decades, a period that David Harvey has described under the rubric of "Neoliberalism 'with Chinese Characteristics'" and in which the Chinese share of global GDP has increased almost tenfold, has been a primary driver here.[20] Cheap consumer goods have been associated with the same processes. Some entrepreneurs have flourished in a world where capital is highly mobile and can be raised with relative ease, especially in Silicon Valley.

But this glimmering surface is illusory. Emphasizing reduced poverty, for example, obscures skyrocketing wealth and income inequality since 1980. Again, the global picture is lumpy, but we are by now quite familiar with statistics about extremely small groups of people owning as much wealth as half the global population. As Lisa Adkins, Melinda Cooper, and Martijn Konings have shown, the neoliberal period has introduced a new logic of inequality whereby asset appreciation, especially but not just in property assets, and relative stagnation of wage growth have both meant that asset ownership, rather than employment, has become the key determinant of class position. Those who don't own have been left behind.[21]

Cheap consumer goods, which we might tend to appreciate at the moment of purchase, are often cheap because they are of poor quality or because they are only a means of locking us into some other transactional relationship. We are supposed to be amazed at the computing power and the relative affordability of the smart phones we all carry in our pockets, so amazed in fact that we forget to complain about how our smart phones begin working poorly just months after we buy them and how, in Canada most especially, having a smart phone requires entering into a contract with a monopolistic telecommunications firm that charges exorbitant rates and, as we learned recently, sometimes fails to provide basic services for days at a time.

The entrepreneurial propaganda of our era tells us that we benefit from the untethered genius of the Musks and the Bransons and the Gateses, and yet as obscene wealth has accrued to these putative innovators, the economic upshot of their projects for capitalism as a system has been an end to meaningful, productive innovation. Some observers have overstated these developments in order to announce the arrival of "techno-feudalism," but overstatements aside, there is truth in the claim that the great entrepreneurs of the neoliberal period are more like rentiers or monopolists than they are like the creative destroyers of Schumpeterian rendering.[22] I could go on and on here: the vices that accompany neoliberal virtues are almost endless.

MCKAY: From my perspective, neoliberalism is hegemonic, and not just because of its intellectual predominance. When you step into a Wal Mart or a Costco, our contemporary cathedrals, you are immersed in a worldview as much as you are a retail facility: and that worldview not only tells you that the point of life is the acquisition of more and more things but has marshalled a vast army of people around the planet to make that eminently political concept a material reality, one brought to you by an invisible legion of workers. In this context, "creative destruction" applies primarily to communities and classes that once functioned locally and, in important ways, limited the scope of market relations. Not to take away from your point about the parasitical rent-like qualities of much entrepreneurship in the neoliberal era, but I would not want to underestimate the atomizing, alienating force of contemporary consumer capitalism and its destructive impact upon local communities and the subjectivities of people living in them. How can we unsettle neoliberalism as a hegemonic project if its everyday praxis has achieved such a material hold on our shared experiences?

PENNER: Without wanting to suggest that I have the answer to this very difficult question, I would posit that neoliberalism features a very "tight" hegemony. I think Wendy Brown describes this, but perhaps I can try to put a similar point in alternative terms. To explain the tight neoliberal hegemony, I would note how rare it is for people living in neoliberal conditions to think about social life in social terms. Instead, we are encouraged to think in almost wholly individual terms. When I encounter, for example, an axiom about the importance of balanced state budgets or a polemic in favour of fiscal austerity, I am supposed to ask what these positions mean for me (lower taxes, perhaps) rather than what they mean for the society in which I live (atrophied services and diminished public life). In this way, I'd say confidently that neoliberalism has seen a furtherance, perhaps even a "qualitative radicalization," of what you've called, in the context of Canadian liberal order, "the epistemological and ontological primacy of the category 'individual.'"[23]

I think the blinders of individualism serve the neoliberal project very well, even and especially to the extent that the project is an ad hoc one. With each foreclosed-upon social possibility, it becomes harder and harder to think outside the hegemony of individualism, and this becomes self-reinforcing. One exciting thing about the present crisis, at least, is that it pokes a great big hole in the idea that we can live in perpetuity as isolated individuals rather than as a collective society. Indeed, I suspect quite strongly that, just like the present crisis, future crises will tend to cut against the continuing hegemonic aspirations of neoliberalism. I don't want to suggest an automatic relationship leading to the emergence of neoliberalism's gravediggers, far from it, but I think that nascent conditions of counterhegemonic possibility are here. Turning counterhegemonic possibility into counterhegemony then becomes a political or strategic question.

MCKAY: Turning now to Covid-19, some people have seen in the pandemic a dire, perhaps terminal, crisis of neoliberalism. Many speak of "deglobalization" and note that without the very global capitalism neoliberals have relentlessly promoted since the 1990s, the coronavirus would never have spread so far and so fast. From their perspective, the pandemic illustrates the most negative aspects of the neoliberal order. State cutbacks, for instance, meant that, the core neoliberal states, the US and UK in particular, were unprepared and disorganized in the face of this challenge. What is your assessment of the prospects of globalization? Do its opponents not risk falling into forms of nationalist narrowness—calling for protection behind stronger borders, for instance, at a time when capitalism has rendered such scheme atavistic? Is the antidote to neoliberalism really a return to the 1950s?

PENNER: The coronavirus pandemic, if ostensibly a global crisis of public health, has been experienced more broadly as a generalized crisis of human living. Restrictions and changes made in daily life, justified as the necessities of public health if not actually and always made for those reasons, have reverberated into all spheres of our collective existence. National or regional contexts have conditioned the experience of the pandemic, for sure, and speaking of a generalized crisis does not imply that the consequences of the crisis have been experienced equally. Far from it.

The global character of the pandemic follows from its causes. All life on earth is collectively entangled, yet unequally implicated, in the operations of capitalism.

One consequence of this is that there is now a very real sense in which nothing, at least nothing with "-ism" as a suffix, is possible in one country. While talk of deglobalization has become increasingly frequent in the age of the coronavirus, these conversations are more about prediction than diagnosis. Every day, we continue to see just how global our economy really is and what that means. Inflation, supply chain breakdowns, war, and so on—each such disruption (to use a very mild phrase) reveals the continued interconnectedness of the global economy, even if they all equally suggest the acute risks of such extensive interconnection. In general, then, the Covid-19 crisis is best viewed not as an isolated event but as an acute flare up of a chronic global condition that we call capitalism.

Turning now to some of the specifics of your question: First, the deglobalization idea, whether in the form of detached prediction or advocative prescription, strikes me as a dead end. And I think you are right to imply that it runs a serious risk of manifesting as little more than parochial nationalism, which could always lead to a world characterized by competitive nationalisms. Among other things, surely the war in Ukraine is showing us the incompatibility of global crisis-fighting and belligerent nationalism.

On the flip-side, with regard to the prospects of globalization, I think it is worthwhile to step back and take a broad view of the Covid-19 pandemic, which has been experienced broadly as a generalized crisis of human living across the globe. Restrictions and changes made in daily life have reverberated into all spheres of our collective existence. And this global character of the pandemic follows from its causes. The work of Mike Davis, for example, shows that the pandemic is traceable to the operations of global capitalism, which have fundamentally deformed our relationships to nature and thereby ushered in a climate crisis that, among other things, makes pandemics like the current one a very likely prospect. All life on earth is collectively entangled in the operations of capitalism.

Undoing that collective entanglement, even if there are reasons to think it desirable, would be a task not just Herculean but Sisyphean. Taking the insight that the pandemic is traceable to a broader ecological crisis, which in turn is traceable to two-plus centuries of industrial capitalism, we must conclude that all of us share in the same broad crisis conditions. We are not equally responsible for those conditions, not even close, and we are not all equally vulnerable to them. Indeed, the less responsible, as a rule, are the most vulnerable. But in any case, even if the boulder of deglobalization were pushed to the top of the hill, the reality of the crisis we face would see it tumble back down.

From where we stand, I think there is scarcely an *ism* of any kind that is possible in just one country. Nationalism, today, is illusory at the very best. We face inescapably global problems, and in the face of those problems, internationalism ought to be the order of the day.

MCKAY: I am struck by how much of the left has responded to pandemic-era movements, commonly (though I sometimes think mystifyingly) labelled "populist," as those of "lumpen" people harbouring primitive ideas and ill-considered myths (and, to reference the Freedom Convoy in Ottawa in January 2022, being so gauche as to provide bouncy castles for their kids). The pejorative term "redneck" (or "beauf" for francophones) often crops up. Book after book about conspiracy theories tell us about stupid people falling for dumb ideas.

The left signed up massively for lockdowns and derided those who opposed them. Many dwell upon the homophobia, racism, sexism, and narrowness of their fellow citizens. The *gilets jaunes* movement in France, the assault on the Capitol in Washington, D.C., in January 2020, the Freedom Convoy in Ottawa, the enraptured fellows of Bolsonaro in Brazil are all grist for this liberal mill, and we are urged to pathologize as "illiberal" all those who get involved in these populist movements.

I agree with the thrust of many of these polemics. Yet, overall they seem a bit simplistic and even dangerous. This way of handling many of the everyday people who have been mobilized by rightists strikes me as counterproductive and, in many cases, damaging because unless we pry millions of such people away from the ideologies that have attracted them, our own chances of changing the world are slim. Much of today's antipopulist discourse ironically echoes Victorian liberalism in its distrust of the unwashed masses, and in an ironic way, also in effect agrees with the neoliberals who sought to encase the global management of trade and production from the importunate demands of the *demos*. And some of the populist suspicion of expert knowledge, whether applied to opioids or lockdowns, seems to be warranted—whereas many leftists seem to echo a "just-trust-the-experts" line I would not expect to hear from them. As someone living in Alberta, home to many right-wing partisans of "freedom," how do you evaluate the left's handling of those it categorizes as its enemies? And when did it become left-wing dogma to rail against the critics of liberalism?

PENNER: This question has to be answered in a general register, which will mean that I ignore some things and highlight others. So forgive me, but yes: the right has been the most successful at using the pandemic for political mobilization, and the response from what I might call the "putative" left has routinely featured little more than dismissive opprobrium. The issue of expert knowledge is a case in point. For understandable reasons, much of what was posed as expert knowledge over the course of the pandemic was actually expert estimate. Against some framings of science as a more or less static body of unquestionable knowledge and insight, the pandemic was an exercise in learning along the way. In the process, many experts comported themselves in such a fashion as to earn some, but surely not all, of the skepticism they garnered from the right. And the right, broadly speaking, was quite successful at mobilizing around that kind of skepticism.

I reference a putative left in order to suggest that, today, when we talk in broad terms about the left, it is often not all that clear what exactly we are talking about. A major part of the reason why the pandemic has mobilized the right most forcefully is that the right is better organized. Even as the pandemic has laid bare the myriad irrationalities baked into our way of living, the right has been able to organize people around a backward-looking desire to return to "normal," a desire that addresses itself both to public health measures and, more importantly, to all sorts of reactionary ideas about an idyllic past. The popularity of right-wing slogans that end with the word "again" is telling.

MCKAY: I would imagine your vantage point in Alberta has offered you ample opportunities to reflect on the paradoxes of contemporary populism.

PENNER: Alberta is a great place from which to think about this dynamic. It was insufferable here during the Freedom Convoy, which, of course, had an Albertan manifestation at the Coutts border crossing where a blockade was established and largely maintained over a period of almost three weeks. Blockade supporters all over the province were highly visible every day. And what was the response? Counterprotests here and there, for sure, but beyond that we saw exasperated pleas for police action against the blockade and critiques of the muted response from government.

On the left, there was little gained from the ordeal, while on the far right there were martyrs and new political stars. Indeed, the protests arguably hammered the final nail in Premier Jason Kenney's political coffin and initiated the process that will deliver us our next premier. Kenney, who had governed entirely from the right (corporate tax cuts, slashed budgets, backwards education policies) was somehow not conservative enough. I hope the new premier won't last long but am far from sure that she won't.

The left can't chide its way into power. It is crucial to have a positive vision in order that we can provide an organizational, as opposed to merely discursive, opposition both to growing movements of the right and to an intransigent liberal mainstream that continually deludes itself about the nature of the problems facing the world and about the mechanisms that might solve those problems. Some polls suggested that almost half of Canadians were supportive of the Freedom Convoy's aims, even if people were much less likely to support its tactics.[24] Writing off, say, 46 percent of the people in the country as lumpen is not a good place from which to begin building a left politics for the coming era.

MCKAY: If we define "the left" as all those forces hoping for and working towards an egalitarian postcapitalist future, it is hard not to agree with your critique of a very loosely-defined putative left, which seems unable to present everyday people with much in the way of a concrete alternative to a resurgent far right. Don't leftists have to reflect much more intently upon what it is about contemporary leftism that is simply not registering—and not in a "blame-the-victim" way that gives us an easy alibi? With reference to the academic left, I am particularly struck by how little most of it is connected, even potentially connected, to the concerns of people who are struggling to survive in a hostile world, surely the left's natural constituency. One finds a legion of would-be leaders haranguing empty lecture halls (or, these days, shouting at each other online in ways unlikely to produce new ideas about anything). And, as you point out, we also find leftists calling out for more aggressive and repressive handling of demonstrations, even in terms that, as Naomi Klein and others rightly point out, could be brought to bear against any and all labour demonstrations. I confess I don't have a ready solution to this deep-seated and complicated disconnect between leftists and the people they purport to lead. Do you?

PENNER: To begin with, I suspect it is worth saying that the political projects of left and right are up against qualitatively distinct challenges. As Wendy Brown and others have pointed out, neoliberalism has been not just accommodative but actively helpful for the far right and its antidemocratic goals.[25] The contemporary right's goals strike me as entirely compatible with perduring capitalism, even if capital, broadly speaking, is not always at the ready to support and further the politics of reaction. The left, on the other hand, by seeking what you call an egalitarian postcapitalist future, has to chart a tougher course.

To the extent that the present, and many "past presents," seem to accommodate the right more than the left, it is understandable, if not excusable, that the left would struggle to realize the kinds of transformative movements that it imagines. Along these lines, it may still be useful to invoke, as leftists have done periodically over the decades, the concept of "left melancholia." The idea comes from Walter Benjamin, who used it to describe the elevation of ideals, and failed ideals, over and above the material project of seizing present conditions in order to change them. I think this is about what you are describing when you mention haranguing lecturers and vituperative exchanges.

To overcome this left melancholia, I would again point to the importance of a positive political vision connected to present conditions and the associated concerns, anxieties, and interests of the people who would make up the movement. This vision won't appear out of the ether, and so the other side of this coin is the kind of left organization from which such a vision could materialize. My sense is that in parts of the world outside North America, perhaps especially in Latin America, this is much closer to being a reality than we sometimes appreciate. Within North America, the supremacy of electoral politics continues to be a stumbling block. Even as, say, the Sanders campaigns in the US were massively mobilizing and represented an unequivocal advancement of the continental left, it is still worth questioning whether established political parties (the Democratic Party in the US and the New Democratic Party in Canada) are the best organizational bases from which the left can operate. Mike Davis often speaks of an "organization of organizers" and I think there is something there.

All of this is easier said than done—but ease surely isn't what we're looking for.

MCKAY: Do you share my sense that populism is one of the more overworked and mystifying terms in contemporary political discourse? I often read descriptions of populists—i.e., "people who suspect a small elite of powerful people is setting a particularly narrow agenda for the governance of the planet"—and say to myself, "Well, factually, is that not the case?" When I read routine denunciations of the notion of the "Deep State," usually couched in terms that make those populists who place any credence in the notion seem crazy, I reflect, "Yes, I can see that this critique is being marshalled by neoliberals opportunistically accessing libertarian ideals and firing up a popular base without any intention of challenging the structures and relations that are actually oppressing that base. Yet, the notion that there is an institution called 'the State' that operates over years and decades to impose a certain shape to social reality, one that privileges the rich and hurts everybody else, does not seem that far-fetched or 'populist' to me."

PENNER: Oh, very much so! To be sure, there are scholars and intellectuals who study populism in some way or another and use the concept to make what strike me as helpful historiographical or political interventions. But the term has this whole other life, as you suggest, in public discourse. There, I agree that the term is routinely asked to do more work than it can, with mystifying results.

In the sense of the term that you invoke—that is, a narrow elite is calling the shots—I am likewise fairly close to agreement, but only when the view is articulated in those broad terms. So-called right-populists, it seems to me, proceed to fill in the view with referents that are misguided and misleading. And moreover, the right-populist theory of elite dominance seems totally absent. Why and how is a narrow elite in a position to impose and perpetuate its self-serving agenda? I don't think a right-populist has a good answer.

The right's inability to fill out its populism with anything like a theory of the society in which we live has ugly results. Instead of an "actionable" description of the structure of our political and economic lives, we get scapegoats and all of the "culture war" rubbish that passes for politics on the right. In other words, I suppose I'm saying that right-populism is an enabler of other resurgent and hostile *isms* that are really the "main event" of the politics that we describe (at least when we see them on the right) as populist.

A form of left populism that would actually describe the mechanisms of elite dominance and state power in order to undo that dominance and wield that power towards emancipatory ends would sit just fine with me. But then: I would rather call that politics, simply, socialism.

MCKAY: You have been much influenced by Andreas Malm, undoubtedly one of today's major left intellectuals, who argues Covid-19 is related intimately to the global climate crisis, and to Aaron Benanav, theorist of a "post-scarcity world." These would seem to be radically divergent theorists with very different points of view—the one laying out the case (carefully) for acts of industrial sabotage against pipelines, the other for a postcapitalist utopia. How can they be reconciled? What might their respective places be in an emergent politics of resistance?

PENNER: Yes, I certainly think that both Malm and Benanav have much to offer. And yes, their political visions are quite disparate. Reconciliation of their views might not be entirely possible, but I can point to the complementarity of their analyses and suggest how they might work together. It is worth pointing out, as well, the connection between this exercise and the issue of a left political vision that we've been discussing.

In *Fossil Capital* most especially, but in other, shorter works as well, Malm is brilliant on the relationship between capitalism and fossil fuels.[26] In the briefest possible terms, Malm's point is that the dominance of fossil fuels is a direct result of their discovery and exploitation in the context of capitalism. The capitalist logic of profit-making and growth led directly to the dominance of fossil fuel sources and thus led in turn to the ecological crisis that we presently face, a crisis that is characterized most especially by the present and future threat of climate change. In *Corona, Climate, Chronic Emergency*, Malm is clear to the point of being syllogistic: capitalism caused climate change, so halting climate change implies stopping capitalism.[27] Malm's radicalism is all about identifying and going after root causes.

Benanav comes from an entirely different angle. His book, *Automation and the Future of Work*, is addressed to debates in "automation theory," the proponents of which envision a future of unemployed and immiserated masses as technological development furthers the automation, or robotification, of labour. Benanav's counterpoint is that, thanks to decades of economic stagnation, the core labour problem of our time is more like a persistent "underdemand" for workers, not an absolute receding of demand. In this context, we should not expect a future of mass joblessness but one where labour is persistently devalued, meaning that workers will mainly be poorly and inconsistently paid rather than not hired at all.[28] Cheap labour ought to suit capitalists, who in this sense are in fact likely to be discouraged from implementing technological alternatives to human labour.

Both Malm and Benanav then move from their analytical positions to propose commensurate politics and, especially with Malm, accompanying tactics. On these issues Malm is a keen provocateur. His two most famous prescriptions are an embrace of "war communism" in *Corona, Climate, Chronic Emergency* and, as you've alluded to, a call for widespread industrial sabotage against fossil fuel infrastructure in *How to Blow up a Pipeline*.[29] In both cases, for sure, Malm is actually quite persuasive. His provocations are far more considered than they sound when I render them in brief here. But still, especially in the case of *How to Blow up a Pipeline*, Malm has come in for warranted criticism.[30] And in any case, provocations that will strike the vast majority of people as completely far-fetched (if not actively unappealing, until they are explained in more depth) mightn't be the best kind of provocations around which to build a political movement.

Benanav, contrastingly, uses the crisis of persistent underdemand for labour to imagine utopia. Benanav's post-scarcity world is described in terms of what Marx termed "a realm of necessity" and "a realm of freedom." In the former, we carry out the tasks necessary for our day-to-day lives. In the latter, the realm of freedom, human beings are able, on the basis of successfully handling life's necessities, to craft identities and pursue projects that express their human potentials and capacities. The sharing of labour in the realm of necessity, and a related reduction in the amount of redundant labour that is currently performed every day, would mean that our collective work would not take that long—maybe three to five hours of work for each of us on any given workday. In such an arrangement, all of us would have substantially more free time than we do currently, and the benefits of technological innovations aimed at reducing human labour would accrue broadly to us all instead of narrowly to capital.

The contrast here should be pretty obvious, though it is worth saying that both Malm and Benanav are committed to the idea that something like state planning needs to be on the table. Addressing climate change makes planning of some kind a requirement. For

Benanav, some kind of collective global effort to address the climate would need to take top priority at the initial step towards utopia. For Malm, addressing the ecological crisis requires taking control of and redirecting the broad "capitalist state." Only the state can martial the kinds of power and capacity necessary to transition past fossil capitalism. So, we should bring the state, especially those parts of it most responsible for current predicaments and most intransigent in their face, under public control and impose an alternative authority on would-be resisters.

The question has to be, I suppose, what are we planning for? Malm seems to think that climate change is such a dire predicament that utopia is effectively off the table. Survival would be a more appropriate goal. Even if Malm is rightly pessimistic, as it were, I am not sure that such a limited horizon will mobilize people as it must. Indeed, the call to sabotage could be read as an admission of relative political and economic powerlessness. Benanav's utopianism is more exciting, but it lacks the kind of urgency that Malm so rightly insists upon. This is the point at which the reconciliation of these thinkers, such as it is, can happen. We can still appeal to a better future, but we might not be able to do so for much longer.

There are "potentialities" in the present crisis and while the powers that be march along in the same old ways, at best aiming to live exactly as we live now (just "greener," or some such), it is imperative for the left to make the case that by living otherwise we can actually live better. And, that we'd better hurry up.

MCKAY: Has Covid-19 fundamentally altered the terrain on which politics takes place? Throughout Covid-19, many states—at least those with the fiscal capacity to do so—expanded dramatically, seemingly ripping up the neoliberal playbook as they in effect renationalized important sectors, offered wage supports, facilitated vaccine development, and so on: if neoliberalism meant the state should have a limited place in corporate boardrooms and a minimal interest in supporting its citizens, it might be considered over and done with. Yet, it doesn't seem to be. It seems to have a zombie-like capacity to survive, its conventional rhetoric little impaired by the deaths of a mere fifteen million people (and counting). In the absence of an effective global left, how do we transcend the limitations of a stance that, having rigorously analyzed our still-persisting capitalist order, then lamely gestures towards nonexistent "armies of redressers" (to recall a phrase from E.P. Thompson) who might challenge it?

PENNER: I do think that the political terrain has been altered fundamentally, but Covid-19 isn't the lone or ultimate cause. The pandemic is only an acute flare up of a chronic condition (our deformed relationship to the natural world, a result of centuries of industrial capitalism). In this way, it reveals our reality more than it changes that reality.

This question goes to the debate about the end of neoliberalism, which you reference, especially the participants in that debate who, for a time at least, saw neoliberalism giving way to more progressive forms of politics and economics. In the earliest days of the pandemic, political possibility could be seen everywhere. Could the "essential worker" category prompt a broad reconsideration of work and its value in places where, for decades, labour had been under attack? Could the massive mobilization of state institutions across the globe induce a renewed look at state capacity and the ends to which it could be put? Could collective vulnerability to the virus lead to a questioning of the individualistic doctrines that have featured so prominently in the political arenas of capitalist countries? Could unequal vulnerability to the virus lead to a serious effort to combat the widening of the gap between rich and poor both within and between states? All these questions were on the table shortly after the beginning of the pandemic. And while it would be short-sighted to announce that all of these political opportunities have passed us by, they have run into familiar challenges and obstacles.

A major part of the reason why these seeming possibilities haven't got very far off the ground, as it were, is that so much political energy has recently been subsumed by the desire to "get back to normal." Take the Freedom Convoy, which, if we squint a bit and ignore some details, was something like a mobilization in favour of a lost normality. This, I would submit, is why the aims of the blockaders and the truckers were as popular as they were with the Canadian public. A certain exhaustion had set in. So, if the early period of the pandemic was defined by political possibility, the most recognizable moment of the latter phase was a testament to narrowed horizons and atrophied political imagination. The end of neoliberalism? Or maybe we can just settle for grocery shopping without a mask?

Despite the apparent appeal of normality, there is still very little evidence to suggest that "normal" is a meaningfully available option. Even as the same old ideas and interests doggedly persist, they do not seem capable of returning us to something that we'd recognize as normal. What this means is that, as the desire to return to normal seemingly restricts our collective political imaginations, the conflict between that desire and reality will widen them again. There are, importantly, no built-in tendencies here. So much is on the table. If status quo capitalism all but guarantees a future of never-ending crisis, something has to give.

Any politics that takes us beyond the cascading crises of capitalism will be made real by people, in whatever organizational form, who act collectively to make the impossible possible. I agree that those people have not, as yet, assembled, at least not in any nonlocalized way. But, to return to the themes of our discussion about the historical nature of neoliberalism's emergence: if we generalize that discussion, we could say that political-economic transformations are always historical processes; they are never, even in moments that we'd call revolutionary, pure acts of heroic agency. Even as I'm skeptical about pronouncements of neoliberalism's demise, I think the instinct to make such pronouncements follows from an accurate sense of nascent historical change. Our "rigorous analyses," such as they are, may be in the early process of encountering the historical conditions that can turn analyses into movements. In the current conjuncture, just a little (impure) heroic agency might go an awfully long way.

AN INTERVIEW WITH
ANDREAS MALM
27 MAY 2021

Andreas Malm is an associate professor of human ecology at Lund University in Sweden. He is the author of several major books, including the prestigious Deutscher Prize–winning *Fossil Capital* (2016), which is a significant study of the transnational history of coal and capitalism; *The Progress of This Storm* (2018); *How to Blow Up a Pipeline* (2021); *White Skin, Black Fuel* (2021; with the Zetkin Collective); and *Corona, Climate, Chronic Emergency* (2021), which is one of the most stimulating interpretations of the pandemic.

MCKAY: By my count, you have, since the 2016 publication of *Fossil Capital*, produced three books, several major research articles, a range of interviews, and you have also devoted your time and energy to parenting two children. My questions would be (a) what do you have for breakfast? but also (b) is there a tension between such activist scholarship that you've been pursuing lately and the immense labour of research that went into the 488 pages of *Fossil Capital*? How do you reconcile being a scholar and an activist at the same time?

MALM: That's a very good question. I would not say that that is an easy combination and it's not one that I master particularly well—primarily because I'm not really an activist these days, in the sense of being an organizer. I was an organizer in the climate movement fourteen to sixteen years ago. My activism nowadays is limited to my academic work, with occasional participation in demonstrations and in climate camps when I have a chance to attend those. But yes, I think that, if you're working on the climate crisis as I've been doing for some time and given the magnitude of the crisis, its severity, the depth of it, it would be strange to just produce knowledge for the sake of knowledge without any kind of attempt to make that knowledge useful for movements that struggle with these questions and to be politically relevant. This is certainly something that I struggle with.

In the spring of 2018, I was really immersing myself in nerdy historical research of the kind I really enjoy doing for its own sake, but I was freaking out towards the end of that spring. I felt that I can't really justify this kind of research when the world is catching fire and all of that. And it actually *was* catching fire in the summer of 2018, here where I live. We had the extreme summer with droughts, and wildfires, and unprecedented heat waves—that then prompted Greta Thunberg to start her school strike. So, I told my publishers that I can't justify to myself doing this kind of work. Part of that became a volume that's just been published called *White Skin, Black Fuel*, on the danger of fossil fascism, which I wrote together with the Zetkin Collective.[1] It is unlike the *Corona* book that you mentioned and *The Progress of the Storm*. It is based on prodigious research, but research done by twenty people in a collective. So that has been my main research project over the past couple of years, and it's been a very collective project. It's been very explicitly conceived as a kind of activist scholarship project, and we had a conference that was for both activists and academics working on the political ecologies of the far right to feed into an emerging conversation around the intersections between racism and climate and justice.

MCKAY: You've really made the "metabolic rift" a core idea of your own scholarship. Scholars like Mike Davis, Rob Wallace, and a lot of other people are really seized with this metaphor, which in a sense originates with Marx and *Das Kapital*. I was wondering if you could tell us what is so important about metabolic rift from your point of view? What *is* it (for people that may not have encountered this before)? And why is—and I'm going to the book that you wrote called *The Progress of This Storm*—a conceptual distinction between humanity and nonhuman nature not only intellectually but politically important?

MALM: The theory of the metabolic rift (I have to say that I'm not sure that I have used it that much in my own writings—I'm not even 100 percent sure the term appears in *Fossil Capital*; I can't really remember if it does) has proven to be a tremendously fertile research program and a very productive and generative model of environmental destruction. It's derived from Marx, but it's really the product of John

Bellamy Foster and his fellow colleagues. The basic idea, as I understand it, is that a metabolic rift is a rupture in metabolic flows between humans and the rest of nature or within extra-human nature—various types of biogeochemical cycles—and this rupture is caused by the disruption coming from capitalist property relations. This is how I understand the model. It's been applied to lots of different environmental problems, from the nitrogen cycle to overfishing, to climate change, and lots of other things.

Now, there's been a debate within ecological Marxism where, very notably, Jason Moore has argued that the theory of the metabolic rift is guilty of Cartesian dualism because it makes a distinct and analytical distinction between what's natural and what's social. What I did in *The Progress of This Storm* was to defend the theory of the metabolic rift against that charge. I think his and others' idea, that any kind of analytical distinction between nature and society or the natural and the social is guilty of Cartesian dualism, itself reproduces the separation between the two realms that is at root of environmental destruction. I think that his argument is flawed. I think the theory of the metabolic rift is obviously not an attempt to say that nature and society are two realms apart, that they are separated. The thrust of the theory is of course exactly the opposite. Nature and society are always intertwined and fundamentally united, but there are destructive relations that can tear the flows apart and lead to various kinds of environmental problems.

Now I also think that it's crucial, analytically and politically, to maintain a distinction—an analytical distinction—between what's natural and what's social. If you look at this pandemic for instance: it's something natural that pathogens, including coronaviruses, circulate in wildlife populations such as bats, the natural reservoir hosts of coronaviruses. That's natural; it's not something that humans have created over time. On the other hand, it's a social phenomenon that you have wildlife trading or certain kinds of conspicuous consumption patterns. That's something that has developed in a particular moment in time in history through a very contingent development of relations between people. Likewise, it's a distinctly social phenomenon that you have global supply chains that cause very destructive deforestation in tropical forests, probably the main driver of zoonotic spill over (all of these new infectious diseases that jump from those animal populations into humans). The political value of maintaining that distinction is that it allows you to say that we as humans should change in our social relations, in our society, so as to avoid causing this disaster again. We can't do anything about the fact that coronaviruses exist in nature and travel on the bodies of bats. (Well, we could potentially eradicate all bats, but that probably wouldn't be a wise solution.) What we can do differently is that we can modify everything that's social, including global supply chains, how we deal with wildlife, crackdown on wildlife trading. I think this is the value of the analytical distinction.

MCKAY: I thought one of the most fascinating moments in *Corona Climate Chronic Emergency* came with two graphs that are really brilliant in terms of showing us that, in many ways, when we look at natural hazards, we put them in this black box and we call it "Nature." And we say, "Okay, it's going to generate these 'black swan events,' but we human beings just have to respond to them." You point out that, in many ways, looking at it as that black box is misleading because within what we're calling "nature" are nonnegligible prime movers that are generated socially. The social, you write, has "saturated the hazards themselves"[2]—so that, in the case of the coronavirus, what we're responding to is a set of natural hazards that are also social themselves. Could you elaborate on that theme?

MALM: This is an argument developed in dialogue with the work of Ben Wiesner and his colleagues, and that work was absolutely foundational in the 1970s and '80s in the development of a kind of critical vulnerability or critical disaster research. What preceded it was a very simplified geophysical view of disasters, which held that disaster is the result of some kind of a natural hazard striking a population that is vulnerable because it lives close to a fault line, or in an area prone to drought, or whatever. Wiesner and others pointed out that the vulnerability of people to a natural hazard is always differentiated, and it depends on the assets that people have, the buffers that can protect them from the impact of a natural hazard. It's been shown in many cases that earthquakes strike much more painfully if people live in ramshackle housing, in slums, for instance, then if you have solid houses because you're reasonably affluent. Some have even called earthquakes "class quakes." I'm not objecting to this, but I'm pointing out a limitation of that model—which is that in it, the natural hazards themselves are considered to be caused solely by natural forces and processes, whereas all the social factors are placed on the side of the impact where the vulnerability is constituted.

My argument is that, now, you find the social drivers existing not only on the side of vulnerability but in the very production of the hazards themselves. For instance, there was a recent report that came out that said thirty million people around the world were internally displaced last year because of extreme weather events—representing 75 percent of the internally displaced people around the world last year. More people had to flee because of hurricanes, droughts, and flooding than because of war and conflict, and this is apparently the first time you have that clear a distribution. This is not exclusively due to the fact that people in the Global South are vulnerable to extreme weather events. It's also because the extreme weather events themselves become more intense, frequent, and ferocious, and that curve is a product of social processes, around fossil fuel combustion in particular. The same argument applies to zoonotic spill over and pandemics.

MCKAY: As a historian, what I find encouraging about your work is that it opens up a pathway that had been blocked by the postmodern turn in the twentieth century. Basically, historians were left with the idea they are telling stories that are almost arbitrarily selected from the past. We're not really expected to be preoccupied with causal factors or serious analyses of them. I see your work as opening a new vista. Historians are responsible for rational reconstruction, for evidence-based interpretations of the past with implications for the present and the future. Do you sense that new horizons are in fact opening up for historians who have this kind of structural perspective in mind?

MALM: I've had this feeling or idea that global warming in a sense lifts a veil on the import of what's been going on for two centuries in that it's only with this crisis that it becomes fully apparent what it really meant to establish large-scale fossil fuel combustion and burn fossil fuels. Global warming raises new questions for historians, and I think also sends us looking back at things that have happened with new eyes.

It's part of what we're doing in this *White Skin, Black Fuel* book on the danger of fossil fascism. We look at how classical fascists, the Mussolini regime in Italy and the NSDAP regime in Germany, dealt with fossil fuel technologies. Against the background of what's happening today (with the far right positioning itself as the kind of most aggressive defender of business as usual), it's quite significant that the interwar far right, the classical fascists, were so extremely fetishistic about cars, airplanes, and coal combustion.

So, yes, I think in the light of the climate crisis, there is a lot of work for historians to do. We're putting together a volume with texts by people in the Bolshevik regime, primarily in the 1920s, discussing the drawbacks of oil and some advocating for solar power and things like that. Ecological discussions in early revolutionary Russia really take on a new importance in the light of what's going on today. And this can be applied to very many different historical fields over the past centuries.

MCKAY: I thought your coronavirus book posed an interesting historical question when you wrote that there's been such a dramatic state response to the coronavirus, with lockdowns (and the Chinese response being perhaps the most dramatic of locking down vast cities in a way that I don't think has ever really been attempted at that scale before)—and that's all in stark contrast to how the climate crisis has been unfolding. People and diplomats gather together every couple of years, pass impressive resolutions, and CO_2 levels keep rising. There seems to be a marked contrast between willingness to take state action on the one side—quite dramatic state action—and on the other side, dithering and passing resolutions that are basically ineffectual. How would you respond to this contrast between these two moments of our polycrisis: coronavirus and the wider climate crisis?

MALM: My argument, to begin with, in the *Corona* book is that there are certain differences between the climate crisis and the crisis at the moment of the outbreak of the pandemic that account for the differences in state responses. One is that this pandemic struck out of the blue, and it travelled with lightning speed into the affluent core of the Global North, whereas the climate crisis has been going on for a long time, and it's always been distributed in a way that the primary victims are people in the Global South. Decision-makers in the Global North have become almost inured to the idea that there is this climate misery always going on in the Global South, whereas we are the main beneficiaries of business as usual, so we can keep going. When the pandemic hit northern Italy (jumping from China and then to Iran), that was really the moment when it was constituted as a global crisis and when there was a panic reaction in Europe and governments started closing down and likewise in the US. It had a different temporal process and a different profile when it comes to the distribution of suffering. That might be one explanation for the differences in reaction.

There are many others, of course. Another is that all the measures taken were advertised as temporary. It's not like on the climate front where the fossil fuel industries would have to be shut down forever. Here all the lockdowns and the restrictions were proclaimed to be just temporary measures that would then be taken away and we would go back to normality.

In the latter parts of the book, my argument is that, if you look closer, in fact the differences are not that great, because what states have showed themselves capable of doing on the pandemic front is to combat the symptoms, the effects. All the discussions, all the policy-making, the decision-making around the pandemic, have stayed at the level of symptoms—as in, how are we going to manage this crisis, what kind of social distancing should be imposed on people, when do we get the vaccines, how do we distribute the vaccines?—and so on and so forth. There's been no initiative (that I know of) to go to the root causes, the drivers of zoonotic spillover. In fact, deforestation in the tropics accelerated massively in 2020 and reached the third-highest level since comprehensive measuring began in 2002. The year 2020 was absolutely disastrous to tropical forests around the world, particularly in Brazil. I don't know of any concerted remedial effort from any advanced capitalist state or from any forum for collective bourgeois class rationality. One would imagine that the World Bank, the IMF, or the G20, or something like that would ask themselves how we make sure this doesn't happen again. How do we avoid another pandemic a few years down the road? And how do we address the causes of this problem?

That discourse is entirely absent. The passivity in relation to the drivers of zoonotic spill over corresponds pretty well to the passivity in relation to the drivers of global heating. There's almost more talk about doing something about climate change than there is about doing something about the things that cause zoonotic spill over.

What you see states capable of doing on the climate front, again, is to deal with symptoms. When you had flooding in New South Wales earlier this year, for instance, a year after the wildfire inferno, you had government evacuating areas, closing down roads, telling people to work from home, taking measures very similar to those taken to combat the pandemic so as to deal with the symptoms of global heating in Australia. But the Australian state has done nothing to address the drivers of the problem. In fact, Australia is still the world's largest coal and gas exporter, and the government of Scott Morrison did everything to keep that structure in place and expand it. Australia looks like it's bent on burning and drowning itself to death. So again, the business-as-usual approach on the climate front corresponds to business as usual on the pandemic front.

MCKAY: You point out that even in Sweden the connection between environmental activism and the pandemic is almost invisible. I guess that we need to work harder to make people understand that these two phenomena are connected, because one would have thought, in Sweden, that this would be an easy sell?

MALM: People have a misperception of Sweden, this welfare state where people are reasonable and rational. Don't get me started on the politics—they are getting more and more extreme by the day. This country is unfortunately not a bastion of rationality.

We need to work harder on making the connections. I think one of the reasons those connections haven't been made or they at least haven't percolated into the public discourse is that there's been no movement mobilizing around this throughout the pandemic. The social movements directly related to the pandemic have mostly been protesting the lockdowns that we've had in both Europe and North America. But there has been no movement mobilization around things like deforestation. (We need to get the supply chains under some kind of public control to make sure they don't raze tropical forests.) No movement has really pushed that onto the agenda. That is partly, I think, because the climate movement went into a coma when the pandemic broke out, and the general environment movement did as well. The climate movement in the Global North reached its peak so far of mobilization in 2019 and then it just completely fell off a cliff when the pandemic broke out.

MCKAY: I really like the discussion in your book relating to E. Ann Kaplan. The argument is that people right now are living in a kind of "pretrauma." They're traumatized before the event because they can see that they're living in a world with a very uncertain future and an unreliable natural environment. This pandemic has clarified some of the harshest features of the capitalist world that we inhabit.

Sometimes I worry that the left is becoming a kind of collective Cassandra. We quite reasonably and realistically pile up these existential crises threatening humanity, but I wonder if that doesn't induce in traumatized people (or pretraumatized people) an almost suicidal sense of living in the End Times. When I raised that question with Mike Davis, he said in effect, I think with an element of sternness, "Well we are living in an age of apocalyptic capitalism and it's the job of the left to tell people the facts." I can see the truth in that. But I still do wonder if we don't need to be respectful of where people are right now, which for many of them is this pretraumatized state. I wonder if frightened people aren't going to be impelled to do irrational, frightening things. Where would you would stand on this question?

MALM: My own take on emotions in relation to the climate crisis is that the one emotion conducive to collective action and social movement organizing is anger. There is this research on climate psychology and this debate about how we get people to act. Do we give them hopeful messages about how good things can become—or do we give them alarming messages about how bad things are and how much worse they're going to get? The one, amply supported, conclusion is that anger is the emotion that really makes people act. Look at the

George Floyd uprising. It wasn't fear, it wasn't despair—it was outrage over the murder of George Floyd that brought those tens of millions onto the streets in the US. And most social movements historically seem to have worked that way.

I think the task of the climate movement is to articulate climate rage and that's not very difficult—at least it shouldn't be difficult. There are all those insane projects for expanding fossil fuel infrastructure still going on around the world that people should be angry about. There are reports such as the one that came out last autumn from the Stockholm Environment Institute and Oxfam that said the richest 1 percent of humanity has emitted twice as much as the poorest half of humanity since the 1990s. (If you add investments, the disparities are even greater.) How can you respond to a figure like that with any other emotion than anger? It should inflame people. It doesn't. And that's the problem. There is a deficit of anger. That's the deficit the climate movement needs to fill.

MCKAY: How do we mobilize, how do we create that historical subject that can change this situation, and who will that historical subject be? Since the world-historic defeat of the left in the 1970s, it's very hard to think of a large social force that can actually change this trajectory. And yet it's also hard to think of changing that trajectory without a large social, class-based force.

MALM: That's the one big existential question for all of us, I think, and we're really groping around for an answer. So far, every candidate for a substitute for the organized working class hasn't really been able to fill in the shoes of that class. You can draw various conclusions from this on the climate front. Some would argue that the only chance for the climate struggle is to resurrect the organized working class and make it climate-conscious. Make trade unions and labour (working-class) parties the subject of the climate transition again, just as they were the subject of socialist politics in the twentieth century. I'm not entirely sanguine about the prospects for doing that, and I don't really think the organized working class in the Global North is in a position to be the driver of the climate movement right now. There could be a massive upswing in class struggle in the Global North that might change this picture, but I don't see that happening right now.

The big climate mobilizations we saw in 2019 in the Global North were not based on class, they were not based on gender, and they were not based on race. They were based on age. It was, very distinctly, a youth movement. And that tells us something about what a possible subject in the Global North could look like. Now, in the Global South, where you have mass climate suffering already playing out and unfolding, it's a little bit different. The problem there is that these people are not close in space to the source of their misery. The source of their misery is cumulative emissions over time that have primarily happened in the Global North. It's very hard for them to put up a fight. Palestinians encounter their oppressors every day and know exactly who's the source of their misery. But it's very different with the climate injustice that plays out across the globe.

Now when you think about these matters—and I'm banging on about this in every context I'm in since I closed the book—the most wonderful resource for thinking about those things that I know is the novel *The Ministry for the Future* by Kim Stanley Robinson, where he really outlines an incredibly compelling scenario for climate struggle emerging from the Global South after a hyper lethal heat wave hits northern India in 2025 killing twenty million people in about a week. And after this extreme cataclysm, enraged and embittered people in India form a group called the Children of Kali and start attacking fossil fuel infrastructure around the world. That's obviously a work of fiction, but I think he sketches a future that's not inconceivable.

MCKAY: "In many ways," you write, "a global struggle to suppress CO_2 does not sit naturally within the framework of the nation state."[3] I was wondering if that gestures toward an agenda of creating stronger transnational state institutions capable of responding far more effectively, not only to future pandemics, but also capable of transforming the social drivers that are now perpetuating this metabolic rift. Yet, this will require the global left to really shift gears from what I would loosely call a kind of anarcho-libertarian stance to an older left emphasizing state planning and rational management of humanity's metabolism with the natural world. Do you think the left needs to undergo a rethinking of the anarcho-libertarian politics that has fired up so many leftists over the past four decades?

MALM: Yes. I'm a recovering anarchist. I was an anarchist for a time in my youth, but I started recovering from that around the age of 20. I guess the ecological crisis should be an incentive for people to get rid of that anarcho-libertarian hangover that so many of us have had since the collapse of the Stalinist states and realize that, whatever we think of the state, it's incredibly difficult to see any other actor than the state being capable of doing something like cutting emissions by 7 or 10 percent per year. It requires, just as you say, comprehensive planning, allocation of resources, regulation, enforcement of certain orders, nationalizing of companies. We can't have a freedom for capitalists to extract fossil fuels and sell them at a profit. The fossil fuel industries should be nationalized and transformed into something completely different and so on and so forth. This is not happening because the state apparatuses that we live under are beholden to dominant class interests. But it's very hard to see anyone else than those institutions even hypothetically being capable of doing this. It's only that they would have to be torn away from dominant class interests and forced by mass pressure to do what's necessary. But the idea that we can accomplish these feats of transition through some kind of horizontal networks or local initiatives, or mutual aid networks, is to me extremely unconvincing.

MCKAY: To just conclude with the pandemic. Since you wrote your book on the pandemic, in many ways the evidence for your position gets stronger with, say, the shambolic vaccine rollout, which will end up privileging the Global North over the Global South, or just the absence of any effective world body that can tell Bolsonaro, in effect: "No, actually, you can't do that. You have to take a more responsible position not only with vaccinating and protecting people but also in deforesting the Amazon—these policies are not allowable." To my eye, it calls for some sort of transnational state authority that can actually defend humanity.

QUESTION FROM THE AUDIENCE: You just made a comment about the transnational kind of organization, and I feel like that's kind of a mistake that we've made. There kind of is a "transnational organization" led by the United States. I think the local population like Brazil (or any country actually) does not want deforestation. The majority of the population of many countries are ecologically knowledgeable, and the world needs to kind of get out of people's way and let Brazil figure it out themselves instead of incentivizing them to exploit their own resources. I don't know if anybody has thoughts on that.

MALM: You're absolutely right. The deforestation that happens in Brazil is tied to global supply chains, and Bolsonaro is opening up the rainforests for entrepreneurs that serve those chains. Despite all his nationalist rhetoric, what he's really doing is opening the rainforest to the advanced detachments of global capital, to put it perhaps a little bit crudely. When it comes to the state, I think the Brazilian case is interesting because there was a period not that long ago when Brazil was the shining example of reduced deforestation. That was during the early period of Lula[4] when the state actually started cracking down on destructive deforestation in the Amazon and installed monitoring, set aside reserves, punished illegal loggers with fines. It managed to reduce deforestation to a fraction of what it was before Lula. Bolsonaro is the latest wave in a reaction to the not-revolutionary-but-reformist progress that Lula presided over. The reaction began already under Dilma, then after the 2016 coup, it has accelerated under Bolsonaro.

This really is just one illustration of what the state can do, potentially, if it's aligned with interests such as the majority interest in Brazil, which would presumably be to preserve the Amazon and not to wreck it entirely. The state can limit destruction. On the other hand, you can say that the Lula case once again shows the shortcomings of reformism because the backlash wasn't prevented. The forces Bolsonaro represents were biding their time and just waiting for the opportunity to seize state power again and destroy everything that had been achieved. This is the tragedy of incomplete revolutions that Rosa Luxembourg and others have pointed to. In the case of Brazil and other countries in the tropics, deforestation cannot be brought under control without this kind of state intervention. It probably needs to be more radical than what happened under Lula, but his early achievements are maybe the best case of what can be done.

QUESTION FROM THE AUDIENCE: Well, I want to introduce the dragon in the room. I want to look at the other end of that supply chain, namely China. So, China—Global North, Global South? And how does it play into your prescription of a radicalized, environmentally conscious working class?

MALM: That's a good question. China *is* the dragon in the room, and China inaugurated the equivalent of one new coal-fired power plant every week last year. There's no way we can get these problems under control without a radical change of trajectory in China. I don't know Chinese politics; I wrote a little bit on the emissions in China and the situation in the Chinese manufacturing industry and the strike waves and things like that back in 2010, but I haven't really followed developments since then very closely, so I'm not in a position to say whether the Chinese working class is even a potential subject for change and whether it's showing signs of some kind of proto-environmental consciousness that could perhaps drive change.

Now, the emissions explosion that's been going on in China since the turn of the millennium is clearly a globalized phenomenon in that (and this is what I wrote about back in 2010; it's one of the last chapters in *Fossil Capital*) this explosion happened because so much of global manufacturing was relocated to China to make use of the supplies of cheap and disciplined workers. They're not so cheap and disciplined any longer, perhaps. But it's still very much the case that the coal explosion there is deeply tied to supply chains that cross the globe, and it's a mistake to attribute everything that's going on in the Chinese economy to China itself because so much of it entails American, Swedish, British, Italian, and Australian companies moving their factories into China or having moved them there for a couple of decades.

QUESTION FROM THE AUDIENCE: Andreas, I'm from Sweden too, so this will be a question from a little bit far up north. You talked a little bit about the need of anger to change things with people. That we need to muster up our anger and our will to change to make people change and to make politicians change things. And you talked about the summer of 2018, and I remember it too and it was pretty close to me where this big fire was. When that happened, you could see a spike in the Green movement. You could see it. You could see the anger. You could see a spike in the people wanting to vote for the

Green Party. But then it just faded away. Something is needed more than the anger. Have you thought anything about that?

MALM: I agree. Unfortunately disasters, such as the one that happened in summer of 2018 in Sweden and other parts of northern central Europe, will become more frequent and will become more intense. It wasn't even a very serious disaster. I don't think even a single person died in Sweden in that summer (or very few). For us, it was a shock because we've never seen our country burn like that. This will happen again. We don't know if it will happen this summer or if it will happen the next or the one after that, but it will happen again, it will get worse, and there will be other events of this kind. It would be a little bit similar to the George Floyd situation in that you get those incidents piled upon each other. If the intervals between disasters are an obstacle to the formation of climate anger or an obstacle to sustaining it, I think that *that* problem, unfortunately, will be solved. These disasters will become more and more regular occurrences. The problem, of course, is that the more regular they become, the later in the day it will be and the harder it will be to do anything about the process. The challenge for the climate movement would be to fan the flames of anger before you have wildfires every month.

I think the climate movement made some headway on this in Europe in 2018 and 2019 because it actually kept growing and drew more people onto the streets for quite a long time after that summer—all the way up to the outbreak of the pandemic. So, for a year and a half almost. The problem then was that the pandemic shut down that whole wave of mobilization.

Another problem that is very conspicuous in Sweden (but this goes for other countries in Europe as well) is that people tend to forget about climate and be obsessively focused on immigration. It's the one political question that always pushes climate concern down to the bottom of the agenda again and again and again. Swedish politics nowadays is only about the "evil of the immigrants." Immigrants can be blamed for absolutely everything, from poor results in school tests to segregated unemployment, everything. It's the same in France and many other countries in Europe. If we want to keep climate in focus, we really need to find a way to convince people that the threat to their existence is not people who are not white and have come to live in their countries but global heating.

MCKAY: A concluding comment that takes us back to where we started, which is the urgent necessity of integrating scholarship and activism. I think about Antonio Gramsci's "Modern Prince," and imagine a modern prince of the twenty-first century capable of both educating people about the climate and about pandemics but also channelling their emotion usefully. Gramsci would warn against wars of manoeuvre, perhaps like physical attacks on pipelines, rather than wars of position, in which you're slowly, soberly trying to change the fundamentals of the situation. You're trying to create a new historical subject—very well-informed and very well-equipped, scientifically and culturally—that can take on so many of the so-called experts who basically have paved the way for this present catastrophe. Do you want to respond to that?

MALM: I agree with that. The only problem is the word you used: "slowly." There is very little time, and we need to act very quickly. That's not to say that war of manoeuvre is the only path forward. But, maybe there needs to be some kind of a dialectic between war of manoeuvre and war of position rather than emphasizing war of position alone.

MCKAY: In your guts, you're very skeptical of gradualism, I sense?

MALM: The problem is that a gradualist climate politics could perhaps have worked if it had been commenced for real in the 1990s, when there was still plenty of time (well, plenty of time is perhaps an exaggeration, but more time than now). The paradox here is that the more the dominant classes succeed in postponing the break with business as usual, the sharper that break will eventually have to be, if it ever happens. The longer you wait, the more revolutionary will the rupture eventually have to be. And that's a result of defeats we have suffered over these decades. When we eventually win, our victory will have to be very sharp and abrupt because climate change is a fundamentally accumulating phenomenon. It's a result of everything that has been emitted. If you continue to pile emissions on the ones that have already been made, temperatures will rise. This is the logic of the carbon budgets and all these things. That means that when the carbon budget is finished, and when the cumulative emissions have reached a certain level, you have to stop completely unless you want to pass certain thresholds. And stopping completely is an extremely abrupt thing to do.

MCKAY: In some ways there's a parallel with the pandemic. When it started in earnest in January 2020, the right response turns out to have been the most radical and far-reaching one. As a senior official of the World Health Organization said, "You move fast, don't look back — yes you're going to make mistakes, but you cannot [look back], there is not time to waste."[5] In many ways it's very hard for Canadians to think that way because Canadians are almost gradualist by definition. We just love being in the middle of the road, we love taking very carefully modulated steps. But the climate crisis isn't that kind of crisis. It actually does call for this kind of real change—and not over decades because there aren't decades to spare.

QUESTION FROM THE AUDIENCE: As the pandemic continues on, how do we deal with the fact that Covid-19 is quickly becoming a Third World problem? Some countries will never be able to obtain the number of vaccines First World countries can.

MALM: This clearly is a massive problem. It prefigures the worst scenarios for climate adaptation, where rich countries protect themselves behind walls of affluence while leaving others to fend for themselves. How do we deal with that? Well, I have to admit that I have not followed the developments with regard to vaccine distribution very closely, so I don't really know what the negotiations and struggles look like around the companies, the various vaccines, the WHO, all of these things. Clearly the vaccine nationalism advanced capitalist countries are guilty of is obscene and has to be fought one way or another, but I don't know exactly how to do it.

QUESTION FROM THE AUDIENCE: I'm also in Canada, and I'm not totally in agreement about Canadians being not prone to move into action. My experience in British Columbia, twice in the last thirty years, in 1983 and then again between 2003 and 2005, tens of thousands of people moved into action around attacks and opposing attacks on union rights, social spending, a whole bunch of other related neoliberal attacks. But my understanding of what happened in those cases when people moved was that in order to get large numbers of people in motion, it wasn't just anger that moved people. It was being afraid and then being angry about it, but also having a feeling that there was some chance of succeeding. Because in both of those cases, when the unfortunate leadership of the movements called them off in full spate, the mobilizations wound down very quickly. People concluded that their chances of doing anything had evaporated.

I'm involved right now in taking a course about how you organize in a trade union situation for getting a new collective agreement or getting a new certification. The people that are talking to us are saying that one of the things you have to do is not just throw out general messages to your entire population. You have to do some analysis. Who are the people that are most likely to move? Who are the people who influence other people? Who are the people that have some connections outside the plant or the workplace? You have to do some analysis, and then you have to start talking about how to get people in those certain places to start moving first. The only class of people I can see on the planet that can move simultaneously in a bunch of different countries have been the youth. Unfortunately, youth don't stay young. In a certain economic and social situation when they're young, they move. They get a little bit older, and they wind up getting connected with jobs or poverty or whatever else, and they don't have those universal characteristics anymore.

Anyway, I'm wondering if there's someone who has started looking at how we can put together people or at least doing an analysis to get different groups in different countries to start connecting internationally, to form some kind of an international of struggle?

MALM: I think there are quite a few initiatives of that kind underway. The Fridays for Future movement, for instance, is fairly global in its reach. Likewise Extinction Rebellion. Internationally, there is the Progressive International. But the problem with these various initiatives and networks, in my view, is that they are almost exclusively based on social media, and social media have, in my assessment, been a disaster for the left. They have further entrenched the kind of anarcho-libertarian mindsets that Ian referred to as a kind of default way of doing politics. Because mobilizations based on social media are very easy to get going. It's very easy to respond to a Facebook call to come to a square or a demonstration or something like that. But it's just as easy to drop out and disappear. Social media–based eruptions of protests tend to have this extremely effervescent way of drawing a lot of people. But then such an eruption just completely fizzles out and leaves no trace in any kind of solid, more-or-less institutionalized organization or political project. It just evaporates. That's been the tragedy for so many campaigns and movements of the past decade, starting perhaps with Occupy, which happened just when the whole Facebook/Twitter/social media universe started taking over. That's not to say there is a ready-made alternative (as in party-centred projects like Syriza, Corbin, Sanders, or something like that. These projects have had their own shortcomings and haven't really succeeded). I'm not saying the left should just opt out and delete all social media accounts and leave it to the devil. But there has to be a way to make those movements of mobilization more enduring in their effects.

AN INTERVIEW WITH
MERRILL SINGER
17 AUGUST 2022

Merrill Singer is a medical anthropologist and professor emeritus in anthropology at the University of Connecticut and in community medicine at the University of Connecticut Health Center. He completed his PhD at the University of Utah in 1979 and served as researcher, then director of research, then associate director at the Hispanic Health Council in Hartford, Connecticut, from 1982 to 2007, after which he moved to the University of Connecticut. He is well-known within medical anthropology for introducing such concepts as "syndemics," "oppression illness," and "pluralea." His publications number in the hundreds.

MCKAY: Our conversation today will be based primarily on just two of your many writings, *Introduction to Syndemics* (2009) and *Anthropology of Infectious Disease* (2016), supplemented by some more recent titles. We'll focus on the concept of syndemics, which some authorities, such as Dr. Richard Horton, editor of *The Lancet*, Britain's leading medical journal, argues has particular significance in our time of Covid-19—because the pandemic has underscored the importance of keeping three core themes in mind: "the virus, the chronic conditions that make people more susceptible to it, and a situation of deepening poverty and inequality."[1] Joining us is also Dr. Ann Herring, emerita, Department of Anthropology, McMaster University, an expert on the anthropology of infectious diseases and epidemics, who has collaborated with Dr. Singer and can offer us knowledgeable insights into the syndemic approach.

Could you give us a sense of the core ideas and principles propelling your prodigious scholarship over the past three decades? One senses that your involvement with the Hispanic Health Council in Hartford was fundamental to the distinctive ways you have approached medical anthropology. Would one be correct in thinking that it was in response to conventional biomedicine's partial understanding of the challenges thrown up by the HIV/AIDS crisis in this community that you developed your distinctive approach to the experience of diseases among subaltern populations?

SINGER: Well, I'm not sure if I have a completely unique perspective. I share my approach with various other people. The Hispanic Health Council was an incubator of ideas I had already had, before I got there. I already viewed society and the questions of anthropology from what, ultimately, I and my colleague at the University of Melbourne, Hans Baer, called "critical medical anthropology." I already had that perspective when I arrived at the Hispanic Health Council. But the Council provided a context, a location, a social role, to try out those ideas in accounting for the health crises of the inner-city poor of Hartford, which is a good percentage of the population, and for developing critically applied interventions to try to address their issues, among which was, with the rise of AIDS pandemic, trying to prevent the virus from spreading—initially, among street injection users and gay men and commercial sex workers and other populations. We could see on the ground how people were put at risk by social inequalities, discrimination, marginalization, and how we could try to address the issues that put people at risk.

MCKAY: One way of grasping what you mean by "syndemic"—and various related terms, such as "ecosyndemic," "syndemogenesis," "countersyndemics," and "supersyndemics" and such phrases as "the syndemic approach," "syndemics theory," and "syndemic interaction"—might be to begin by describing the paradigm it critiques. Could you give us a sense of the conventional "biomedical model" and why you feel it often comes up short in its handling of particular diseases?

SINGER: Building and acting on a critical biosocial model of health and treatment would significantly improve the quality, affordability, and patient experience of biomedicine. But let me start off by saying that there is a lot that's good about the reigning biomedical model. I use biomedicine. The issue is, in terms of its limitations, that there are the ways it could be improved. Many medical doctors appreciate this. Our recently lost colleague Paul Farmer, both a physician and a medical anthropologist, understood these limitations very well.[2] I coauthored a book about another doctor who also took this social medicine approach.[3] So, within social medicine, this understanding exists.

Unfortunately, it doesn't easily translate into the day-to-day practice of medicine, given the dominance of medicine by major institutions, including the insurance companies, hospitals, and biotech companies. They limit what is possible in medicine. For instance, there is political opposition to lowering the cost of insulin for diabetes patients. It's very clear that people's health and health care in general are very much political-economic and social phenomena. They reflect the fault lines of society. Just look at the rates for Covid-19, heart conditions, cancer, you name it. These diseases reflect social inequality—who gets sick, when they get sick, and, if they get better, how much damage they'll suffer: all of these things are about social factors.

Right now, for example, I'm writing the foreword to a book by a colleague of mine in Pakistan about the spread of measles. His book makes it clear that entrenched social factors are what's driving the measles epidemic *and* the resistance to vaccination. Building a fuller biosocial model of health helps us grasp why people might take up that position, both in Pakistan and here in the United States.

MCKAY: Turning now to defining "syndemic." A succinct definition of the term from your 2009 *Introduction to Syndemics* is "a concentration and deleterious interaction of two or more diseases or other health conditions in a population, especially as a consequence of social inequity and the unjust exercise of power."[4] In more recent work, you specify that syndemics have three components: "(1) sequential, co-occurring or clustering diseases or other health conditions; (2) adverse biological interactions between these diseases/health conditions (biological-biological or bio-bio interaction) and (3) social/political, environmental factors that cause or exacerbate disease (biology-social or bio-social interface)."[5] Even more strictly: "the term 'syndemic' describes various disease-disease interactions caused, exacerbated, or intensified by adverse social conditions and environments."[6] You distinguish this stricter notion of syndemics from looser usages such as those that merely add up harmful comorbidities without pondering either their actual or potential interactions or exploring their social origins. What is at stake in this definitional tightening up of the term syndemic from your perspective?

SINGER: From my perspective, all of those components were there from the beginning. If there's been some tightening up—and I guess that's a good way to describe it—it is because, after my initial publications in the early and mid-1990s, on syndemics, a couple of people at the CDC [Centres for Disease Control] picked up the concept and started a website to which people could contribute and then began speaking about syndemics. That was great because it really publicized the idea.

But as the term spread, people started adopting it for things I hadn't meant when I introduced it. There is an ongoing struggle to make the term as clear as possible, so it isn't misused, in the interest of conceptual clarity. Richard Horton came across the idea at Georgetown University in DC, where Emily Mendenhall teaches. They met and got to talking. That led to a special publication that she edited and to which I contributed. He certainly made the concept better known because of his stature.

But he also misused it in a certain way. For instance, he speaks of Covid-19 as a "global syndemic," when both Emily and I, together and separately, tried to make it clear that we're talking about a group of syndemics that have Covid-19 in common but may have other different diseases involved in different places and different populations and different risk factors. So, the configurations vary from country to country. It's not one global Covid-19 pandemic. It's a group of syndemics.

That distinction is important. You need to know what's going on, on the ground. If you're in Italy, old age was a key factor; in Mexico, with a much younger overall population, diabetes and some other factors were involved. To mount an effective syndemic response, you need to understand the local syndemics, not just have this emphasis on the global.

MCKAY: Is another factor in the definitional tightening up an emphasis on interaction between distinct diseases and health conditions? If you don't have that interaction, it's not syndemic, right?

SINGER: Right. There are these two fundamental components—the bio-bio interaction (two diseases) and the biosocial interaction (the interaction of these two diseases with social factors that drive the interaction).

MCKAY: Turning now to the present pandemic: What do you think a syndemic treatment might add to our understanding of it? People have seen in the syndemic concept a way of thinking about Covid-19 holistically, both as a mirror held up to the inequities and inequalities of our social order and—partly because we shape the virus as it shapes us—an active force intensifying those patterns. Are they right to do so? What is new about this approach, compared to those we find in the mainstream today?

SINGER: Well, for one thing, it brings social factors immediately into the discussion. (While that's not unique to syndemics—there is a social determinants model that exists beyond syndemics—syndemics at least immediately draws it right in.) In any given population, there are always other diseases. Within any individual there could be multiple diseases at play at the same time. Syndemics asks: Is that interaction critical to what's going on?

I'll give you a current example—the possible interaction between chickenpox (which in older age represents itself as shingles) and herpes simplex, which is very widespread. There's now new thinking that there might well be interaction between the two. And this interaction might be one of the critical forces driving Alzheimer's disease. You wouldn't normally link infectious disease and Alzheimer's. And then, when you look at who has the highest rates of Alzheimer's, lo and behold, it reflects social inequality. African Americans have disproportionately high rates, the poor have disproportionately high rates. Also, Alzheimer's has been connected to stress. Social inequality and social discrimination and class oppression are shown, very clearly, by William Dressler and others, to be stressful.[7] So, the question I'm exploring now is: Is there an Alzheimer syndemic? What are the social causes involved here, in this rise of cases? What other diseases, what social factors, might be involved? That's the value of this approach.

MCKAY: And it also raises, to my eye, radical questions about the very identity of the "diseases" you're talking about. When we speak of the HIV/AIDS epidemic in North America and Africa—well, for sure the disease has commonalities the world around. Yet it unfolded in such distinctive ways, in different locales and in different sociocultural contexts, that its profile is dramatically different. I know you don't want to be too aggressive in your critique of the biomedical model in the abstract, but doesn't this highlight the limitation of saying, "Here is disease X with symptoms Y to be treated with measures Z"? The disease is treated as though it were a static thing, something you can pin down, whereas in the syndemic approach, it seems to treated more like a dynamic process that changes according to its context. Syndemics seems to say: "You think you grasp this disease, but without understanding its context, you don't. It cannot be effectively treated just in isolation from everything else." Is that a fair interpretation?

SINGER: Yes. Syndemics does not treat disease as a narrow biological event. A disease is a biosocial event. How we know it, how we respond to it. We come to know what it is in the course of responding to it. The history of an infectious agent is shaped as much by society as society is by epidemics.

For example, drug-resistant TB reveals a pathogen adapting to the changing conditions effected by inoculations. Pathogens change in response to what people do—and not just with respect to vaccines, but how they live, how they interact with each other, even how they bury their dead. In the case of Kuru, for example, among the South Fore people of New Guinea, who practised mortuary cannibalism, because of the eating of the bodies of the dead, the prions (deformed proteins that spread in the brain) associated with the disease were passed on in the ritual, killing, disproportionately, the women and children. So, the pathogen itself would not have created an epidemic had the social practice not existed. You can't think of diseases in isolation.

Diseases are real. Yet, while they're real, they're not just biological. They're entwined, ongoing biosocial phenomena.

MCKAY: As a historian, I notice how thoroughly models of 1918–20 have affected our understandings of (and hopes about) the future evolution of Covid-19. And Professor Herring has enhanced our understanding of this pandemic in Canada and in Hamilton, in addition to her work on the syndemic concept.[8] You underscore the limits of the doctrine of "commensalism," according to which "the less-toxic strains of a pathogen will prevail when it is difficult to move from host to host because it is evolutionarily disadvantageous to damage or kill the host before the pathogens have time [to] spread to others, given that reproduction and spread are the driving forces of microbial (and other) life forms."[9] I suppose that's what most people are hoping for now—a replay of the earlier pandemic, with the disease becoming progressively milder and ultimately becoming an endemic part of our modern lives. Would it be fair to say that much of the official readiness to declare Covid-19 over and done with stems, not only from wishful thinking, but also from this misleading doctrine? And don't we have to recall that influenza, for the millions afflicted by it every year, is not necessarily a minor thing?

SINGER: And not experienced equally. Rates of infection and death are higher in minority populations around the world.

MCKAY: It seems, to my eye, incautious to predict that Covid-19, a very different pandemic than the one that unfolded between 1918 and 1920, will necessarily follow its script. It could be commensalism doesn't apply in this case. We've been trying to declare this pandemic over and done with, and we would love it if indeed it was getting milder and milder. But, might we not be deluding ourselves with an attractive model from the past that doesn't really apply in the present?

SINGER: Let me start by pointing out an interesting point. The 1918–20 influenza global pandemic was explored by a now strangely controversial figure, Anthony Fauci. His research suggested that what may have been at play there was an interaction between a virus and a bacterium. That is what made it such an explosive influenza pandemic. As you rightly point out, there have been some other bad ones—periodic major jumps in influenza harm, and disproportionately so across minority communities.

On the issue of what's going to happen with the present virus [SARS-CoV-2], one of the things we have to keep in mind is that it *isn't* the case that viruses necessarily become progressively milder in order to ensure their biological survival and reproduction on the grounds that "it's in their best interests." Sometimes making people really sick is to the evolutionary advantage of the pathogen. That helps spread the disease from one person to another very quickly. It really varies by context and disease. With influenza, it keeps coming back, but in somewhat different forms, so we need to keep adjusting our vaccines every year and hope that the one we receive blocks the major variant for that year. We're living in a new era with Covid-19. I don't know if these patterns will hold.

There is now such political resistance to, and a political defining of, vaccines. Even now in the wealthiest country with the largest supplies of available vaccines, more than 15 percent are unvaccinated against Covid-19. So, even if we have a new vaccine against a new variant, if a substantial number of people aren't vaccinated, that will also influence how the disease spreads.

I agree with you: people are tired of the pandemic. Some of that tiredness has resulted in people just ignoring it. Emily Mendenhall wrote a book on Covid-19 about her small hometown in Iowa.[10] She quarantined there with her husband and her kids. She went there to be with her family and her brother—they could all hang out in a bubble. And she realized, as she drove across the country from Washington, D.C., that there were fewer and fewer masks as she went west. By the time they got to Iowa, they weren't seeing hardly any at all. People were living as if there was no pandemic. Her town became a hot spot for the spread of Covid. That *still* did not lead to widespread masking. Her brother-in-law is the public health official trying to push masking. She had this window on her neighbours and their resistance and the public health institutions and the Iowa government, which opposed social distancing and other measures.

We've created a social crisis that will drive new waves of infection. Right now, we are lucky, in a sense, because the dominant variant is not the same as its predecessors. There is not the same horrible relationship between infection and hospitalization and death. There's been a drop in death rates, for the time being. But, there are going to be more variants. We just don't know when the next variants will come on the scene and what they will entail.

MCKAY: In the British case, it seems many authorities, both medical and political, were almost mesmerized by the legacy of 1918–20. They seemed to say, "we can just get through this little flu" with a stiff upper lip and ample supplies of elbow-grease. It will be over and done with quite quickly, was the line. In my view, lives were lost because of the power of that historical model. Whereas, where other models prevailed, as in much of Asia, with a more vivid memory of the recent SARS outbreak in 2003, in places like China and Vietnam, they had a more accurate grasp of the virus they were confronting and the urgent measures needed to fight it. There was, I think, a sharp disjunction between these two approaches, in which the "memory of 1918–20" played a key role.

HERRING: I could just jump in here. There was this assumption that the present pandemic would follow the pattern of 1918–20. As Merrill suggests, it had been forgotten—there even is a well-known study called *The Forgotten Pandemic*.[11] But, what was really interesting to me was the pervasive assumption that everyone was going to be affected. No one had any resilience or resistance. We would just all be infected and then it would be over. That ignored a lot of the literature that had emerged about how social inequality influenced how the Great Influenza Epidemic actually spread. It didn't hit everyone equally. And everyone was not equally susceptible. In Canada, in places marked by poverty, with visible minorities living lives under very different conditions, inequality and infection went hand in hand. To me, it was curious to need to be telling this story again so many years later.

MCKAY: I got the sense that the history of 1918–20 was often being presented in a very reassuring way. The tone of much of it was, here are some "fun facts" about the past, without any real bearing on the current tragedy. There was an almost sepia-toned nostalgia to some of it. That doesn't really serve us well in a time of crisis. In some ways, we couldn't really access the historical knowledge we urgently needed.

HERRING: One of the things that generated so much viral panic around Covid-19 was the fact that we in the western world and in the biomedical tradition have been raised to think that infectious diseases were a thing of the past. All these emerging interactions only happened in countries that didn't have good medical systems and poor economies and so on. So, this was a major shock. People were struggling to find what we can compare this to. And so, they turned to 1918 as their reference point. It served as a kind of anchor.

MCKAY: I find it so striking how thoroughly the message about the Great Influenza Epidemic was disseminated—"We haven't been through anything like this since 1918!" Yet, well, surely the AIDS epidemic, killing an estimated thirty-three million people worldwide by recent estimates, counts for something? It's certainly not the case that this is the first global pandemic we've experienced since 1918. There was a drastic foreshortening of historical memory. Something in me suspects that's not an entirely innocent abbreviation of this history.

SINGER: One thing's for certain: it's going to be a little while before we can ever return to the way of thinking that held that contagious diseases lie in our past. You know, we've had HIV/AIDS, and influenza epidemics, and Ebola, and Zika, and now Mpox. You have to have real blinders on not to see that, in our time, it's one epidemic after the other after the other. And they're overlapping now. And I'm sure we'll see super-syndemics as these various diseases interact in specific places.

HERRING: One hears now of the re-emergence of polio in some of the larger cities.

SINGER: Meanwhile, one member of the Kennedy family was applauding the fact that vaccination rates among children were dropping—coincidental with the rise of polio!

MCKAY: Ecosyndemics are syndemics promoted by the degradation of the natural environment, with, for example, "respiratory risks to human health . . . on the rise around the globe, not least in part because anthropogenic environmental changes are increasing and multiplying the likelihood of respiratory disease comorbidity and disease interaction."[12] I sense, especially from your recent book *Climate Change and Social Inequality*,[13] that you are sympathetic to critical approaches that emphasize humanity's metabolic rift with the rest of nature, humankind's almost suicidal behaviour in the way in conducts itself in the natural world, mismanaging its metabolism with it, undermining the equilibria intrinsic to its functioning, damaging it irreparably in quest of profits. Is humanity entering an era of "supersyndemics"; that is, "synergistic interactions among two or more previously independent syndemics"? And do you in fact find this "metabolic rift" approach congenial?

SINGER: If you search through my work on climate change, especially the collaborate work with Hans Baer, you'll find we use that concept of metabolic rift fairly regularly.[14] We don't take the position that it's something about people per se. All species make use of their environment. Our argument is that under certain social and economic configurations, the human impact is enormously magnified. That is, under capitalism, we have this driving engine for production, a constant cycle of need and want, and a definition of the planet as a limitless resources that can be endlessly exploited, as well as a built-in plan for not taking responsibility. So that you can build cars that release pollutants into the atmosphere, but that's not part of your production costs. The damage to health that you produce is not included in your costs. The industry operates on the assumption that such costs are "external," independent of the process itself. They're not responsible for them. The result is this rapid increase in damage done to the environment. Now we're living it.

We're living with the consequences. The drought in the western United States, forest fires across Canada and the US, the heat wave in Britain and Europe—you name it. The damages are spiralling. And these changes in the environment interact with and drive disease interactions and syndemics. Climate change is going to significantly accelerate the spread of infectious diseases, given the ability of vectors to live in new places leading to new disease interactions. We've already seen it. Take tick-borne diseases. Climate change has allowed different tick species to move to new places where they interact with other tick species, leading to new syndemics. Some of them have significant health consequences. So, unfortunately, in addition to all its other problems, one of the results of climate change and environmental degradation is a rise in infectious and other diseases.

MCKAY: You critique the tendency to weed out patients with comorbidities from many randomized control trials, which proceeds from an approach that seeks to limit variables and which skews our understanding of particular diseases by encouraging medical professionals to treat each disease as a free-standing entity. You suggest that it's problematic to separate the diseases from the people actually experiencing them. Elsewhere you note that such comorbidities as obesity or diabetes can in themselves be considered diseases of poverty.[15] Do you share these misgivings about Covid-19 and the present discourse around comorbidities? What difference might thinking syndemically mean in this context?

SINGER: The starting point is the emergence of the concept of comorbidity, which is really not all that old—it dates back to c. 1973, I believe. It was used initially to describe the coexistence of two diseases without consideration of interaction. And the problem there is that it allows people to think, "Well, there are these other diseases present, but we can just conduct clinical trials, just focus on the disease of concern or the disease that we really want to fight" (often because that's where the big money is from a pharmaceutical perspective). We get "cleaner data." We don't have all the messy complications. Science always wants to control experimental conditions, for understandable reasons.

But if the controls so distort what's seen that it's different from reality, there's going to be problems with the medicines that ensue. If the interpretation you produce is at variance with the social and environmental conditions under which diseases develop and become worse and so on, they are inevitable. Interacting diseases within the population of concern should be a central part of the clinical trial picture—that would be the syndemic argument. If the population that you want to use a particular drug also suffers from this other disease—which we know interacts with the disease of concern with adverse outcomes—then it only makes sense, from a medical standpoint, that this be taken into consideration in the structure of the clinical trials.

MCKAY: Going back to the HIV/AIDs context: it would be simplistic simply to address the virus in question in isolation when in fact it interacts with many other social patterns and pre-existing conditions. There was a very different shape, thanks to them, to the pattern of the disease in Africa and that in North America. And aren't we finding the same "syndemic" patterns in India today, where Mucormycosis (a rare fungal infection) is flourishing alongside Covid-19, or in North America, where both obesity and diabetes have also been identified as important considerations in explaining Covid-19's epidemiological patterns? It could be a misstep to call Covid-19 itself a "syndemic," as you suggest—but doesn't this evidence suggest that disease enters into syndemic interactions all around the world as it interacts with existing diseases?

SINGER: With respect to HIV/AIDS: in South Africa, what a number of people, myself among them, have pointed out is the interaction between inadequate diet and HIV. So, if you create vaccines but don't consider that the population that might get them is malnourished, the vaccine will be less effective. If you create a vaccine, maybe you simultaneously have to create programs to address hunger. That's the context you have to create to make your vaccine or your medicine effective. You have to address other interacting factors that would diminish its effectiveness. The problem is not just HIV, but HIV and hunger. Both problems have to be addressed simultaneously.

MCKAY: There was, certainly in the case of the HIV/AIDS epidemic, and also today with Covid-19, a certain "blame-the-victim" game going on with comorbidities. If you say, for example, that obesity is linked to Covid-19, self-righteous people will blame individuals for not eating nutritious meals, oblivious to the fact that many poor people live in "food deserts" without adequate grocery stores and, as you point out in your *Introduction to Syndemics*,[16] have grown reliant on food that quickly delivers a lot of energy at a bargain price. If we think in traditional liberal ways, ones that encourage us to focus on the failings of individual agents, we fail to grasp the social origins of those patterns.

SINGER: When I was at the Hispanic Health Council, we started this project for youth. One of its major components was to bring them by bus to an organic farm where they would participate in harvesting various vegetables for the kitchen, which had been set up to show them how you can create meals with these things they themselves had picked. Nutrition was discussed. We thought: "Well, this is a good intervention. They get outside, they come to understand how plants grow, where their food comes from, how to make dishes from them." And one day I was talking with the bus driver. "How's it going with the kids on the bus today?" "They're tired out," he said, "now they all want to go to McDonald's. They're always bugging me to go to McDonald's on our way back." Where did they get the idea that good, tasty, satisfying food comes from there? Well, from McDonald's.

MCKAY: Along with many other recognitions of your contributions to medical scholarship, you received the Rudolf Virchow Prize in 1991, named after one of the world's most renowned advocates of public health in the mid-nineteenth century. Virchow is often considered the father of modern pathology and the founder of social medicine, and he is well-remembered for the often-quoted adage: "Medicine is a social science and politics is nothing else but medicine on a large scale. Medicine as a social science, as the science of human beings, has the obligation to point out problems and to attempt their theoretical solution; the politician, the practical anthropologist, must find the means for their actual solution." [17]

In the Virchow model, doesn't defending public health mean opposing extremely powerful interests in the world of medicine—such as Big Pharma, funding agencies, and ultimately, in the North American context, all those driven by possessive individualism rather than inspired by holistic understandings of the social order? All the people instructed by a culture of consumption and possessive individualism that a Big Mac is nutritious and satisfying? Is it not hard to row against so powerful a current in our society? How do you feel about reconciling activism with scholarship? Is it not difficult for the activist and the scholar comfortably to cohabit in the same mind?

SINGER: Well, they certainly cohabited in my mind. I started as an activist. My first political involvement was as a high school student when we walked out of my high school. And then I started college. The next year, I helped to lead a boycott of the school cafeteria in support of the United Farm Workers' movement. I was a card-carrying union member for five years. I headed one of the boycott offices for the union.

When I came to anthropology and to scholarship, I was an activist. The Hispanic Health Council, where I was located for twenty-five years, was a community-based organization that implemented research and orchestrated interventions—but also participated in community activism around city health issues (like the failure of the city to address the rat problem: the Council participated in a march in which people carried dead rats). We took part in many struggles to change how Latino families, poor families, were treated in the ICU. That was part of the culture of the Hispanic Health Council. We saw ourselves as part of the community and involved in the community's struggles. And the Council was seen as a place where people could meet. I have always had that perspective.

Critical medical anthropology is a *praxis* that brings together sound social science and a recognition that that science is useful if it's applied. I support basic science. But you also have to think about how that science is used. Who dominates the science? It was the AIDS movement, coming out of the LGBTQ community, that changed how the medical establishment responded to the disease. It's interesting to read what Anthony Fauci said about what he learned from AIDS activists.[18] They changed how he does medicine.

MCKAY: A related question. I share your sense that knowledge should be about something and it should really feed contemporary struggles. At the same time, I worry about the mood of depression I sense all around me. When Greta Thunberg says, "I want you to panic," part of me warmly agrees.[19] But another part of me reflects, "Panic-stricken people can do things that aren't necessarily progressive." The more we enter into this atmosphere of dread and fear and ambient panic, the more I fear the demagogic right can profit far more readily from it than the rational humanistic left. Do you share these misgivings?

SINGER: She was addressing the big institutions, the powerful people. She's trying to shake them. And, you know, she's talked about hope. If she didn't have hope, she wouldn't be doing what she's doing. If there's nothing that can be done, there would be no need to create a youth climate movement and dedicate her life to it, inspiring young activists around the world. You have this tight problem: if you don't have hope, you don't have action; but if you have too much hope, you don't have enough action. It's a tension.

Every time I write about the climate crisis, I struggle. I don't want it to be just so negative that all it does is depress people. On the other hand, I want to be honest enough to say things are *really* bad. Not "kind of bad" or "sort of bad" or "maybe it will get bad." No—people are dying in increasing numbers right now. This will only get worse if we don't change. It's hard to find the right balance between the two.

I'm glad to see these young activists, not just in Sweden but in Africa and Asia, South America and the Caribbean, in the minority communities across the developed nations, coming together around climate change. And that will lead them, quickly, to realize that climate change doesn't happen independent of war and social inequality and so on. These are patterns that, if they were addressed, would make life for everyone a lot healthier.

HERRING: I would like to ask Merrill what the main changes are that you see happening over the years you've been thinking about syndemics? Other than tightening the definition?

SINGER: Well, initially, the focus was on violence, drugs, and AIDS. It was clear in our interviews with drug users who were also suffering from tuberculosis at high rates. And sexually transmitted diseases. And endocarditis. And skin infections. So, we knew from the beginning, it wasn't just a question of the three phenomena, substance abuse, violence, and AIDS.

And so, over time, I grew interested in exploring the broader patterns of syndemics. My *Introduction to Syndemics* talked about multiple other syndemics. So, there was some expansion of syndemic thinking. And when you write multiple papers and books on the same subject, you are constantly challenged to say things a bit differently. How can I develop the same theme without being boring? And so one tries to find new ways to conceptualize and express a pattern that has, for me, been relatively constant. Then other people contribute ideas and that's positive. There is that kind of evolution. A colleague of mine, Nicola Bulled, and another former student, Bayla Ostrach, looked at the evolution of the concept of syndemics. We looked at the literature to learn how the concept is being used. Sometimes it was being used for phenomena we would not define as syndemics.[20] We had to develop this typology of other concepts that are "syndemic-like" but not syndemics. The struggle for clarity is ongoing.

HERRING: For me, the power of the concept has remained the same, in the sense that it asks for people who are investigating any kind of health condition to consider everything that's going on in the community. You have to look at the other conditions that people are coping with medically. Do they have enough to eat? Can they get to a grocery store? What kind of work are they doing? Are they in factory settings, where they are in contact with many other people? What is the history of the community? Syndemics really asks researchers to do ethnography, to struggle for a holistic approach. That kind of research takes years and years. It's my impression, and I might be wrong, that there wasn't as much take-up as one might like of this powerful idea because it requires a lot of different kinds of research work. Am I wrong?

SINGER: You're not wrong about that. Syndemics urges researchers not to have narrowly defined questions and to look at what they're interested in, relative to context. But, on the question of the take-up of the model: from my perspective, it's been pretty large; from the perspective of medicine as a whole, pretty small.

For me, watching it grow from the ground-up, the take-up has been amazing. If you look at any of the mechanisms there are for seeing the number of articles on particular topics, syndemics have a steady rise over the years, spread across many disciplines. Doctors, nurses, epidemiologists, historians, even dentists have adopted the concept. It's broken into major journals. And it's been picked up (and then dropped again) by the CDC. I used to read, fifteen years ago, things in the media that would say, "It's not in any dictionary." But now there are many dictionaries that do define it (not all of them by any means). It's a process. It clearly takes time.

PART TWO
SACRIFICING THE SUBALTERNS

PART TWO
SACRIFICING THE SUBALTERNS

AN INTERVIEW WITH

NORA LORETO

25 MAY 2022

Nora Loreto is a Quebec City–based activist and author. Her works include *From Demonized to Organized: Building the New Union Movement* (2013) and *Take Back the Fight: Organizing Feminism in the Digital Age* (2020). She is the editor of the Canadian Association of Labour Media and also co-hosts the podcast "Sandy and Nora Talk Politics."[1] She has written for such publications as the *National Observer* and the *Washington Post*. Her new book is *Spin Doctors: How Media and Politicians Misdiagnosed the Covid-19 Pandemic* (2021).

MCKAY: In April 2020, Nora began compiling a spreadsheet tracking Covid-19 deaths in LTC facilities (as senior citizens' or old folks' homes are termed in Canada), a task, remarkably enough, not undertaken by any government authority—which suggests, perhaps, the level of confusion and interjurisdictional rivalry characteristic of the country's response. She also got her children through the pandemic while still managing to produce "the 3,000 words I had to write that day."[2]

Thank you for *Spin Doctors*, which many of us will regard as an indispensable reference book on the first thirteen months of the pandemic in Canada.

Before we get to the pandemic, I wanted to ask you about one of the key themes of *Spin Doctors*: that's the extremely procorporate, ideologically hidebound media landscape in Canada, which often reminds me of a quip once attributed to Dorothy Parker on the subject of Katharine Hepburn: "Let's all go to see Miss Hepburn and hear her run the gamut of emotions from A to B!"[3] In this case, one might say: "Let's all go to the ranking Canadian media sources and savour how they run the ideological gamut of nineteenth-century liberalism, from the hard-shell 'up-with-markets' liberalism of Herbert Spencer to the *somewhat* softer liberalism of John Stuart Mill." From A to B, all within the framework of liberalism—and, in Canada, generally, nineteenth-century liberalism at that. Certainly, when I watch the CBC or read the Toronto *Globe and Mail* and *The Star* or Montreal's *La Presse*, I am conscious of being in a liberal universe 24/7, whose individualistic assumptions about property and progress and identity go almost entirely unquestioned. Is this your sense, too? How do we change this very limited media landscape in Canada?

LORETO: We have been talking about media concentration in this country since the mid-1990s at least, when we started to see the consolidation of a lot of daily newspapers. We once had a news ecosystem that, while still flawed, was far more robust than what we have now. And, in talking about concentrated media ownership in this country, we often neglected to talk about what that would do, or what that has done, to the quality of journalism.

And so, not only do we only have a handful of major owners, but the owners are virtually indistinguishable from one another. I can encounter an article from CTV or the CBC or the *Montreal Gazette*, all owned by different owners, and have a hard time figuring out where it's coming from. Not only do we have fewer people actually calling the shots, but there's been this incredible convergence, solidification, of ideology, within Canadian media. The only voices that are a little outside the norm are the far-right sorts of things we find in the *Toronto Sun* or *Ottawa Sun* or *Postmedia*. During the pandemic, anybody with a critical voice was basically shut out of mainstream media.

That meant that average people were trying to understand what the heck was going on—trying to figure out what the daily statistics meant, or what they should be doing to keep themselves safe, or whatever. They only got one message, whether they're listening to the local radio station or reading their newspaper. It was all the same message. As someone outside the establishment, my primary goal was to break through that wall and try to present them with a message that was a bit different. Over the course of my work, I think I did fewer than twenty media interviews in the two years I was undertaking that research.

MCKAY: One of the great contributions of your extremely useful book is the attention it pays to the effect of the pandemic on the Canadian media landscape. It got worse. In retrospect, I think we might say that was one of the big transformative impacts of the pandemic. It shoved out a lot of independent voices from the media. And a lot of local newspapers bit the dust.

LORETO: It also accustomed us to seeing things from more centralized perspectives. The immediate reflex of national broadcasters was to centralize all television in Toronto. If I were running the public broadcaster, my immediate reflex would have been *don't* centralize—get people to pay attention to local data, talk to people on a first-name basis, speak with the experts within the region, and start reporting locally. And then have a team in Toronto that can bring in the national perspective. But not only did we have [coverage] localized and centralized in Toronto, we *still* didn't get that national perspective. Rather than a national perspective, what we got was national reporting that was just about Ottawa or was just about federal politicians.

And so, on any given day of the pandemic, people lacked local information. Where are the hot spots? Where are the cold spots? What does the testing look like? There was just nothing. Instead, we had stenography on all the major news networks. When Prime Minister Justin Trudeau sneezed, the sneeze would be broadcast across all the platforms. It was incredible, the extent to which the mass media controlled the message so well.

This was the whole theory behind the "crisis management" of the pandemic: control everything. Not necessarily in a sinister way. All it took was a daily briefing at eleven o'clock, which all the journalists covered. That's all it took.

MCKAY: I love the term you just used: "stenography." A point you brought out so well in the book is that as newsrooms get more and more overburdened, with many underpaid, [precariously situated] journalists, it's very hard for them to acquire any independent outlook from what they're being fed by powerful actors. Mass media end up being mere stenographers for the powerful. And that's a tragedy in a crisis like this one.

LORETO: I've been reading articles about Covid-19 every day, right? Every single day. You came to realize that, out of thirty articles, fifteen were the exact same article.

MCKAY: One of the core unifying themes of your book is that the state and most of the media continued to pound home this individualizing message throughout the pandemic. I personally found one of the strongest chapters to be the one you devoted to the "Lie of Personal Responsibility." So many of the arguments we heard throughout 2020–22 were essentially founded on the doctrine that it's our individual responsibility to keep ourselves safe.

Even the federal government's app was premised on this doctrine (which was, perhaps, one reason why its approach to contact-tracing failed so conclusively). Young people were blamed for getting sick through their "reckless behaviour," which dovetailed nicely with the mantra of personal responsibility. Much propaganda was dedicated to staying at home, but governments did almost nothing to mitigate Covid-19 spread inside those homes and proceeded as though normal Canadians all live in detached suburban houses. Those who were unhoused were subjected to state violence. As you put it, the "personal responsibility narrative" worked to erase "the causes and therefore possible solutions necessary to slow the spread of COVID-19."[4]

In the form of liberalism hegemonic in Canada since the 1840s, the "individual" has always been the irreplaceable principle of economic, social, and cultural life—so, in a way, this individualistic thrust (which you trace in many other chapters as well) is perhaps not that surprising. Yet, I thank you for bringing out this individualistic theme so powerfully and so well. Can we also ask you for your suggestions as to how this liberal individualism became so omnipresent—and how might we transcend this pattern?

LORETO: That's the struggle that faces all left-wing people in this country—and anybody who understands that every single one of our social issues is only going to be solved by some level of collectivity. This is the biggest challenge. That's the case when we look at climate change, housing, any number of issues. I think what was very interesting with the pandemic is that it was often a radicalizing moment. People talk about how leftists have to do education, and education is really important. You have to teach people certain things and give people the words or the understanding of whatever they're experiencing.

The pandemic was a crash course. There were a lot of things that were taught during the pandemic that we don't have to sit down and explain to people. We don't have to go through this process of education in a theoretical way. Many people now have had this direct experience.

So, that's positive. But it's very difficult because there are no mainstream political parties, there are no mainstream corporate entities, no mainstream media entities that want us to see ourselves as living in community. Margaret Thatcher won, right?[5]

The biggest struggle for the left is: How do we inject community back into our communities? How do we break that isolation?

And this is where the left has really failed in the pandemic. It was coded as being a progressive, enlightened, pro-science position to follow what the politicians were doing. We were fed the line that vaccines would get a lot of us out of all this. It was coded as being the correct response to hide in your homes, wait for the vaccine, and Covid-19 will all go away. There was a lot of good advice wound up in that. There were lots of reasons to self-isolate. But the left never tried to experiment with ways to build community outside of online spaces that would actually break through some of that isolation.

And then, even worse, a lot of people refused even to consider the question, "How far do we push our risk tolerance?" There were a lot of voices in 2020 on the left *insisting* that it was still dangerous to be outside when it was pretty clear that it was *not* dangerous to be outside.

We just lost so much ground, especially to the far right, which used this time to create the community everyone is so desperate for while keeping ourselves safe. Pushing boundaries.

We find ourselves in 2022 with the left lacking any experience in building such spaces.

Then came a bunch of truckers [in the Freedom Convoy] who say, "We're going to build these spaces. And we're going to build them outside, so the risk of Covid transmission is pretty low." They seized the initiative. We did not. It was a real missed opportunity.

So how do we rebuild after this? Well, we have to be bold. We have to stop being afraid. We have to find ways to keep each other safe and in ways that allow for a diversity of involvement that doesn't necessarily mean that everyone needs to always be doing all of the same things, together. We *have* to build spaces where we can come together. It is not enough to take care of ourselves in our isolation, because isolation is not society. We cannot survive in isolation.

MCKAY: Your book looks at how Canadian journalists covered Covid-19, as well as offering us hard-to-locate information about the country and the pandemic. From your thirteen substantive chapters, a reader can find a wealth of material on the long-term-care crisis, the federal government's Canada Emergency Response Benefit (CERB) and its employer-friendly counterpart, and the Canada Emergency Wage Subsidy (CEWS). We are also introduced to systemic racism; schools and Covid-19; migrant workers; the "race for the vaccine"; the pandemic's gendered impact; its effect on the disabled community; and its spread through workplaces. It's almost encyclopedic in its coverage. From your perspective, what is the most important new information your book brings to Canadians?

LORETO: First and foremost, it would be the information and analysis around disability. I structured the book to have a hook, with each of the chapters on a theme. The hook for the disability theme was that we've started a new year knowing Covid-19 existed. So it's the chapter that marks the end of one year and the beginning of the next. It highlights the analysis disability activists brought to everything in the pandemic—how do you survive infectious disease? Why are things happening? Why are people being treated like this? It built on a lot of philosophical and critical thinking about how people in general are treated by health care in this country. I tried to synthesize the chapter from what activists were saying—who are so often ignored. They are just not given the kind of platform they deserve within mainstream media. That remains, maybe, the most important part of what I wrote.

But—just to get everything in the same spot! You mentioned all the chapter topics. You can imagine what it was like to write all that. You've got to add this, you've got to add that. You mentioned the personal responsibility chapter. It was originally going to be the workplace chapter. As I was writing through the personal responsibility side of it all, I thought: "I haven't even mentioned the government app or housing." It's all connected. I wanted everything to be accessible in the same book. You might hate what I write—although not so many people who read me hate what I write, which is great—but if you do, at least you have a resource that explains, for example, the race-based data or the data related to deaths and hospitals. It's a snapshot in time.

Very few of those data are my own personal work. A lot of them are drawn from other people. (The long-term-care data are my own personal work. And the hospital data are my own, generated from my requests for health information.) By and large, what I write about is based on the work of other people. To have all that information in the same location, to have that all together in an analysis you can actually read from A to Z and say, "This makes a lot of sense"—that was my goal.

By the time I started collecting data in April 2020, it was so obvious that the process of forgetting would be intense, that it would be aided by people's fatigue. People wanted it to end. We cannot forget what happened, and I wanted to write the book as it was happening because the analysis would change too much afterwards. If I wrote the book now, it would be completely different.

Frankly, I didn't suspect two years ago that, in Canada, this would stand as the sole substantive English-language book on the subject. That, to me, is ridiculous. Now we have this record. It would have been very difficult to recreate it after the fact.

MCKAY: Getting back to the disability chapter, I really liked what you did with the theme of "comorbidity." You did imaginative work with that word. In a sense, the term depoliticizes the inequality of Covid-19 because the "comorbidities" we focus on arise out of the social and economic order in which we all live. By calling a condition a "comorbidity," one implies both that it's the person's fault and that the condition is likely to lead to death. It's a very depoliticized, asocial way of thinking about disability. Coding all the disabilities as comorbidities suggests a very fatalistic outlook.

LORETO: I should give a shout-out to Gabrielle Peters whose thinking on these themes was really important to me.[6] Had we called "comorbidities" "disabilities" from the start, there would have been far more outrage, as there was in the United Kingdom. Britons with disabilities were way overrepresented in the statistics. Canadians were sharing British stories and saying, "Oh, this is horrifying!" But Canadian journalists were just packing the data differently. The government of Alberta had all of these data: 96 percent of the people who die from Covid had one comorbidity and 72 percent had three or more comorbidities. The outrage wasn't the same because Canadian journalists were not packaging the information in the same way as the British. The data were differently arranged. It was very political.

It was gross and disgusting. We weren't having an honest conversation about what this meant. And then journalists would chase stories like "42-year-old man died and had no underlying health conditions," right? But that wasn't the whole story. The ableism that is so omnipresent in reporting on Canadian society was exposed in an incredible way during this pandemic. And that made that section on comorbidities very difficult to write.

MCKAY: Your chapter on gender focused closely on women, yet could one not also say that men, many of them workers, dying of Covid in higher numbers—with an overall global death rate estimated to be about 1.6 times as high as the death rate for women—were also influenced by gender ideologies and gender expectations? Such as the one requiring them to put their lives on the line to feed their families?

Many such men spent the pandemic working in risky and often stigmatized jobs—sanitation, construction, driving buses, migrant farm labour—as well as those who died in such congregant settings as nursing homes. The suicide and opioid-addiction rates among them are also skyrocketing. And gay men, especially the many exiled from their families of origin, have had a particularly difficult pandemic, which coincided with an HIV/AIDS crisis with many more victims, so far, than those of Covid-19. Lots of countries have made it hard to obtain retrovirals. Gay men were already experiencing a (sometimes forgotten) pandemic when Covid-19 arrived, which as a stigmatized group raises all kinds of traumatic memories. Is there room in a feminist gender analysis for men?

LORETO: That was actually the hardest chapter for me to write. It echoes a lot of the book I had just written. I kept thinking, I just wrote a book about this. When I get to the part where I'm talking about our various "Premier Dads," this persona our premiers took on, whether the "Angry Dad" or the "Benevolent Dad," I had more of a blast writing that part of the chapter. Whereas, the rest of it made me feel: "Oh God! Again!"

This is foremost a book of media criticism. Men didn't get that kind of coverage in the media, right? Childcare figures very, very strongly in a lot of it because many women are writing in journalism, so many parents of young children are journalists, typing away while their kids are bothering them. But yes, on deaths from the infection, men were way overrepresented. And racialized men were way overrepresented. I didn't have time to integrate the opioid crisis because it was such a big issue that I was unable to weave it into the narrative. It's definitely something that's missing from the book. And the mental health crisis, which I think is also being felt acutely by men. I touch on this in one of the chapters around CERB[7] in Medicine Hat—how difficult it was for men, especially. That is a huge story that needs to be told.

It was also interesting to see how sexual health took a back seat to Covid-19 testing in so many public health units in this country. As you say, people who are already marginalized, who need to access testing, were totally pushed aside as sexual health nurses and sexual health public health experts or practitioners were seconded to the processing of Covid-19 tests. It just pushed everything else back, with incredible backlogs. People aren't getting tested—which of course means there's going to be more increases in other illnesses. That would all be wrapped up in a new gender chapter, which hopefully I'm never going to have to write.

People will not recover easily from the trauma of the past two years. And from how their state has failed them.

MCKAY: Your work has interesting reflections on sexual minorities. Many sex workers were basically excluded from CERB, right? There was a very heteronormative logic built into what we consider to be "families." The whole New Zealand metaphor of the "Bubble" was perhaps an attempt to get beyond the Ozzie-and-Harriet stereotype of the nuclear family, but in many ways, it too intensified the idea of the traditional family.[8] You felt you really had to justify yourself if you weren't living in such a family, a particular burden confronted by the LGBTQ+ community. The fallback assumption seemed to be that we were all living in heterosexual families in detached houses, following the conventional script. But—lots of people aren't. As your book points out, close to half of Canadians don't even live in detached homes, to begin with.

LORETO: Think of the many people who had to ask themselves: "I've decided to 'bubble' with this person?" Even single people said: "We're going to bubble together to become a family from the perspective of the rules of isolation," right? Or all the stories of mixed and blended families, where parents have no control over what ex-partners or other people raising their children part-time might be doing. And then coming home, and their kids have Covid-19, and they have Covid-19, and it's spread that way.

And then, for the people that did live in standard, nuclear, heteronormative families: there was nothing to help them survive the horror of the nuclear family on overdrive. Isolated with someone whom you love enough—but not enough to see them every single minute of the day!

How many families didn't survive this? What does the postpandemic family look like? So many couples realized during the pandemic: "This is not the person I want to be locked up with."

MCKAY: Am I right in thinking you are a bit skeptical of school lockdowns? You're kind of going up against teachers' unions who were very emphatic that we needed to shut the schools down.

LORETO: Yes, I am. I thought about it quite carefully.

MCKAY: You're not convinced by their argument. Is that a fair summary?

LORETO: Yes, that's totally fair. I'll give you an example. In August 2021, my partner and I decided, "OK, things are safe enough. Not safe. They're safe *enough*. And these kids have to see their grandparents."

So, we took a trip to Southern Ontario. We and every other person we saw on that trip had not had anyone over for almost a year and a half—whether in their yard or the house. And the people who were the most nervous, our friends, were teachers, by a long shot. But I'm looking at the data, I'm seeing who's dying. Not, for the most part, teachers in 2021.

So, I'm sitting down with friends and family. The teachers among them were so petrified. I would explain my research to them. "I'm writing this book. I know all this stuff." And they said: "You're the first person to reassure me that I'm not just going to die when I enter the classroom in September."

My partner is a professor, and some of our friends in Ontario were shocked to hear that he had been back in his lab as of August 2020. He's a science professor, right? "I have to be there. There's no choice." In Quebec, everything shut down. In May 2020, the government announced: "We're going to reopen." I thought, "You're not. No way." Am I sending my kids to school? "No way." Then there were no massive outbreaks in schools. The school season ended really well in 2020.

There seems to be a cultural difference, as well, between my "Anglo-Saxon-ness" and what was going on in Quebec. I talked with a lot of parents. Parks here were never closed. We were seeing people all the time. There was this moment, at the height of an outbreak in town, when out of nowhere this kid appears in my house, and I'm thinking, "Oh, God, I can make a big deal out of this and be scared that this kid has Covid. Or I could just relax and realize this kid probably isn't going to infect us at all. We're OK. The kids can play together." The milieu in which I lived was a bit calming, telling me not to be afraid of everything.

Schools play dual roles. They take kids out of home situations that might be good or that might be bad. And so every time you close the school, you affect them. The only way you can protect children at home is if you have a parent or two parents or three parents who can stay home all the time, and we're isolating at home. That's the only way you can protect children in the home situation.

And so, who do we hear from the loudest? The parents who have that capacity. They say, "Close the schools. We can keep our kids at home. But then support us—because keeping kids at home is really hard."

I could never reconcile myself to the fact there was no safe alternative for kids in informal care situations. They would just be sent back to daycare, then sent back to school. Emergency daycare was needed for the parents who can't stay home.

The movements for better air quality are important, paid sick days for teachers are really, really important. All of that is really critical. But before Omicron, before Covid-19 became exponentially contagious, it was not clear to me that the schools were *the* problem.

But what *was* the problem? No one was talking about the neighbourhoods in which the schools were located. Schools exist in a network. Is this a school where parents work in a meat processing facility? Is this a school where parents are medical workers, where Covid-19 can enter very easily? Is this a low-income school? Or a predominantly racialized one? Almost no conversations like that. Generally, the schools were treated as though they were all the same. Children were all treated the same. There was no appreciation for those most at risk, who were also the ones most affected by school closures.

MCKAY: You'd face a strong argument from some teachers, some of whom told me: "We're all in the soup. Our government (i.e., Ontario's) is giving us such confused and conflicting messages. It announces new spending that sounds ambitious, plans for better ventilation—but, in truth, not much really changes inside the working classroom that makes anyone safer." Social distancing in schools was unenforceable. There was a sort of moral panic induced by the high level of state chaos and confusion. And, as your book points out, the Canadian response was *so* fragmented. We almost don't know how it unfolded in other regions.

LORETO: That's true. We have a right-wing government in Quebec, but it was decisive in its actions and clear about their decisions. It justified them with explanations. So, even if you disagreed with it, there was some public sense about what it was doing. Ontario had none of that, right? And not just Ontario—Manitoba, Saskatchewan, Alberta, BC. There was no public sense to many of the decisions they made.

While I'm highly critical of, and frankly despise, our Quebec government, still, there were not many moments related to the pandemic and schools when I was uncomfortable with what was happening. I always felt there was at least some sort of expert looking at the data and saying, "The benefits outweigh the negatives," and we need to keep schools open for that reason. And in Quebec, we had a very robust shutdown system, which was responsive to local conditions.

In Ontario, the entire system was shut down for six months of 2021. There were parts of the province that had no Covid cases at all, but schools were still closed. What does that do to parents? Just trying to make sense of it makes you feel you're losing your mind, right?

And then that fuels, of course, conspiracy theories and other kinds of things.

There were also teachers who didn't take the power they could have taken. They could have shut down certain schools and they could have reopened certain schools. But instead the message was: "We have to respect the school boards. We have to respect the Ministry of Education."

MCKAY: You write very powerfully against journalists who encouraged panic and pessimism in readers. Still, I think many of them will also put your book down with something like a feeling of pessimism. Here is a Canada so poorly led, and so poorly informed by its journalists, and so under the domination of a corporate elite: isn't pessimism kind of called for?

And, to go back to journalism, your chapter on "One Year in Media Cuts" parallels Naomi Klein's analysis in *Shock Doctrine*: media employers across the country undercut their own journalists with a drastic reorganization (and centralization) of broadcasters like the CBC and Global, intensified corporate control of the Toronto media, and almost no alternative to a fully neoliberalized media landscape.

Then, what message of hope can we draw from your book given that those who might deliver messages alternative to individualism have been so consistently sidelined or silenced? A message that might suggest a future a bit brighter than the events we've just passed through?

LORETO: I've got messages from people who've read the book who tell me it made them feel better. Which is very weird because the book can really be considered quite pessimistic. In essence: the government could have chosen "not destruction" and they picked "destruction." And this is on every single page.

It's still leaving people with a sense of—I'm not sure I've got the right word—purposefulness. A *sense* of what has happened. There's power and there's hope in recovering the sense of what happened.

I've never despaired during this pandemic. I was not surprised by many things. There was no moment when I was shocked by anything or surprised by anything. And one comes away with a clarity of understanding about what needs to be done. It's very, very clear. Of course, *how* we get it done is up for debate and discussion, which we have to engage in. But it is very, very clear what the source of all our problems is, who the sources of our problems are.

I think that is hopeful, because there's a clear path forward. You have to break up monopolies. You have to break up the banks. You have to have public ownership. We have to reassert our power over this fake democracy in which we live. There are movements that people can get involved with. There's resurgence, excitement. In every single community in this country, there are movements that people can get involved with. That's extremely hopeful.

What isn't hopeful is confusion. Why is your CERB being clawed back? Why are you expected to put your life on the line to serve coffee? When you bring sense to it, then you can actually start to do something. We need to unionize. Or, our union's not that great—so we need to fight them or take it over or change unions. Once people are given the path to fixing things, the despair becomes a lot less overpowering. We know what we have to do. I wanted this book to give people that sense.

MCKAY: You've pierced the fog of the pandemic and offered us a glimmer of light as you present the various structural patterns as well as the individual responses to them. Once the pandemic is seen to make sense in terms of structures, the politics will likely change.

I would say that a primary challenge, though, will be to develop media that are more sympathetic to a more critical perspective. (In addition to worthy left-wing sources like *The Breach* and *Canadian Dimension* and *Briarpatch*, all great projects reaching relatively small numbers of people.)[9]

LORETO: Left-wing media are underfunded, they don't reach millions of people, and in general they don't pay writers. This is a huge, huge problem.

On the positive side of the ledger, there has been an explosion of alternative media. You mention *The Breach*, and other examples are *Passage* and *The Maple*.[10] There are a lot of people who have gone on their own with Substack. Or one thinks of someone who is not a left-wing person but whose journalism is driven by a humanity that is lacking in the mainstream media: *The Rover* run by Chris Curtis in Montreal.[11] There are lots of really excellent things happening.

I'm very encouraged to see that in addition to *Rabble* and *Canadian Dimension* there are so many other things people are experimenting with in different models. But as for the mainstream, it is such a disaster. We have to reach more people.

I did an interview with CJAD in Montreal on Christmas Eve of all times, to talk about this stuff, and the journalist literally asked me at the end of the interview: "Where have you been this whole time?" I didn't know what he meant at first. He wasn't asking whether I was based in Montreal or Quebec City. No: "Why have I never heard of you? Why have I never heard anything like you're saying before?" The power to block voices out is so strong. I've been interviewed by the *Globe and Mail*, and literally had the journalist come back and say, "Oh, I'm sorry, I can't actually use that. I was just told."

I don't know how you get around that. Part of the answer is in new kinds of media like podcasting. The audience that we have with my podcast with cohost Sandy Hudson is as big as some of the main newspapers' podcasts.[12] We can build those kinds of platforms, but we need something that's more cohesive. The only way we're going to change any of the big media institutions is from outside pressure. In no way is the CBC changing from the inside.

MCKAY: I really loved your treatment of the *Toronto Star* on the subject of long-term-care facilities. I quite admired their zeal on the crisis. They offered good investigative journalism, I thought. There was a very polemical editorial. Even a petition for readers to sign. The world must change! This must not go on! And then—radio silence. Is that right? They never really got back to the issue?

LORETO: As I say in the book, you can't even easily access the initial petition. I had to search through the WayBack Machine, to use the Internet Archive, to find the original petition that they scrubbed. The funny thing about "investigative journalism" these days: so much of it is often about things hiding in plain sight. There's not a whole lot of digging involved. On the long-term-care stuff, the *Toronto Star* did not even build up its own list of deaths. They just took the government's line.

I guess you can do that. But then you miss every death the government doesn't consider Covid-related. There were people dying from dehydration, directly linked to the pandemic. They should have been included on these lists of deaths. There were also a lot of facilities that weren't formally long-term care facilities where people died. They don't appear on any official list.

So, again, if you're not building your own lists, you're relying on government data that you can't verify. You're not listening to the workers saying: "We pulled out seven bodies today, it wasn't five, like the government says. It was seven."

Even the *Globe and Mail* just did a report on deaths in long-term care facilities and then correlated them with contracts from Doug Ford's government. Copying and pasting from a government document, pasting from government announcements, and then putting it on a spreadsheet. There's no "investigation" to that. It's important work, of course, no one else is doing it. But it's not as deep as we need. And it's certainly not as deep as Canadians expect. That's the state of where things are right now. I'm sitting on data on how many people have died in hospital from Covid. And I just don't know what to do with them.

MCKAY: You conclude the book with a powerful paragraph: "You know how this turns out. You know whether the delta or lambda variants trigger a fall wave in Canada. You know if the omega variant ever comes to pass. You know what October 2021 looked like. You know if Covid-19 sticks around until 2022, if the global death toll hits ten million or if Covid-19 dies out. If you're reading these words, it means you're still alive and there's still enough hope for you to spend any time at all reading books. Your time is precious. Your time is needed. Your time is now."[13]

It suggests to me the promise and pitfalls of writing history as it's happening. So much of what historians write is conditioned by the wider causal patterns they see in the evidence, and as of now, we can't know if Covid-19 will be remembered, like the Influenza Epidemic of 1918–20, as a two-year blip, which remarkably went by with very little commemoration—or, as many Marxist environmentalists contend, one manifestation of capitalism's multiyear climate crisis, of which Covid-19 is but a symptom, the first of many pandemics. How do you assess the promises and pitfalls of writing this form of "contemporary history" of an event whose contours are still unclear to us? We don't even know if we're right to speak of the pandemic in the past sense. This has been a virus full of surprises.

LORETO: I was writing that in November 2020. Then, in 2022, I actually got Covid-19. Triple vaccinated, but still got it. Very mild.

I'm not an historian and I didn't try to write a definitive history, to provide the obligatory way to tell the story of this pandemic. I wanted to write a record, a journalistic record, of the here-and-now. As long as we're able to keep this record so the work of historians can then be influenced by it later on, I think that's the most important thing. The times we're living in right now are very strange. I hope *Spin Doctors* provides a record that will stand the test of time.

MCKAY: I really identify with your dilemmas, as a historian trying to write something about Covid-19, too. How does one tell a coherent story about something that's so full of surprises and is still unfolding? Your own strategy in *Spin Doctors* is to start each chapter off at a particular date, situating the reader in that time and place. And then your chapters tended to flow beyond those chronological parameters.

Providing the record of what happened was important. I think your book will play a significant role in the Canadian literature on Covid-19 because it integrates so much information from coast to coast to coast, something we Canadians find very difficult to do, divided as we are by language, region, any number of other things. We just don't know that much about each other.

As Covid-19 transitions from traumatic memory to recorded history, how do you think it will be commemorated and understood? It was striking to me that there was so little attention paid to the "million-victim milestone" in the US, in contrast to that lavished on the one-hundred thousandth death. At a time of marked pandemic fatigue, a yearning for normality, will people *want* to remember Covid-19? Aren't those keen to preserve an accurate memory of it up against the challenge that, for many people, these are just years to forget? How do we combat that?

LORETO: I think there will be a tendency to *not* commemorate it. There are few governments with an interest in commemorating it. Unless average people commemorate themselves through culture, or music, or some sort of collective production, even people putting up their own monuments—we're not going to see much of anything. You might see a plaque someday at certain facilities where there were mass deaths. Maybe.

MCKAY: So, for you, the 1918–20 scenario—mass forgetfulness—is a likely one?

LORETO: Absolutely. Where I'm situated in Quebec City, right across the street, there was a field hospital for the 1919 flu. There's no commemoration of it at all. Many, many people must have died there. But, when you go into Lower Town, less than a kilometre from where I am, there's a memorial to the five Quebeckers shot dead in the anti-conscription protests, the Easter Sunday massacre. It's important to remember them. Yet, still, literally no commemoration of the hundreds of people who must have died in that field hospital.

What I wonder about is: at least the 1918–20 flu epidemic took place at a time when people still did live in community. There were collective ways of handling the trauma of war. The full impact of it would be felt in the 1930s. There were still families that would make music together, extended families, there were language-groups communicating with one another—in a way that doesn't exist today.

Where does our trauma go in a digital age? We're told the Internet is our community, now. That's really what worries me the most. It will make us far sicker. It will make the trauma far worse, and we will have nowhere to channel it. I think we are in for a post-Covid, posttrauma crisis that is going to be immense. Without a single politician who knows how to fix it, their policies likely making it worse.

MCKAY: I think the one thing your book does, brilliantly, is to weave the theme of individualism through so many discussions. Covid-19 was this paradoxical event—one calling for both individual isolation and collective focus. Everyone who could was supposed to isolate, acting together. I suspect, for many people, loneliness was almost as much a scourge as Covid-19. And think of the way many people were asked to say goodbye to loved ones. Often they weren't allowed even to say goodbye. So, you had a violation of a very widespread human need to commemorate the death of people you cared for, suddenly uprooted by this pandemic.

Your point about trauma is a powerful one and suggests a contrast with 1918–20. This pandemic has been a far more individualizing event. The political and social consequences could be more severe as survivors go in search of community, mythologies, meaning. Some are drifting into very dangerous alt-right channels, ones a bit reminiscent of fascism in the 1920s.

LORETO: That's right. If they go anywhere. Alcohol and opioids beckon—or many will try to swallow the trauma on their own and it will make them sicker. The internal trauma of loneliness and isolation injures and kills as well.

A number of people I talked to said, "Oh, I couldn't go to see my mother's final moments, because I was told to socially isolate." It was very shocking to me in 2020. There was no ban on people doing that. People, in their honesty and in their good faith, assuming governments were operating in good faith as well, trusted them. "This is too dangerous, and therefore I will sacrifice this last moment with my loved one." There are a lot of people I talked to online. I didn't know them personally, but if I had, I would have told them: "Get on the plane. Get a good mask. You'll probably be fine. You probably won't get Covid-19 if you're wearing a good mask."

But there was none of that. People did not say goodbye to people they loved. There was this stoical sensibility: "The government asked us to fulfill this very simple demand—stay home. It sucks that I can't say goodbye to my loved one. But, I'm doing my duty." There's no dignity in that.

When people start to process the grief from those moments, that will be explosive. And then there are all the people who died so quickly people couldn't say goodbye to them. That's a whole other kind of trauma and grief. And that's going to be borne not only by the families but also by staff. I interviewed one personal care worker. She works in a facility in the Kitchener-Waterloo region. She described to me what it was like to wheel out the still-warm bodies of her clients from this facility. There's no state program to deal with that kind of grief. Nothing.

Healing in the current age that we're in often seems like an impossibility. At least in the 1920s there was at least a sense of, "Well, we've got to submit ourselves to God's will, we're going to see everybody in church, we're going to gossip, we're going to live in our communities, we're going to struggle for food, to pay for stuff—but at least in this struggle we have a community." Nowadays, we don't have that spirit at all.

MCKAY: Another significant difference is that this lockdown went on much longer than those of 1918–20. The fatigue is understandable. It hasn't been a month or two. It's been more than two years. I would call the atmosphere one of ambient dread and anxiety. What new disaster awaits us around the corner? Even if one hasn't gone through traumatic experiences in this pandemic directly, one has experienced them vicariously.

It inspires the perennial question: How can we break into this cultural atmosphere and say, "OK, let's do something different." Present a message of hope to people surviving this crisis.

LORETO: I think understanding how things have unfolded in other parts of the world is really important. There's a level of whiteness in many of our conversations: "I don't want to get this kind of disease at all, it's dirty, I don't want to get sick at all." This is not how other people in the world live, because they can't. The circumstances of their lives don't allow it. People go to tremendous lengths to create fake bubbles to keep themselves safe. You can see just how much that is damaging people's minds and their wellness in general.

We also have to get serious about the Internet. The left has been very slow on this. There are still discussions out there along the lines of, "Isn't the Internet amazing because it's bringing us together and we can organize online and it's accessible and all this stuff." Well—no. What the hell are you talking about?

Real life isn't optional. Especially if we're going to start organizing in ways that challenge the state—we're not going to do that on Zoom.

We have to have a very sober conversation about the limits of the Internet. How do we use it? How do we *not* use it? The Internet is a huge problem in all of this. We don't get back what we give to it.

One of the things that exploded during the pandemic was this idea of mutual aid. I grew up in a religious family, I worked for the Catholic church and a lot of it looked like traditional "church-lady" stuff. Yes, it kept people alive, communities alive, fed people, gave people a reason to live. But it's not activism. All of my aunts were feeding the poor. But they weren't changing society. There has not been much analysis of the difference between feeding the poor and revolutionary societal change. We're not insulting people when we say that feeding the poor is not revolutionary.

This is the biggest problem with the left right now. There is a lack of understanding. Even if we've been radicalized around all the structural problems in society, there's a fundamental lack of understanding of social change and of revolutionary change—the distinction between revolutionary change and what is just maintenance to keep people alive. We have to do both—it isn't one or the other. Church ladies are great. We need them. They're not revolutionaries.

MCKAY: I think we're living in a revolutionary age—one that calls out for a revolution if the species is going to survive—but we don't have a revolutionary movement. That, in a nutshell, is our dilemma.

Spin Doctors is undoubtedly the best Canadian book on the Covid-19 pandemic, and you're to be congratulated for bringing it out. It offers great coverage, from coast to coast to coast, of how Canadians experienced this moment. Thank you for it.

AN INTERVIEW WITH
TITHI BHATTACHARYA
3 FEBRUARY 2022

Tithi Bhattacharya is professor of history and director of Global Studies at Purdue University and a renowned feminist scholar whose work on both social reproduction theory and the gender politics of contemporary India has won a wide and appreciative global audience. Her edited collection on social reproduction theory suggests that a full understanding of the capitalist world demands close attention to the preconditions of that world in the often unpaid, generally disregarded—and in a time of pandemic, often very dangerous—work undertaken disproportionately by women.[1] This work is that which makes our social order conceivable.

In 2019, Dr. Bhattacharya coauthored *Feminism For the 99%: A Manifesto*, which argues for the revitalization of left politics based on this practical and theoretical insight.[2] As Dr. Bhattacharya remarks in *Dissent Magazine* in 2020, "Right now when we are under lockdown, nobody is saying we need stockbrokers and investment bankers! Let's keep these services open! They are saying, 'Let's keep nurses working, cleaners working, garbage removal services open, food production ongoing.' Food, fuel, shelter, cleaning: these are the 'essential services.'"[3]

MCKAY: I thought I might start off with a general question about social reproduction theory and about *Feminism for the 99%*. Can you tell us why you and your fellow authors, Cinzia Arruzza and Nancy Fraser, came to write this manifesto, and how is this manifesto being received throughout the world?

BHATTACHARYA: The answer to that question is mass feminist politics. Right now, as we continue isolated in our activities and our pods, that movement and politics seems rather far away. Let me back up a little bit and remind ourselves how the arguments of the book continue to live, despite our pandemic times.

The book is actually a distillation of the political conversations and arguments that emerged through the first wave of feminist strikes. In 2016, there were massive feminist public protests in Poland to oppose an abortion ban and in Argentina against femicide and gender violence. During the winter of 2016, after those massive public demonstrations, many feminists in various parts of the world got together and started having a conversation. What if we revive the feminist strike?

The nightmare of the election of Trump in the United States ended 2016. And so, in 2017, when we got invited as feminists in the United States to an international conversation about a feminist strike, it made perfect sense to us. The failure of liberal feminism to have any anchor in working-class politics in the United States was actually demonstrated by Hillary Clinton's form of feminism (or "girl boss feminism" or "lean-in feminism.") The election of Trump came as severe blow to this kind of liberal feminist politics. So, it made perfect sense to us, as feminists in the United States, to talk about a feminist strike and join in the global process of feminist strike organizing.

On 8 March 2017, we witnessed a massive rolling wave of strikes across the globe. In the United States, we had organized massive demonstrations and work stoppages in all of the major cities. In Spain and Argentina, in particular, trade unions joined in the strike. It was the repoliticization of March 8th (or International Women's Day) like we had not seen in many, many decades. And this happened in 2017, in 2018, in 2019—until it came to an abrupt halt in 2020 with the pandemic.

How is a feminist strike different from a normal workplace strike? One of the very crucial arguments we tried to make was that, whereas a workplace strike was about the stoppage of work in the capitalist arena of profit-making, a feminist strike was the stoppage of all work. It wasn't just that we were urging people to not go to work. We were also urging people to refuse to cook, to refuse to smile, to refuse to do care work. So, all the preconditions that made capitalist work possible, we were refusing to do as well. Those arguments of the street, and those arguments in the various feminist collectives, we tried then to distill and give voice to in that book. So, it's really a book about the politics of the strike, if you like. We hoped that we would bring that politics to a wider arena.

The arguments of the book did really well, in the sense that it engendered a feminist conversation in many, many contexts and countries. The book has been translated in more than thirty languages, and I feel really proud of the feminists who (say, for instance, in China or in South Korea), under tremendous odds, had a study session about the book and then reworked those arguments in their own national contexts and translated the book.

MCKAY: In many ways the *Manifesto* echoes your work on social reproduction . . . I would like to quote just one of its most striking passages: "capitalist society is composed of two inextricably braided but mutually opposed imperatives—the need of the system to sustain itself through its signature process of *profit-making*, versus the need of human beings to sustain themselves through processes that we call *people-making*."[4] I sense that's the core of the idea of social reproduction.

Would you be willing to give people a kind of introduction to social reproduction theory? I know it's a complicated body of knowledge that's accumulated over four decades, but I was just wondering if you could explain to people who haven't heard about it, what does social reproduction mean? And can you tie it into what's happened over the last four decades with neoliberalism? Because I think one argument might be that neoliberalism has systematically devalued social reproduction and monetized virtually every part of life, and that's had a tremendous impact on all those carers, and cleaners, and cashiers, without whom it could not function.

BHATTACHARYA: I would really love to hear from the rest of you as well about how this theory makes (or doesn't make) any sense in your own work or your own life, but I'll just start that with a brief comment.

I think there are two impulses of capitalism as a system. There is a short-term impulse, which is to make profit at any cost. And there is a long-term survival impulse, which is that it has to take care, in a capitalistic way, of the widgets, us, the human beings who make those profits. I say "widgets" because capitalism doesn't really take care of human beings for the sake of taking care of human life, but it has to provide the basic conditions of reproduction of life because otherwise the widgets, which is us, would not be producing profit.

Both of those tendencies go on at the same time. On the one hand, capitalism giveth—it creates minimal conditions for life to continue and reproduce and the working-class family to be continuously reproduced. On the other hand, it taketh away—in that it makes it impossible for many working-class families not just to flourish, but even to exist in many cases. Here I think race, ethnicity, caste come in. We have a disproportionate social reproduction of certain families at the expense of others. In other words, if the worker makes profit possible, then what are the processes, social processes, and institutional processes that make the worker? So, profit-making versus people-making.

Now, there are a couple of qualifiers. The qualifiers are as follows: capitalism will always try to deplete the conditions of life-making so that workers basically are provided only with the very basic minimum of life-making in order to reproduce themselves. That's the one rider, if you like. Every single advantage we have as a society, as a collectivity, has been won through working-class struggle.

So, to go back to the question: Capital is constantly trying to deplete or minimize life-making because any investment in working-class life actually has to come from profit. It has to come from a section of the profits, through taxes and so on, which has to be invested in health care, in schools. What capitalism wants is 100 percent profit, so even a tiny portion of the profit invested in social welfare of the working class is anathema to it.

But then, there is the long-term consideration that the widgets must be kept alive. So a skeletal infrastructure of social care is maintained by almost all capitalist societies—whether they are capitalist democracies, capitalist dictatorships, or anywhere in-between. When people argue, "Oh, but look at the Scandinavian countries, they have very robust systems," there are two things to be said in response. One is that if you look at any country's health care or public education, investment in public care, and if you then look at the rate of unionization, you will see they're absolutely similar. So, all countries that have a unionization rate of 80 percent or above have that robust public social care system. But, this does not make them any less capitalist. If you look at the Scandinavian countries right now, you will see that the minute that kind of an infrastructure brushes against questions of race and ethnicity, then it reveals its capitalist nature. For instance, if you go to Copenhagen, you will see that certain neighbourhoods are segregated for Muslim immigrants (the line seems to be: "Muslim immigrants should not be part of the wonderful urban life of Copenhagen because they're not liberal enough.") So, immigrant children are sent to segregated schools, they're kept in ghettos, and so on. So again, before we celebrate the flourishing of public care in certain capitalist countries, we have to be careful to notice that it is not necessarily the flourishing of universal life but is still a capitalist system of care. And yes, it's better than what we have in the United States, but it is not what we want under socialism.

So social reproduction theory looks at this tussle between capitalist profit-making (that is continuous) and the processes of life-making (that are also continuous). How much can the working class wrest from capital to remake our lives?

This tussle, I have to emphasize, does not have an end under capitalism. The system is set up in such a way that we can never actually all share the fruits of the earth equally. That's never ever, ever going to happen because it is a system built on continuous profit-making for the few at the expense of the work of the many. In other words, if we're talking about actual flourishing of human life—if we're really exploring what human relationships could look like—human sexual relations, human relationships of parental love—we can't do those experiments under capitalism fully. They will always necessarily be partial.

MCKAY: I wonder if I could bring you now to the pandemic that we're going through and some of the ways in which social reproduction theory might illuminate the past two years of Covid-19. I noticed in your very wittily titled essay in the *Social Reproduction* collection, "How Not to Skip Class," that you call attention to the myriad capillaries of social relations "extending between workplace, homes, schools, and hospitals."[5] What impact do you think the pandemic has had on those capillaries?

BHATTACHARYA: I'm going to start with a very cheap example, if you like. The Democrats are in power. We are no longer under Trump. Everything was supposed to go well. Joe Biden proposes two kinds of bills. One bill is the infrastructure bill, which is to pour money into bridges, roads, railways, et cetera. (I am not opposed to that bill—we need more infrastructure.) Then there is the bill about childcare credit, universal childcare, free college, better environment protections, et cetera. That bill has been whittled down from one trillion dollars to almost nothing—and even at that nothing stage, it will be vigorously opposed. Even during the pandemic, you see the priorities of capitalism there.

The priorities of capitalism are still absolutely not about preserving life. We can see this in so many distinct ways. In every single decision capitalism was forced to take, before the vaccines came out, you could see the kind of things the system is capable of. Overnight, hospitals were built, hotel rooms were commandeered by governments to house houseless people. In Britain, everyone was given a minimum wage while they stayed away from work. The system went on a sort of war footing to make sure the pandemic was dealt with. But the minute it stabilized to a certain extent, the whole effort of the system was put into getting people back into work.

In the United States, the question of school closing for K through 12, for kindergarten to high school students, has been all about putting their parents back into work. So, to me, here I think capitalism demonstrates very clearly what its priorities are. And its priorities are: "Yes, there is a pandemic we need to survive, and once we've passed the big swirl, we just need to put people back into work."

To me this is criminal in so many ways. It is going to affect certain populations far more than others. I have a choice, sometimes, to work online. The person who checks out my groceries does not, so she has to go to work every day and she is not given any protection by my local government. So certain populations will simply die off. Disabled people, people in dangerous jobs in the meat production plants (we saw how the virus ripped through them). Union protection is very low in the United States. Even where there are unions, they are often business unions and they do not protect their members adequately.

This is the short-term sort of component of the system coming to the fore: "We need to get people back to work, we need to continue to make profit. Life be damned, we need to get people back to the workplace."

More and more I hear people saying things like, "Zero Covid is not possible." This is the sort of absolute ideology coming from the ruling class. "Zero Covid is not possible; Covid has to be endemic." What does that mean? It simply means that we're just going to have to sacrifice some of our lives in order for us to live with Covid. So, "Zero Covid is not possible; we're not going to stop the profit-making in order for some life to be protected, in order for us to defeat the virus. We're just going to sacrifice some lives in order for us to normalize Covid."

I don't know if the system can be saved. The long-term prospects of the system look really, really bad, not just in terms of profits but also (more seriously) in terms of the climate crisis. This is a case of capitalism playing out as in the *Don't Look Up* scenario: "I'm not going to look at the climate crisis, I'm going to focus on short-term profit-making." Fossil fuels continue to dominate the conversation in all countries. In the long term, the prospects of the system look really poor.

MCKAY: My last question to you and then I will turn it over the audience. I'd like you to shift the focus to India and what you've written about Narendra Modi. His is an extreme form of Hindu nationalism, but you also describe his deep-seated commitment to neoliberal verities and to neoliberalism as a body of thought. Other people depict him as a populist, some people even call him a fascist, and I think to the outside world he's a bit of an enigma. You have the marriage of a fairly strident drive for Hindu purity in India combined with a form of neoliberalism. That doesn't really seem like a natural combination. So, would you basically agree that there's a contradiction between Modi's neoliberalism and his Hindu nationalism? Is India an example of the contradictions of the liberal order as we've experienced them over the last two years?

BHATTACHARYA: I don't think there is any contradiction between neoliberalism and Hindutva[6] as a politics. As a historian, I have to remind everyone that there is nothing called Hinduism per se. This corporate understanding of Hinduism as one, singular religion was created in the nineteenth century. If you went back to twelfth-century India and you asked someone, "Are you a Hindu?" that would absolutely make no sense to them. They would say "I don't know what you mean." If you asked, "Well, what gods do you worship?"—most likely, if this were an ordinary person, they would say, "Well I worship Shiva." So, they would be a "Shivaite." "But what do you do on Fridays?" "Well, I go to the local Sufi saint, and I put a little lamp there." "Really? You go to the Muslims? And what do you do on Saturdays?" "Well, Saturdays, I'm very holy, because I do worship the snake goddess, because I work in the jungle, in the forest, and the snake goddess is very potent, so I worship the snake goddess."

This is what absolutely mystified the British census takers in the nineteenth century. They would go in and say, "What is your religion," and no one knew what that question meant and so they would say, "Who do you worship?"—and they would say "Well, Shiva," and they say, "Okay Hindu" and then they would say, "Well, the Sufi Saint Nāimī." "Oh, then, Muslim." This was how a corporate identity of Hinduism was created.

But to go back to Narendra Modi. There is no contradiction because, actually, Hindutva as a force emerged in the 1980s and the early 1990s as neoliberalism was being consolidated in India. Hindutva is an expression of neoliberalism—and a particular way the Indian ruling class discovered to organize violence and to organize neoliberal production. So, for instance, in 1992 the leading Hindutva advocate was a central government minister at the time, Lal Krishna Advani. He led what was called a "Ratha Yatra."[7] So, he took a sort of mythological chariot from Hindu mythology, and he rode the chariot throughout India. Wherever the chariot went, it sparked riots against Muslims. It was these Hindu fanatics riding behind this mythological ancient chariot—but the chariot was pulled for the first time by a Toyota engine, because the market had just opened up for Toyota cars to come into India. That is the perfect moment, for me, of how neoliberalism expressed itself in India through Hindutva politics.

Narendra Modi as a person is absolutely a fascist. He comes from the openly fascist organization of the RSS [Rashtriya Swayamsevak Sangh], which is a militia group. It does not run elections. It's a street-fighting gang. It organizes branches in neighbourhoods to arm Hindu gangs and basically attacks Muslims and Dalits. The RSS was formed in the 1920s and openly admired Hitler in the 1930s. In its literature, it talks about how Hitler dealt with the Jewish problem, which is how in India we ought to deal with the Muslim problem. These are very open RSS lines. And Modi was a pracharik (or in other words, an organizer) for the RSS. That's how he rose in the ranks of the BJP [Bharatiyia Janata Party], which was the electoral, more civilized wing or expression of the RSS. That's how Modi rose.

So personally, he comes from an openly fascist background. He was the chief minister of Gujarat, which had organized pogroms against Muslims, which included things like Muslim families being burned alive and RSS members organizing and directing that kind of violence on the streets.

There was no question when Modi was elected as chief minister that he was going to Hinduize and turn the Indian state in these authoritarian directions. I think we were all hesitant to call the Indian state fascist when Modi first came to power, but the Indian state is rapidly turning fascist as we speak, and particularly through increasingly authoritarian moves. Journalists are being murdered in their own homes. There are open lynchings of Muslims and Christians and Dalits on the streets. These are all state-sponsored activities.

As you probably know, the Modi government was dealt a decisive defeat by the farmers' movement, which was a months-long movement against the government withdrawal of farm subsidies and policies that would have flooded the market with corporate seeds and so on. I want to say that with Modi, the prospects of democracy in India darken every day, but I also want to say that after the farmers' movement, Modi still hasn't had the last word.

MCKAY: Can I just take you briefly to his handling of the pandemic? To someone who doesn't know India in detail, it sounded unbelievable that the government would give people just four hours' notice before it launched one of the world's most rigorous lockdowns, with almost no provision for people who were going to be thrown into acute deprivation, forcing them to migrate hundreds of miles with many deaths, with no real regard for their welfare. One thinks of that amazing scene in which a whole crowd of migrants was doused with bleach as a visual metaphor of how they're regarded as subhuman.

BHATTACHARYA: I want to say one thing, though. Modi represents an ultimate sort of authoritarian fascist expression of Hindutva, but there has been a continuous escalation of this, and this is where I want to draw attention to the fact that the value of life in India has been depleted and lessened through successive governments of neoliberals.

Yes, Modi is an extreme example. But if you look at faculty from India—in Canada, the United States, and England—I guarantee 90 percent of them will be from the upper castes. I went to school in India, and I studied with almost no Dalit classmates.

So, this kind of lessening of life, this kind of depletion of the value of life, has been a standard practice since the big mass movements of the freedom struggle receded. The story of independent India and the story of the coming of the neoliberal era from the end of the 1970s from the '80s has been a steady lessening of the value of life. The bleach incident was horrible, but I can see a Congress government doing exactly the same thing. (What I can't see under a Congress government is perhaps some of the more extreme things like the "Love jihad" campaign[8] and the murder of journalists in their own home.) But this kind of cheapening of working-class lives and Dalit lives would be perfectly possible under a Congress government.

MCKAY: Well, maybe I can ask a question of Sue Ferguson, in our audience, who has also written a major text on social reproduction.[9] It strikes me how much Canadians have contributed to social reproduction theory. I can list about a dozen major theorists who are Canadian—and without sounding like the Canadian nationalist I'm not, isn't that interesting? Is that a pattern you yourself have noticed?

SUE FERGUSON: So, I have in fact written about that. One of my very early articles I ever published was in *New Politics* and then reproduced in *Critical Sociology*. *New Politics* insisted that I change the title to something like "Canadian contributions to social reproduction theory" or something along those lines. So yes, it is remarkable.

I don't know exactly why, except I would say there was a *very* strong cohort of folks at York University who were not just academics but also had very strong ties to the daycare movement in Toronto. I think connections between their kind of social movement activism and their academic interests really made an impact, and they developed their own cohort. There was a pretty strong tradition of

Canadian critical political economy as well, too. They then set out a set of discussions that feminists wanted to, and needed to, respond to.

I think in the US, maybe, the lack of a social democratic party also made some difference, because I'm not sure the milieu was as strong for putting those questions on the table at that time.

BHATTACHARYA: I think one of the things that maybe Sue you're pointing to (and it's also worth sort of thinking about and thinking through, perhaps) is a tradition of open Marxism. And by open Marxism I mean a Marxism encompassing a freedom to explore Marxist ideas without heresy-hunting. It emerged in the 1970s organically on the street, but from the '80s onwards, it got pushed into certain academic enclaves. York probably was a sort of safe space, if you like, to explore some open Marxist ideas and gained a critical mass. In the United States, it would be impossible to gain that kind of a critical mass in any university for *any* sort of collective Marxist exploration.

To me it's quite significant that when Historical Materialism as a conference space began to emerge from the 1990s, those kinds of conversations came back on the table. People again felt freer outside of Marxist organizational practices to actually explore ideas, explore themes, and most importantly, those kinds of conferences allowed an interface between activists and academics. Those kinds of critical open spaces to explore and think through some Marxist ideas helped cohere some of these ideas. I'm so glad Canada had them.

MCKAY: Sue, did you want to add anything to that?

FERGUSON: I think in the more recent past, what's been so fabulous has been the internationalization of that very same pattern, and I think a lot of that had to do with precisely the strikes that Tithi talked about. I think post-2008, there was just a real uptick in interest. There was a shift away from poststructuralist, postmodernist kinds of explanations. People were frustrated with the lack of a materialist kind of analysis. I think there's much to be gained and learned from thinking through and reading a lot of the poststructuralist, postmodernist work, but I think the lack of materialist analysis was glaring. I certainly know people being a lot more interested in my stuff after that point (I've been writing about it since the 1990s).

BHATTACHARYA: There was, in traditional Marxist circles, constant talk of trying to find the "unicorn," which is workplace struggle. Everything—working-class consciousness, working-class radicalism—was all calibrated and imagined through workplace struggles. But, on the other hand, you actually had a massive uptick of working-class struggles, except they were not always in the workplace. We had housing struggles (as Sue points out), we had struggles for water in Cochabamba, Bolivia, you had struggles against privatization of land, forests, and native rivers and access to water. So, all of these struggles were obviously working-class struggles, but they did not arise in the theoretical register of traditional Marxist thought. I think social reproduction theory suddenly began to resonate when those struggles became more legible for a wider left.

MCKAY: Can I ask both Tithi and Sue a question about intersectionality. The social reproduction collection has a major critique of intersectionality theory by David McNally—a careful critique.[10] It says intersectionality makes a positive contribution, but it has limitations. It tends to treat the "streets" that are in the intersection as fixed and firm entities, without really pondering how these categories came into being, or how they interacted with each other. I think he's sensing a kind of static quality to intersectionality theory. Would you two share that critique? Do you see social reproduction as distinct from intersectional theory or as a complement to it?

BHATTACHARYA: First of all, yes, I share David's analysis of intersectionality. But (and I want to reemphasize what you said) David's is a very careful analysis of intersectionality. It's not a rejection per se of intersectionality; it talks very much about the contribution, especially the contribution of drawing attention to certain categories of oppression and the workings of these oppressions that perhaps had not received the kind of attention they deserve in the world of theory and theorization. But it is in the world of theorization that I think our differences become more prominent, vis-a-vis intersectionality.

In the United States, for young people (and activists in particular), when they say "intersectional politics," they mean "antiracist policies." I would not actually walk into a classroom and say, "I am against intersectionality" because in the street language, in the activist sphere, that would be like me saying, "I'm against antiracist politics." If an activist says, "I want to be intersectional"—it means simply that they are signalling that they want to be sensitive to antiracism. They want to incorporate antiracism in their work. In this, we are absolutely on the same page with them.

David's critique is very much a theorization of intersectionality and where we differ from it. I direct everyone to go read that essay because it's such a carefully laid-out argument, but essentially the argument is that intersectionality as a theory falls short because there is no explanatory framework. It's more of a descriptive framework that says, things intersect. We don't get a sense of why they intersect in particular ways, nor do we get a sense of how these relationships are often modular (and by modular I mean that violence is organized in a modular way under capitalism, but with its own national or local instantiation). For instance, in the United States, violence is organized through race; in India, violence is often organized through caste. Now intersectionality will tell you that violence is organized through race or through caste, but it doesn't give you a sense as to why these modular organization patterns happen over and over again in capitalist society. So, it's a very useful theory if you're describing oppression under capitalism, but it falls short in actually explaining why it happens the way it does.

MCKAY: Sue, did you want to add anything to that?

FERGUSON: I think one of the key differences is that intersectional feminism will resist, often, naming the social power relations of capitalism—as the way social power works through capitalist social relations. So, that's why there's no kind of explanation for how these "modular patterns" appear, to use Tithi's term. Whereas social reproduction theory will say, "Well, we're talking about a capitalist world and it's a capitalist world because we can only make our world through the work that we do (either paid or unpaid) in a society in which capitalism has dispossessed all of us of the resources for the work. This is the terrain on which our struggles are happening." I owe a huge debt, though, to Black feminism, antiracist feminism, intersectionality feminism, whatever we want to call it. Because it is through thinking through their challenges to earlier social reproduction feminists, and thinking about their notion of co-constitution and how our relations are mediated in so many different ways and not just through the labour/capital relationship, that you can come to understand that social reproduction itself is a much more complex thing than just an issue about gender relations. We are always building off each other in those ways. It's not that social reproduction theory has the last word, either. I think some of the things that have already been talked about with the development of more disability theory—those things will expand and breakthrough in different directions in ways that we should all celebrate with all theory. It's not a competition between them.

MCKAY: Tithi, you write, "If the virus passes and we go back to life as before, then this has taught us nothing."[11] As we're entering, very reluctantly, year three of the pandemic, what do you sense of this as a turning point for the struggles that you so deeply believe in? Do you get a sense that pandemic weariness is draining the energy out of many of the hopes that people had in the first year? In the first year of the pandemic, I think, we found a lot of very expansive, almost utopian ideas. After it, there was more bitter realism, so far as I could see. Do you think we're still at a kind of historical inflection point where the left will really be able to gain traction out of what has been an exploitive and cruel experience for so many people?

BHATTACHARYA: That's the million-dollar question. I do not want to end on a low note here. But I also have to be realistic. This has not a been a great time for the global left. We had, as you pointed out, some exceptional global moments of solidarity and protest. Who would have thought that the regular murder of Black men in the United States would acquire this absolutely brilliant powerful global moment of resistance, all the way from the toppling of slaver statues to fighting against the Modi government in India to large demonstrations in Latin America for Black Lives Matter? It was an extraordinary moment—and that was at the height of the pandemic.

So, I do not want to draw too strict a line between the isolation that the pandemic has imposed upon us and the ability to mobilize. I don't think they are as firmly separated as sometimes it may appear.

Having said that, the prospects of the organized left in the Anglo world (as well as in many important sections of the globe) have been very poor and, in a lot of cases, the left has disarmed itself to a large extent. The attack on Palestinian rights and the capitulation of sections of the left to Zionist pressure has been very disheartening for many of us in the Palestinian movement. We are also seeing a reconsolidation of the centre through Biden and centrist politics, which is also disarming sections of leftist mobilization. And of course, the pandemic has meant that authoritarianism continues to march. Bolsonaro still lives on while the Amazon burns. Modi's electoral chances have been affected through these last two years, but I don't think he's going to be toppled anytime soon.

That's the bad news, if you like. I think the good news is that we have no other options left. The reason why millions of people took to the streets around the open murder of George Floyd was because there was nothing more to lose. If the Black community did not show the way at that point, it would just mean a continuation of a regime that was going to actually destroy entire communities and ways of life and entire histories.

All those conditions of oppression and violence continue to exist. So, I do not see a reason why this powder keg that we are living in is not going to have a spark in the future. What worries me is the episodic nature of these protests. So, we're going to see huge bursts of protest, and they're extremely energizing and that's what keeps us going, right, as a left. However, without a strong organized left—and I don't mean necessarily parties but any kind of infrastructure to cohere those protests, to anchor them in workplaces, in communities, to actually build a new generation of activists and train them—without that infrastructure, the protests will continue to remain episodic. That's really the challenge and the danger that I think we face in the coming years.

AN INTERVIEW WITH
CHANDRIMA CHAKRABORTY
15 JULY 2021

Chandrima Chakraborty is professor in the Department of English and Cultural Studies and director of the Centre for Peace Studies at McMaster University. She was awarded the title of University Scholar at McMaster University in 2017 and was elected to the Royal Society of Canada's College of New Scholars, Artists and Scientists in 2019. She has published extensively on Indian nationalism and historical memory in India and Canada, including a major study of the commemoration of the Air India disaster in 1985.[1]

MCKAY: You've written a lot about the ways the "model minority" stereotype has been applied to Asian Canadians. Is it, in a way, the flip side of the old "yellow peril" theme of the period before the 1960s? Iyko Day recently argued that the yellow peril and model minority stereotypes function as complementary aspects of the same form of racialization in which assumed economic efficiency is the basis for violent exclusion or assimilation.[2] Can you elaborate on the connection between what might appear to be very contradictory sets of stereotypes about Asian Canadians? And to what extent has this contradictory discourse worked to divide the racialized themselves, with a so-called model minority encouraged to pride itself on its supposed superiority over others?

CHAKRABORTY: I think, on the surface, the yellow peril and model minority seem like oppositional categories or stereotypes, but they are complementary aspects of the same form of racialization. The racialization of Asian Canadians as the model minority is intimately associated with the relative historical and social positions of Caucasian Canadians, Black Canadians, and Indigenous peoples in Canada.

If you look back, in terms of the nineteenth century, you have the first substantial Chinese settlement in Canada, in British Columbia, as a result of the gold rush.[3] You have large movements of Chinese migrants, recruited to perform much of the labour-intensive agricultural work, or other local industry and commercial work, that the white labouring classes were not willing to perform. Then, with the Canadian Pacific Railway, you have the government actively recruiting Chinese labourers to come in. But soon after the completion of the CPR, agitation began in terms of the Chinese not being quite right for citizenship. There is this momentum to get them out, or at least stop their immigration.

The Chinese are not, in the late nineteenth century, seen just as an economic threat (with the typical argument: "immigrants, they're taking our jobs"). They are seen as "too different," in terms of their bodies, their cultural practices, living habits, et cetera. The Chinese are seen as diseased bodies, as a public health risk. The racialization of Chinese Canadians was not simply a matter of legal exclusion or labour exploitation. Public health policies played a key role in the racialization and creating the stereotype of the yellow peril.

With the 1960s, you see the shift from the yellow peril to the model minority, the discourse that we are most familiar with. It's in the 1960s, with the 1965 US Immigration and Nationality Act, and the 1970s, when you have the liberalization of immigration policies in Canada, that you have this new stereotype emerging as the model minority. These are new groups of immigrants coming in, often not from the labouring classes but middle-class and upper-class Asians. Also, the 1960s is the era of civil rights. So, there are African Americans demanding greater rights, demanding an end to discriminatory policies. You have the model minority now being defined against the "bad minority." The assumption is that, if you work hard enough and you can pull yourself up by your bootstraps, you can rise up to the surface. According to this interpretation, Black Americans are not working hard enough, or they are not doing what the model minority is doing. So, you have this racialization and hierarchization within the racialized minorities.

I was looking into some of the first articles that mentioned the term model minority in the 1960s and all of those articles always end by comparing either Japanese Americans or Chinese Americans to Black Americans. You're being defined against, not just white Caucasians, but other racialized minorities.

MCKAY: In a crisis like this, these fault lines are coming to the surface. If we don't realize the depth of this history, the weight of this history—we're always going to be just responding superficially to a crisis. Yet, I think some people would ask: "What evidence have you got that this is really still up and running the same way?"

CHAKRABORTY: Well, read the news!

MCKAY: One of the things I really liked about your piece is how the term Asian American or Asian Canadian is, in a sense, a confection of the 1960s itself. Remembering that Asia is a vast area with a huge diversity of cultures, in the eyes of a xenophobe, there nonetheless is no distinction between one Asian and another.

CHAKRABORTY: Absolutely. Think of the 1982 beating up Vincent Chin, right, which most folks are aware of.[4] A Chinese American who's constantly called a "Jap," he was beaten up by white autoworkers. So, to the white gaze—Japanese, Taiwanese, Filipino—it doesn't matter. To the mainstream gaze, a person just seems "Asian."

With Covid-19, the discrimination and the exclusions we saw with the global pandemic are not just against Chinese Americans. All Asians are viewed as a monolith. You forget the class differences, you forget the geographical differences, you forget age, gender, all of that. There are so many intersectional identities that create a heterogenous "Asian subject."

MCKAY: You touch on Sinophobia, the heightened fear of China or things associated with China, and you write,

> During the COVID-19 pandemic, many Chinese Canadians, especially those working in low-wage precarious labour sectors bore a double burden, facing increased risk of COVID-19 infections as essential workers (manufacturing, warehouses, retail stores, sanitation, and health care) and increased risk of racisms at workplaces and in public spaces. Well-paid professionals often escaped the first risk but remained vulnerable to the second, encountering persistent anti-Chinese racisms in their everyday life. Several surveys and polls point to this exacerbation of anti-Asian racism during the COVID-19 pandemic.[5]

To what extent do you think anti-Asian prejudice has been fed, not just by age-old yellow peril-ism, but by the new Cold War that is coming upon us in which the Chinese are depicted as a monstrous "Other"—and not just their regime, but Chinese civilization as a whole?

CHAKRABORTY: A global competition between two superpowers involves episodic confrontations and shows of might and power. So, the US administration introduces tariffs on Chinese imports, saying that the Chinese are stealing US technology and intellectual property. China retaliates with its own tariffs. The Trump administration, as we know, has asked that foreign-made telecommunication equipment should not be used because it threatens national security. We know that a Chinese foreign ministry spokesperson, without any evidence, claimed that the US military brought the virus to China. Trump claims it's a Chinese virus, repeatedly, even after the World Health Organization's best practices seek to dissuade us from assigning viruses to places and ethnicities. And then we know the effects of that in terms of the intense escalation of anti-Asian racism both in the United States and in Canada.

MCKAY: I'm really taken by how much metaphors of war and militarism are suffusing even discussions about the virus itself, which is seen as an invading force. It's really interesting to watch how even supposedly objective reports about the virus start drifting into a very militarized vocabulary. And I'm also wondering about the lab leak theory that's been broadcast all around the world, claiming the virus leaked out of a "Chinese" lab. Yet, the lab in question had extensive American funding. Covid-19 is a story in which national boundaries don't matter as much as global supply chains. Had Wuhan not been a key centre within global supply chains, we would probably never have experienced Covid-19 globally. In the zeal to make it all about warring nation-states, we're misrepresenting reality. It's happening within an interconnected world.

CHAKRABORTY: So true.

MCKAY: I really liked what you said about the racist treatment of Dr. Theresa Tam, Canada's chief medical officer. Derek Sloan, the

Conservative candidate, actually asked, "Does she work for Canada or for China?" in his most ominous tone of voice. You critique the mass media's admiring comments about Dr. Tam. They kept playing up how graciously she responded to this race-baiting, and you critiqued this.[6] Can we expect less polite responses to such race-baiting in the future?

CHAKRABORTY: I'm glad you brought this up. To me, reading the media coverage brought up the image of the ideal minority, the model minority. A member of such a minority not only works hard, but works hard while keeping their head down. Theresa Tam's response to that was something like, "I'm just not distracted by noise. So, I'm not going to get into this. I have work to do."

But anger can be marshalled for justice to create multiracial alliances and solidarity. In an essay I read a long time ago (for a very different project I was doing on India and the cultivation of hate and anger against minorities) by queer feminist theorist Audre Lorde, called "Uses of Anger,"[7] she drew a distinction between anger and hatred. The object of anger is transformation. Hatred is about destruction—about death—and it is taken up by those who do not share our goals. I find that really instructive in terms of thinking about building alliances and prompting structural change.

What structural change could be the focus for our anger? I have multiple responses. For me, personally, the first thing would be an overhauling of the educational curriculum so we see our own privileges and complicities while educating new immigrants to Canada about Canada's racial history, so that we don't buy into white supremacy and perpetuate colonial mythologies and racist stereotypes.

Perhaps in terms of terrorist attacks and sort of the coverage that I was looking at in *Remembering Air India*, I would say the need for a more diverse press room, so that diverse stories are told, and told not just from the perspective where Asian Canadians or racialized minorities are always victims whose plight is being depicted, but including stories of activism, of advocacy, of triumphs, of survival—those kinds of stories, too. And for that, you need a diverse press room.

I would also say, perhaps, resource- and knowledge-sharing among different racialized communities and groups so they can share their experiences of anger and grief, learn from each other, as well as engage the wider public in calls for solidarity and alliance. So, I think there are so many different things we can do to bring about changes in the structure. There's a lot of work to be done.

MCKAY: I thought some of your most striking evidence was drawn from some Angus Reid polls, which showed that majorities of Asian Canadians are changing their daily work patterns so they steer clear of racism; over 60 percent reported having experienced racist comments. Some have been spat upon. Have you experienced any manifestations yourself?

CHAKRABORTY: Well, I'm privileged by class. I'm privileged by education. I'm privileged by religion. I'm privileged by heterosexuality. So, I'm protected in many, many ways, right, and I have had the privilege of working from home throughout the pandemic. Not the same for, say, small businesses that had to close their doors, or cashiers in retail businesses, et cetera.

So, my experiences are not the same. I am protected, but at the same time, my experience of racism is different because my research and public advocacy (over more than a decade) has been on the 1985 Air India bombing. I've written lots of op-ed pieces, public-facing works critiquing Canadian multiculturalism and all of that. So, I get my share of hate mail, saying that I should be the "grateful immigrant." I'm not the grateful immigrant I am expected to be. I get my share of that. And then, of course, in the classroom, I teach materials that are bringing up hazy, inconvenient histories (both for my Canadian-born students but also for South Asian students) who grow up with particular versions of the past. So, my takes on the Partition of British India or the Air India tragedy often do not match up to the stories told to them within their families or their communities. And at those moments, of course, my gender, my age, my brown skin produce difficult encounters.

MCKAY: I think one of the major themes that we're seeing from this Covid-19 pandemic has been the intersection of class and race. The "Color of Coronavirus" project in the US keeps coming up with these startling statistics of how many more Black Americans are contracting the disease and are dying of it. Huge numbers of them don't have health insurance. Basically, Black and Latinx Americans are three times as likely as their white neighbours to become infected and nearly twice as likely to die from the virus.

There are very similar data coming out of the United Kingdom. In Toronto, racialized residents accounted for 83 percent of cases, although making up just 52 percent of the population.[8] A major theme—and you've already alluded to it, but maybe you could say a little bit more—is just the power of class and the job market, one so structured that many of the highest-risk occupations (like PSWs, meatpackers, migrant agricultural workers) are made up of racialized minorities. So, I was wondering, as your study of race and Covid-19 goes forward, how much importance will you yourself assign to class as well as race as an element in the subaltern experience of the pandemic?

CHAKRABORTY: That's a great question. I don't think we can talk about the differentiated effects of the pandemic without talking about class or even gender. The pandemic has unfolded differently for lower-class, racialized, or minoritized communities. Class and race are enmeshed in the context of the global pandemic. So, I don't think we can talk of one without the other. It's not just the "racial subject" but "classed, racial subjects" who are bearing the burden of the global pandemic.

MCKAY: So much of scholarship buried class as a category of analysis sometime in the 1980s. To be interested in labour was no longer fashionable. That's likely going to change after this pandemic.

CHAKRABORTY: I hope so. We are designating particular groups of people as essential workers, but those essential workers are the ones who are in precarious employment, bearing not just the burden of contracting the virus but also discrimination, racism, no sick benefits, all of it. The transportation industry, manufacturing industry, as you said meatpackers, Mexican immigrants who are doing much of the work in Niagara, all of those are "essential." So, I hope so, because I don't think you can talk about just race because that would not give you a full understanding of the context unless we bring in class.

MCKAY: My last question. You've pondered deeply the politics of commemoration and really focused especially on the public memory in

Canada of Air India Flight 182 in 1985, which blew up with 329 people on board and yet came to be sidelined in Canada, never really considered a "Canadian event." It never got to be considered a Canadian disaster. It was always something happening to "others."

I sense a kind of parallel—not a precise one—between that tragedy and the tragedies that we've been experiencing this year. Such events are intrinsically global. They transcend the boundaries of the nation-state. Yet, so much of the apparatus of public history and commemoration remains firmly in the hands of public nation-boosters (we might say) who have atavistic (often very atavistic) ideas about race and belonging. Have you ever seen so many references to "Churchill, our great hero," never pondering his ideas about race and belonging? He's just, unqualifiedly, "our" hero. They're trying to drum up a nationalist feeling around the pandemic.

So, I wonder if you have considered how Covid-19 could be appropriately commemorated? Must these commemorations be inevitably bound up with the complexes of myths and symbols particular to particular nations, or can we imagine a transnational form of commemoration around Covid-19?

CHAKRABORTY: Even at the level of the Air India tragedy: yes, it's a national tragedy, but it is also a transnational tragedy because the bombs on the Air India plane were put in in Canada, but the plane blew up in Irish airspace. So, there is an Irish memorial and Irish investment in the tragedy. Some of the Air India family members who were Canadians just could not live in Canada anymore after they had lost their entire family. Many have gone back to India. So, it's a Canadian tragedy; it's also an Indian tragedy; and it's also an Irish tragedy. And on that plane there were also other people; there were some British, some German, et cetera. So, it is a national tragedy, but also a global tragedy.

And I think the same could and should apply to this pandemic. This is a global pandemic. We can see similar kinds of treatments of minorities across North America and beyond. And I've been deeply interested in questions of public memory and cultural history. What gets scaled up to the level of the national or the global, and what always stays at the level of the local?

With the global pandemic, I think the losses are multifaceted. Many have died quietly, many have been grieving in isolation, many families have not been able to perform last rites and rituals that provide solace to the families, many have not been able to see family members who died in another city or died in another country. It will be important to remember those losses—all those who died without an appropriate funeral or memorial service and their families and friends.

But there have been other kinds of losses too. Losses of jobs, losses of employment, housing, and the loss of national belonging (if you think of the anti-Asian racism that we are talking about and the effects it has on mental health: the racial grief of nonbelonging, feeling nonsecure in your citizenship.) Those are losses too—and deep losses. They are not just bound within the family but spill over into communities and children and transgenerational memories. So, the losses are multiple, I think. It is a public health crisis that has demonstrated the inequities in our societies, and we have to acknowledge all these different kinds of losses if we are going to learn from this critical movement of history. There cannot be one way to commemorate this because there are shared losses, but some losses are also very particular.

MCKAY: One optimistic reading of the crisis we've gone through is: maybe it's been a harsh lesson in global citizenship. We have to acknowledge the humanity we share with people all around the planet because national boundaries don't make the same sense they used to make, even forty years ago.

CHAKRABORTY: I keep saying that if there is one thing Covid-19 has taught us, or perhaps should teach us, it's how interdependent we are. I can be well if my neighbour is well. I can be well if the person I'm sharing public transit with is well. I can be well if the person I'm working in the office with and who shares the cubicle with me is well. Interdependence has become so critical. A better understanding of our interdependence and our shared coexistence—perhaps that could be a lesson.

QUESTION FROM THE AUDIENCE: Vaccine nationalism is so intense. Could you comment on that?

CHAKRABORTY: I am thinking of India, where there's not enough vaccines. I have close friends that I have lost as a result of Covid-19 because there were not enough beds, not enough ventilators. And they were living in the capital city, Delhi! I don't think there will be a willingness to share vaccines until countries have made sure their own populations have been vaccinated—even though, until everybody's globally vaccinated, we are not safe.

MCKAY: It reminds me that not only is class coming back into the analysis, but so is imperialism. So much of what happened in India was reminiscent of the imposed famines by the imperial power of the past century.

CHAKRABORTY: Also misgovernance. We can't just blame imperialism. There's been intense misgovernance by the Indian government. Complete mismanagement.

QUESTION FROM THE AUDIENCE: You made a few comments earlier in your talk about needing to modify our teaching. We have a lot of international students. In introductory history classes, we have lecture halls full of two hundred students, and you're hoping to get students to interact with each other, or even in their tutorials with thirty students. But, they're often all going off in their particular separate cultural groups. Do you have any thoughts or recommendations on how we as educators in the classroom can combat that? So that we're actively working not to promote those kinds of divisions?

CHAKRABORTY: Unless the structures on the outside change, can you as a TA in one classroom effect that change? One way of doing that might be to look at what kind of materials we are using in the course. Can we have a conversation say, for example, between Black Lives Matter and anti-Asian racism? If we can build in those conversations throughout the course, so that we're not replicating those divisions we see in the classroom, and if we can bring out those intersections, then the students might also see those intersections. I might not have racial kinship with somebody, but I might have class kinship. Or I might have the same kind of immigration history or educational interests. If you see a lot of people hanging out together, maybe open up opportunities for those students to share so they see themselves as knowledge creators and not just knowledge recipients. That might be a way to also create cross-cultural conversations.

QUESTION FROM THE AUDIENCE: Even in the darkest of times I've seen the development of this truly impressive, amazing interconnected analysis [in Hamilton], coming mostly from youth activists. Health justice is houselessness justice, is disability justice, is defund-the-police, is Palestine, is land-back. Activists are seeing connections. I've seen it in this city. The moment of despair—and the anger that produces change. Your thoughts?

CHAKRABORTY: I am a pessimist who's also an optimist. I take a lot of lessons from Roger Simon, the political scholar who was doing this amazing work on historical memory and trauma. And he kept holding on to hope—hope of the possibility of justice through public education. I see the classroom as a site of radical possibility. There's a lot to be hopeful about. There are seedlings there that will mature into big trees that will shade themselves, and us.

MCKAY: I think we're in a moment of deep crisis in which so many of our presuppositions and assumptions about the world around us have been shaken. And many conventional ideological grooves have been upset. What emerges from that is going to be decisive in the next years. Will people retreat back to their quest for normality? Do they really want to go back to the way the world was? Or, can they retain insights into the deep structures of racism, the deep structures of class? Can they retain those insights? This is what Gramsci called an organic crisis of the ruling order, a tremendous moment of opportunity, and of danger.

CHAKRABORTY: We seem to be moving from crisis to crisis. It's overwhelming. We seem to be constantly moving from grief to grief to grief. It's a crisis in so many different ways. The question also is: Is the past the past? For some, the past resides in textbooks, and monuments, and museums. But, what if the past is your daily present? The long history of racism, the long history of classism, the long history of sexism all need to be grappled with, as disturbing and inconvenient as they might be. Unless you acknowledge those histories, and recognize them, I don't know how we can move beyond them.

AN INTERVIEW WITH
MERLIN CHOWKWANYUN
19 MAY 2022

Merlin Chowkwanyun is the Donald H. Gemson Assistant Professor in Sociomedical Sciences at Columbia University, New York. Dr. Chowkwanyun has just brought out a book, *All Health Politics is Local: Community Battles for Medical Care and Environmental Health*, with University of North Carolina Press. In a close examination of health politics in New York City, Central Appalachia, Los Angeles, and Cleveland in the 1960s and '70s, Dr. Chowkwanyun argues that bird's-eye views of health politics in the US, often reliant on "large aggregate, nationally representative data sets," tend to lose sight of fundamentally important local phenomena and edit out all the local activists and local experiences that "challenged the paradigms of more powerful actors working on the national level."[1] Dr. Chowkwanyun is currently at work on another book about political unrest at medical schools and neighbourhood health activism. He was also the principal investigator on a research grant for ToxicDocs, where one can find millions of pages from once-secret documents pertaining to industrial toxins.

With Adolph L. Reed, Jr., he recently published an article in the *New England Journal of Medicine* cautioning against the subtle re-emergence of myths of racial biology, racial stereotypes, and the stigmatizing of entire territories in seemingly objective statistics that help to frame Covid-19 as "largely a problem of minorities."[2]

MCKAY: I'd first like to start out with the meta-question about the methodological and disciplinary challenges that relate to your stance as a historian of public health. In 2011, you brought out a really interesting paper on the "Strange Disappearance of History from Racial Health Disparities Research"—about how history has completely dropped out of many public health discussions. Historians had played a central role in discussions of public health in previous times; nowadays they generally do not. Here you noted that, although the field of racial disparities research in public health is booming, "what is missing . . . is a deeper understanding of how and why these social determinants of racial health matter so much, the long-term *process* through which they came into being, and how they might have been avoided." [3]

To put this less diplomatically: It seems to me a lot of contemporary discussion of the politics of public health drowns the reader in wave upon wave of descriptive statistics that don't really give us any idea of the context. Citing Robert Aronowitz, you suggest that many mainstream investigations privilege the quantifiable and the "properties of the free-standing individual" in order to squeeze data into preestablished equations, thereby neglecting fundamental forces and processes that can better be grasped holistically and historically.[4]

So, here's a three-part question. (1) In the ten-plus years since you published this critique, have you noticed anything shifting in what we might call this pattern of simplistic positivism? (2) Are there indications that the chasm between critical historical intelligence and model-driven medical science is closing? (3) Do you find some sympathetic audiences for your call for the recognition of history as a "fundamental policy science"?

CHOWKWANYUN: That's an excellent set of related questions. In broad general terms, I don't think much has changed. So, my critique, I think, still stands.

And I'm not surprised by that. Anybody who has studied organizational inertia and how science is produced knows that those big dominant funding agencies, the ones that give out the most influential kinds of grants that really shape research agendas and how universities operate—they're very, very, very slow to change (*impervious* to change, sometimes). They are often dominated by people who are embedded in the same tight social networks and who often think the same way. So, it's not surprising to me that, even if I do see the occasional currents suggesting we have to be more expansive about how we think about this, it's very slow for the funding agencies themselves, who are some of the most important stakeholders, to change. Often, studies have to be proposed to them in a kind of "A is on this side and B is on that side" format—with the independent and dependent variables all clearly demarcated in the framework.

I'll give you an example. Lead poisoning continues to be a scourge in the United States in some communities (and I assume in Canada as well). You are much more likely to be funded if you can count the number of people who have been exposed to lead poisoning and the adverse health effects that they've experienced. That's an important thing to continue cataloguing, of course—I'm not saying it is not—but, ultimately, we are dealing with what some would refer to as "downstream" effects. And I think what was often missing in that research (despite a lot of rhetoric saying we need more of this) is the "upstream." How did the lead get there in the first place? And why is it *still* there—even though remediation, in the grand scheme of things, is not that expensive an undertaking relative to other things we spend lots of money on?

So, I think that kind of outcomes framework, whether it's qualitative or quantitative, is still there, but I do see some signs of change. There are people who don't derive their funding from the big science world—medical anthropologists, sociologists, historians like myself. They are advancing some really provocative questions on much lower budgets. But the thing that worries me is, essentially, we have two kind of discourses going on. There's the one that's produced by those more traditional quantitative researchers. And then there's the scholarship produced by those who study institutions, legal regimes, historical processes, and so forth.

I do sense some restlessness with just presenting the same general story over and over again about racial health disparities and not much beyond that. I especially see it with students of colour. They say a lot of this research is actually bothersome to them because the only depiction that comes forth from it is that they're a bunch of damaged people. That's all that's presented to them. They actually want a story that tells them more about the kinds of power dynamics and political arrangements that create this damage—not just a damage story itself. So, I do see a lot of energy from the student perspective. But, you know, it's hard for those old paradigms to change.

Here's an example of how some of the funding agencies, especially after the tumultuous events of the past few years, are operating. They signal, "OK, we have to expand our agenda, a little bit." It's also an example, at the same time, that shows that that instinct has some limits. After the summer of 2020, the National Institutes of Health

(NIH) issued a call for proposals for research on "structural racism" and health. Now, whatever you think about this term, I think that was pretty eye-opening to a lot of people. NIH (at least in the United States) tends to stay away from terms that have a sort of normative critique embedded in them. And "structural racism" is, I think, such a term. Some people were heartened that the NIH was interested in studying things in this way, was interested in structures and institutions.

Still, the NIH listed the sorts of projects that are *not* eligible in bullet-point form. Here's one of the bullet points: projects that are exclusively qualitative or that only use individual-level data. The second I could understand, but to just dismiss exclusively qualitative projects just because of the data type—that seems very, very questionable to me. And a second bullet point really stuck out for me: "projects that do not examine the impact of structural racism and disparities on health-related *outcomes*." There's that obsession with, or fixation on, outcomes. They're important, but they're not the only thing you can study.

The arc of how society affects health is a long one. Measuring outcomes is an important part of it. The stuff that gets you to the outcome is also important. I think this is an example of how I do see signs of change—but institutional structures are very tough. Still, I see, from the younger generations of students, a lot of foment, and I'm very optimistic about that.

MCKAY: It's really interesting you're starting to see push-back from students of colour against some of this portrayal of them as damaged people living in damaged communities. My second question relates to that theme. In 2012, with Adolph Reed, you published "Race, Class, Crisis: The Discourse of Racial Disparity and its Analytical Discontents." This is a very strongly-worded piece. Here you indict as "interpretive pathologies" many analyses of disparity made in the wake of the 2008 financial crisis, arising from a "distinctive, *pro forma* narrative structure": "Quantitative data, usually culled from large aggregate data sets, [are] parsed to generate accounts of the many facets of apparent disparity along racial lines with respect to barometers of inequality such as wealth, income and economic security, incarceration, employment, access to medical care, and health and educational outcomes." You add,

Among those pathologies are a schematic juxtaposition of race and class that frequently devolves into unproductive either-or debates; the dilution of class into a cultural and behavioural category or a static (usually quantitative) index of economic attainment that fails to capture power relations; sweeping characterizations of white Americans' racial animus and collective psyche; ahistorical declarations that posit a long and unbroken arc of American racism and that sidestep careful dissection of how racism and, for that matter, race have evolved and transformed; and a tendency to shoehorn the United States' racial history into a rhetorically powerful but analytically crude story of "two societies," monolithic and monochromatic. [5]

Along with such scholars as Adolph Reed, Touré Reed, Barbara Fields, Karen Fields, Michele Mitchell, Kenneth Warren, and Joanna Wuest, you raise profound questions about how one ought to navigate a very complicated situation. In our time, the scientific reputation of "race" as a useful category of biological analysis has all but collapsed. Yet, in much of the everyday world, race has never been more pervasively invoked. The paradox is that even though the scientific credibility of race as a concept has eroded, in much of the world race has never been more prominent as a category of analysis. You hear of it every day.

For the Fields, for instance, placing so much weight on race as a master-category can be likened to stubbornly insisting that crop failures are the result of spells cast by witches—a holdover from the Victorian "race science" that offered so much ideological cover to Jim Crow in your country and equivalent policies with respect to Indigenous peoples in ours. For Wuest, "even when older schemes of racial classification are seen as outdated and false, the proposed solutions wind up retaining the logic of racial aggregation."[6] Do you see your work as a contribution to this school?

CHOWKWANYUN: Generally, yes. I use the qualifier "generally" because I'm always cautious about terms like "schools." You and I know, as historians, that there are intellectual schools that are very tightly bound, and they try to hold the line. The head of the school tries to get the mentees to propound a given thesis. In this case, I don't think there's a line or anything. In fact, among all those people that you mentioned, many of whom are colleagues, teachers, friends of mine, there are probably some subtle differences among us (and maybe some not-so-subtle differences). To the extent we have something in common, it's the conviction that we should not make race and racism static, reified categories that are timeless and contextless and always the same, no matter where you are on earth and what time period you're in.

So, unlike a lot of academics, including some historians, I'm pretty averse to *any* kind of generalized statement about how race works and how important racism is or isn't to larger patterns of inequality. Those are empirical questions, ultimately, to be investigated. And the answer to that investigation varies a lot just depending on the phenomenon you're looking at—whether it's health or housing or something contextual, such as the time and the place you're in.

You know, our students use social media a lot (for better or worse) and not just to share pictures of themselves at concerts or whatever, but, increasingly, to learn about politics. One of the things I've never really liked about this (although I can see some benefits to it) is the diffusion of aphoristic statements on little squares. So, you know, one statement might be: "Racism is the fundamental force United States has been built on and always will be built on." It's true enough but also vague and general enough that it doesn't really actually explain things like what vectors the racism is running through, where it came from, if it ever changes, how it cuts across other axes of inequality, and so on.

I generally just don't like statements like that. Even if they seem self-evident and true (at least initially), I'd rather be very contextually specific. I think that's what probably unites those scholars you mentioned.

Race is part of a genus of a larger set of ascriptive categories and labels that people have fixed to each other. In the United States, that label happens to correlate very closely with phenotypical characteristics. In other societies, it might correlate with language, religion, the town or village you grew up in, tribal affiliations, whatever. So, I view it as an item on the menu of many different categories. The interesting puzzle is to figure out why some items on the menu seem to be more salient in some societies or in some eras than in others.

There's a book that actually influenced me a lot on this, Charles Tilly's *Durable Inequality*.[7] He was trying to figure out why inequality forms and why it seems to really stick. And what are the mechanisms that make it so that people fall on one side or the other in a society? Now he *could* have written this book and focused it on just race alone, but he intentionally doesn't do that. He instead uses a huge litany of examples from around the world and different time periods. The one thing in common with all of these examples, heterogeneous as they are, is that, basically, in societies, lines (i.e., categories) form. And you're either on one side of the line or the other. It can be a gender line, a racial line, a professional/nonprofessional line ("You're in this tribe, not that tribe," et cetera). He calls this process "categorical inequality." That's always how I prefer to think about racial inequality, ultimately: a manifestation of a broader process underneath called categorical inequality. The onus is on us to figure out exactly why that version of categorical inequality arose.

MCKAY: You write that, "at its most simplistic," a bird's-eye quantitative analysis of race can leave the reader with

> figure after figure illustrating disparity and not much else, or only slightly better, a series of plausible just-so stories that attempt to fill in the explanatory black holes post hoc. Simplistic use of race as the key analytic category . . . suggests intra-racial class uniformity and encourages thinking in monochromatic dyads. Much of the problem rests with the almost exclusive reliance on quantitative data sets, which usually limits researchers to pre-defined administrative and demographic variables while ignoring consideration of forces not captured by that data.

Further, you argue, there can be a neoliberal agenda active in such formulations, as signalled by such expressions as "equal opportunity" or "American Dream" or "level playing field":

> These red flags confirm that the agenda at work here stems from a concern to create competitive individual minority agents who might stand a better fighting chance in the neoliberal rat race rather than a

positive alternative vision of a society that eliminates the need to fight constantly against disruptive market whims in the first place.

And you are emphatically critical of the "constantly expanding panoply of neologisms—'institutional racism,' 'systemic racism,' 'structural racism,' 'colour-blind racism,' 'post-racial racism,' et cetera—intended to graft more complex social dynamics onto a simplistic and frequently psychologistic racism/anti-racism political ontology."[8] Here are some more phrases from this piece: "analytical sloth," a "stifling, ready-made narrative," "superficial," "self-righteous," "lazy-minded." One might fairly say, your article does not want for fighting words. Some will fight back, saying your current of antiracist thought, if we agree it *is* a coherent current, disregards the grievous injuries of racism. Does it?

CHOWKWANYUN: I don't think it does. In fact, quite frankly, I think it does the opposite. I'll explain why.

Sometimes, criticisms of that sort are based on the point that we just don't put up in neon lights a very general polemical slogan about how racism explains *X* and *Y*: *X* and *Y* are "racist outcomes" explainable with reference to "racism." That's kind of tautological. I think you have to drill a little deeper than that. What we were trying to do in that article is take a term like "race," often used as a kind of static variable, and disaggregate it down to its component parts. And, most important, to get to the processes underlying it, whether those processes are tied to the labour market, the housing market, finance, land use, or whatever else. We want to know what chain of institutions and laws and public policies and collective actions resulted in that.

Some writers criticize prior generations of researchers for not labelling this racism. There are a number of papers that have come out in health policy journals in the past couple years saying that racism needs to be a word that is explicitly used in these articles. For me, I actually find this not particularly satisfying and a little beside the point, because declaring those outcomes "racism" doesn't actually elucidate the various specific forces through which that racism operates and of which it is a by-product. So, I would argue for placing more emphasis on the *processes* that constitute what you call racism. I think that is the opposite of disregarding it. It's actually trying to probe more concretely what it is, beyond just using what is actually a pretty elastic construct of racism.

For a similar reason, I'm also a little averse to constructions like "structural racism," which has seen an uptick in social science and health literature. This is actually an interesting term. It's traceable to the late 1960s, when more and more activists and academics started realizing that racism often (not always, but often) was more than just the psychological hearts-and-minds problem of individual prejudice. Even if you changed many hearts and minds, why are racially disparate outcomes still intact? The answer was that many institutions or societal structures, sometimes even without nefarious people in them, could still perpetuate aggregate outcomes that were racially disparate.

That's a very interesting idea. And I think that is indeed how a lot of society works to produce those kinds of outcomes. But, I also think not all racism works that way. Sometimes it *is* very much just the result of prejudicial beliefs or, more commonly, the consequence of many individuals collectively holding those prejudicial beliefs and then acting on them. I think the task for us as researchers is to figure out exactly what flavour of racism we are dealing with. But having that "structural" adjective in front of it nudges you in that one direction. You don't want to actually take your constructs and stuff your theses into them. The constructs are supposed to serve (in my view) as heuristics that help guide the inquiry—not answer the inquiry before it starts.

MCKAY: Does your emphasis on the local case study and the problem-solving engaged in by elites as they wrestle with public health questions preclude looking at global, transnational patterns? For some scholars—here one thinks of Loïc Wacquant—one of the major deficiencies of much US work on race and racialization is that it narrows our understanding of the phenomenon, transforming the outlying American case, with its "one-blood rule," into the measure of all of humanity, in a perverse form of American exceptionalism.[9]

A less parochial approach is one that suggests, for example, the analytical possibilities offered by comparisons of various kinds of racism in various places. Some are drawn to the seemingly very different, yet also oddly comparable, stories of US racism, with its foundations in chattel slavery and Jim Crow, and the caste systems of India, based on age-old Hindu cosmologies—yet strikingly similar in its consequences for subalterns, at least as perceived by such organic intellectuals as Martin Luther King. Do you consider this "transnational turn" a promising one for students of racism?

CHOWKWANYUN: I'm not a transnational scholar. I'm very much bound, for better or worse, to a nation-state framework. I'm very humbled, often, reading this very ambitious transnational scholarship. My general inclination is to say, absolutely. But, you know, I guess the qualifier would be, I don't fetishize scale for its own sake. Transnational history was a very hot thing when I was starting graduate school in 2005. It's since become a little less hot. You can do transnational history really well; you can also do it really sloppily and badly. For example, taking categories of analysis, particularly around race in the United States, and imposing them elsewhere. You can also do it from a brass tacks perspective—really superficial stuff with surface-level landings in a lot of places.

But, that said, from the best of that work, I have learned a tremendous amount. The Latin American work offers us so many counterexamples to the "one drop-ism" of the United States. Again, it shows you that race in many cases is a lot more fungible and anchored fundamentally in particular places with unique histories. You get that with well-conducted transnational analyses.

I've also been interested in the circulation of racial ideas. One of the insights from comparative analysis is that, actually, the race idea in the US looks nothing like other categorical regimes in some other place or nation-state. That's one big insight from that comparative work. Yet, that stands in some tension with other transnational work that looks at the circulation of racial ideas. I am very interested to see whether or not the American idea of race, which seems so exceptional and parochial in many ways, was in fact transported and exported to many other places.

Now, my case for the local is actually grounded a lot more in the field of public health. Among public health researchers, research has been very top-down. It's still dominated by the language of statistical aggregation. It seems somewhat disconnected to me from the block level, the neighbourhood level—which, wherever you are in the world, is where, ultimately, public health policy is implemented and enacted. So, I wanted to restore that.

The major political project of our time, right now, is to speak to people on the ground in the context of their real day-to-day lives while also realizing that their real day-to-day lives, even if they don't necessarily see them this way, are very much structured by huge processes at all levels of society. I'm not saying that the local is the only optic we should all be switching to. Keep your eye on every single level.

MCKAY: And the paradox surely in the American case is that some people even dispute whether there *is* a national public health system. There's so many local actors and disputing jurisdictions, so much chaos and confusion. Yet, at the same time, we're given all these statistics that make the pandemic appear very uniform and understandable from a bird's-eye view of the process—with elegant looking waves and endless pseudoscientific measurements of them. There is a kind of illusion to it all. Through the pandemic, one almost had the sense that "someone is in charge"—if not the Centers for Disease Control, then somebody else behind the Wizard of Oz's curtain. But, I'm not sure there was anybody behind the curtain.

CHOWKWANYUN: That's something that's particularly difficult, I think, with the United States versus some of the other OECD nations or nations in general. Our governance system is federated, especially, in sharp contrast to countries in which there's a more centralized function.

You're absolutely right that a kind of fracturing is built into the system. It's been especially difficult, over the past two years, not to have that kind of central coordinating system.

MCKAY: Turning now to the pandemic, your piece with Adolph Reed in the *New England Journal of Medicine* argues that, although disparity data can be useful, "Disparity figures without explanatory context can perpetuate harmful myths and understandings that actually undermine the goal of eliminating health inequities."[10] Can you offer examples of this pattern from the Covid-19 years?

CHOWKWANYUN: I have a couple. One is something people are more familiar with and one is maybe something people are a little less familiar with.

We're all familiar with data visualizations of curves and models and things like that. Another one of those things is, of course, the "dashboard." Every municipality and state has a dashboard. The country at large has a dashboard. And on this dashboard you can usually disaggregate the figures by race and you can see the rate at which white people versus nonwhite people got Covid-19 or died from Covid-19. *The Atlantic* magazine also had what I thought was a pretty admirable project called the "Covid Tracking Project."[11] It was an attempt to scrape all the data sets from a bunch of different municipalities and levels of government together in one convenient place. But they also had something that I thought was a little less admirable: the "Covid Racial Data Tracker," which lets you take those data and disaggregate them by racial demographic variables.

What's the problem with doing that? If I show you those racial charts, without any kind of explanatory context and facts next to them, people can just start making up "just-so stories" to explain them. Often there is no evidentiary basis to those stories. They also often stigmatize the various populations that these graphs show are on the short end of the stick.

I know you had said earlier that the biological notion of race is discredited. More so in academia, less so with the person on the street. If I go to the person on the street and ask, "What makes me Asian?" I think we would find many people would just start spouting off stuff like blood and genes and stuff like that. "You've got Asian genes" or "You've got Chinese blood" or whatever. It's very ingrained at the folk level, if not at the academic level. So, people tend to pivot when they see these figures without any context and imagine, "Oh, there must be something just intrinsically, biologically defective about those people that makes them weaker and unable to fight off Covid." And a second default narrative is also very powerful. It's the notion that there's a racially specific culture, and that there are certain populations that just don't follow rules and hygiene practices. So, the reason they have Covid-19 more is because they haven't been following public health directives, and so on and so forth. Again, it often takes the form of a "just-so story."

Lots of numbers, without any context for them. I think they can be dangerous. I've seen a lot of that during Covid.

Another, more obscure example of how these narrow post hoc narratives can often substitute for explanation: In the first year of the pandemic, when Black Americans were experiencing higher rates of Covid, at large, there was this strange narrative going around about Vitamin D. The claim was that Black Americans, because of complexion, don't have enough Vitamin D. Therefore, this is the reason their immune systems can't fend off Covid. Again, there are all kinds of holes in this analysis, including not a lot of unambiguous evidence about why Vitamin D was related to Covid to begin with. In these kinds of narratives, you just put out stuff without actually giving some explanatory context to them.

MCKAY: What kind of response did your *New England Journal of Medicine* article generate?

CHOWKWANYUN: We have been surprised. My strong sense is that people have been frustrated with just seeing a bunch of tables that tell us sad (sometimes depressing, sometimes outrageous) stories and then leave them hanging with nothing more. Not only is that analytically unsatisfactory, but it's actually potentially dangerous. Our article seemed to resonate. Both Reed and I have been giving a number of presentations about this paper, including to medical students and residents.

It hit in some unexpected ways. One of the things I always encourage historians who want to see more history in the public health arena to do is to infiltrate those specialized publications. We could have presented this critique in some science and technology studies journal but far fewer people would have read it. Putting it in a venue like the *New England Journal of Medicine* means a more challenging audience, in many ways—and a more skeptical audience, but it is ultimately more consequential.

MCKAY: With respect to Covid-19, there were all these attempts to say that elevated Black levels in the US were related to nonworkplace-related customs, such as funerals, weddings, church services. There was far less attention to the workplace conditions that were, in all likelihood and in most places, of far more causal significance.

CHOWKWANYUN: In our article, we suggested a variety of explanatory contexts, but the one we didn't stress was occupation. I have no idea why, in retrospect. We didn't do that, and that's still what I think is really missing from this conversation about Covid and inequality: the workplace. The labour movement, and interest in labour, especially in the public health world, has really declined in the past twenty or thirty years. It's actually been hard to find a lot of scholarship on occupation and Covid risk, even though I believe it was the most important factor other than age.

MCKAY: Some people might say, given how much the race talk has been abused throughout the Covid-19 period, wouldn't it be a good idea to abandon the term "race" altogether? It's become such a loaded, complicated, and in many ways toxic term, used, often in the most damaging ways, to oppress people. Might it not be a good idea, as I think the Fields argue in *Racecraft*,[12] to just set this politically-charged, damaging word aside? Yet, remembering an earlier point in our conversation, "race" may have collapsed as a scientific category for much of biology, but it still seems to be going strong in public discourse. By attaching ourselves to this old term, do we not, in a sense, elevate it? Do you see a way out of this trap?

CHOWKWANYUN: If we embargo the term (or make it so that every time you use it, you have to have like a long qualifier about how it's just the label for a construct or an idea people invoke for various purposes), your writing starts to just get kind of cumbersome. On a practical level, we're probably stuck with it.

But, I do think we can enhance the ways we use it. One way is to, again, teach people that race is a label, one of many different labels. Sometimes it's the most salient label in society and the most consequential. Other times, it may not be. And at other times, it may work in tandem with other kinds of labels and other kinds of mechanisms for marginalizing, stigmatizing, and separating people. If you understand that race isn't just this static thing but actually a kind of technology that is used and applied to sort people, I think that's the way to go about it. It's definitely a social artifact that's there. One thing to worry about if it's simply dropped is that you play into the hands of people with certain political persuasions who want to make a problem disappear by disappearing the ways we can measure it. That's not what I think should be done at all.

It is a term doing category work. Thinking about it that way has helped me, in some ways, deprovincialize and de-exceptionalize the term and see it as one of the many categories Charles Tilly was talking about. Latin American scholar Mara Loveman also argued for this categorical approach to race.[13] Not race as this kind of exceptional category, even though it often seems that way in the United States—but as one of many categories.

MCKAY: A skepticism of identity politics characterizes many of the works I would associate with your current. In Adolph Reed's words, "identitarians" seem convinced that the basic units of a radical politics "should be groups formed around ascriptive identities that relate to one another on a principle of recognizing and preserving the integrity of their various differences." From this perspective, the lengthy exposés of one's positionality one associates with intersectionality solidifies divisions between people by "reading coherent group perspective unproblematically from common identity" by "giving them an elaborate theoretical foundation."[14] For you, the rigorous exploration of distinct localities in which subalterns wrestle with the legacies of capitalist deindustrialization and pollution offers progressives something much more valuable than predefined and often simplistically dualist notions of racial politics in the US. Where would you align yourself with respect to intersectionality?

CHOWKWANYUN: I have a pretty high bar for concepts in general, and the coinage of new terms, and I'm quite conservative on this. There's a basket of terms and, for the most part, I'm not sure we actually need to be inventing more of them. An issue with intersectionality is that the definition of it has morphed so much, so that you actually don't often know what exactly people are talking about when they invoke it. It refers to everything from having multiple ascriptive identities that reinforce oppression in some people to an approach that refers to the ways everything just kind of operates simultaneously. We have to look at every kind of variable you can think of, not just race, gender but also sexuality, class, et cetera. There's such elasticity to the term that I wonder about how useful it actually is. That said: if one of the key claims of the term is that we should be examining people's life chances and power from as many axes as possible, my answer is absolutely, yes. But I'm not sure the term is really needed to do that. People were doing this before the term arrived.

The original version of intersectionality as it was elaborated was a pretty interesting thought experiment in legal studies examining how antidiscrimination law is supposed to work when you could potentially file an antidiscrimination claim around either racial discrimination or around gender discrimination (because, in American courts, it's often very hard to make the case for both). A very interesting thought experiment. I *have* noticed, though, that in some of the definitions of intersectionality, class is either missing or is minimized. My issue with that approach is that class fundamentally operates in a different way than those ascriptive labels. If intersectionality means to be more holistic, I'd like to see more class analysis in our understanding of categorical differences.

What do I mean by class analysis? Three things, and it's worthwhile describing each of them.

Many of my colleagues, especially in the quantitative social sciences, tend to define class in a way that is most measurable and most operationalizable but perhaps is less analytically fruitful. That's the socioeconomic status (SES) approach. This approach is to measure one's education level or the amount of money someone has either stored or that's coming in a flow as an income. Sometimes, occupational status. So, there's the SES approach, focused on quantitative measures of stratification. I do think that it provides a lot of insight. But, I don't think that is all that class is. A second approach is based on your relationship to the labour market, including not being in the labour market. Are you a boss? A petty owner of a small proprietorship? A worker? A third approach looks at class as a process, particularly a process whereby a number of goods in society, especially essential goods, get commodified. Access to them is determined by ability to pay the price of the commodified good.

I would like to see these three aspects of class enter the racial disparity discussion in the United States. I don't view these as mutually exclusive juxtapositions to race and other kinds of ascriptive difference. I view them as often working in tandem. I find race-versus-class kind of debates, especially in a quantified form, to be incredibly frustrating. I think both of these processes are working at the same time and in different ways. They're not things you should butt against one another.

MCKAY: Can you tell me a bit more about the distinction between ascriptive and other differences?

CHOWKWANYUN: One is ultimately a label that gets put on to you. And then that label generates meanings. And those meanings result in different kinds of life chances and the way people treat you and even policies that dictate that if you've got this label you get this and if you have that label you get that. Whereas classes entail a set of economic processes having again to do with those things that I mentioned—the relationship to the labour market and the commodification of social goods. Often I find people treat class like an "ascriptive" category like race, especially if you just flatten class to "what did you make on your most recent pay cheque?"

If you start from those considerations, you can very quickly get to all kinds of other things like immigration and flows of people around the world and justifications using labels of coercive labour systems—which is how race arose, at least in the US, where it was used to justify bondage and slavery and say: "You've got this label on you. This is why you are an enslaved person."

Sometimes categories are not anchored to the economic system as well. You can get into a kind of "Robo-automatic Marxism" thing whereby you think absolutely every single kind of label is anchored to the capitalist system. Often it is, but sometimes it is not. Perry Anderson, in an interview many years ago, remarked, apropos of Frankfurt School analyses of capitalism and antisemitism: sometimes antisemitism is just antisemitism. Sometimes racial animus is not really anchored in labour and economics, even though we do realize it often has been.

MCKAY: That reminds me of a point you raised earlier, when we were discussing the treatment of the peculiar, outlying concept of race in the US as a generalization about the world. Might not the same point also apply to class? It's far easier to talk about class in other contexts in the world—in some, it's not all that controversial. In France, once speaks quite readily of the bourgeoisie, the petite bourgeoisie, the workers. Obviously, this can come with risks of oversimplification. Yet, generally, people grasp that class is so much more than income and "status" level. In American discussions, though, class is almost always quantified and treated in terms of social status. Sometimes, as in discussions of the opioid epidemic, people treat having an education as a proxy for class.[15] That doesn't seem adequate to me at all.

CHOWKWANYUN: I moonlight as a historian of McCarthyism and have written a few pieces on its legacy, particularly with respect to the American medical system. The scars of McCarthyism are still with us. Even though you had versions of red scares all around the world, I think it was most pronounced in the United States, especially on social science. Different ways of thinking about class, particularly on the left, got sidelined. Social science in the United States became highly quantitative in the 1950s and 1960s. This pattern started to reach its zenith in the Cold War period. There's a reason for that. Of course, there are places where you have the resident "house Marxist" or something like that. But, generally speaking, class analysis is very, very off-limits. I think this is very much traceable to the red scares in the United States.

There's a very interesting book called *The Second Red Scare* by Landon R. Y. Storrs.[16] She identifies a number of people in a number of professional spheres, especially people who worked in government who, after they touched the Red Scare, started to thin out their views and move away from leftist ones. McCarthyism really had a lot of career consequences and chilling effects. I think they're still here, today.

MCKAY: In the wake of the 2008 financial crisis, and now as we grapple with Covid-19, aren't we experiencing a moment when economic structures and social structures are just so glaringly important that those who downplayed both (coming for instance from postmodern or poststructuralist positions, influential since the 1970s, with their characteristic emphasis on the ambiguities of experiences and subjectivities) have been fundamentally challenged? Recalling your point about individualism in the medical literature, it's hard to see how either crisis could be understood without a robust concept of structure. And both are unreadable, I would say, without an understanding of class.

CHOWKWANYUN: I agree. I mean the one thing I would say, from an organizing perspective, is that one has to work with what is presented before them. And so, you know, I understand why that individualistic kind of discourse is appealing to people. It's often your first way of making sense of your life. I think you can hold the two in your head at the same time.

MCKAY: One of the most striking aspects of the pandemic recently in North America was the muted way we recently observed the passing of a significant milestone in the US: a million deaths (far more than that, when you look at the world). When we got to a hundred thousand there was a commotion; five hundred thousand—quite a flutter. A million? Not so much.

For me, it seemed to say a lot about the subaltern, disrespected lives of those who passed away. What would have been unimaginable before the pandemic—the deaths in North America of over a million human beings, many of which might have been prevented by governments less myopically focused on the needs of business and more intent on ensuring the survival of their citizens—was crowded out by other events and stories, as though these million lives have been erased from our memory, much like those lost in the first Great Influenza Epidemic of 1918–20.

We're starting to see the first drafts of history coming out. And isn't it also telling how zealously defenders of a neoliberal order, including so many model-builders and quantifiers, are rushing to bring out accounts of Covid-19 that seek to show they were right all along? Do you sense that, as it passes from memory to history, Covid-19 is going to challenge their seemingly still very buoyant positivism—their utter faith in "the numbers" rather than in the close and rigorous examination of historical processes?

CHOWKWANYUN: That's a terrific question. Which model-builders?

MCKAY: I follow the British debates, and there we find quite a few model-builders defending their models and predictions.[17] Often the tone of the discussion is very defensive: "We were right all along! I didn't cause 50,000 deaths! It's not my fault!" I imagine the first historical takes on Covid-19 around the world will have that super-polemical quality. "Don't blame me! I didn't do it!"

My question is, once this moment passes, will we really be able to remember this event accurately? And within the requisite time frame? Many critical scholars say we're confronting an era in which pandemics have been made far more probable by the ongoing capitalist assault on the planet. We don't have decades to polish our interpretation. But the results of the current and pervasive comic-book-level of discourse can be quite dangerous.

CHOWKWANYUN: Covid-19 has shown how many things in the society are broken. You wonder if people are going to shove the broken pieces under the carpet and pretend they're not there. There are so many things, ranging from the credibility of experts and eggheads to (still) a lack of occupational health protections and quality ventilation for people who are at most risk for Covid.

I've always been curious about which large-scale tragedies society chooses to remember and which it chooses to forget. Why are some genocides remembered and commemorated every year, while there are others nobody knows about? It will be interesting to see which side Covid lands on. When my students ask, "What the heck is the point of studying history?" I recall a powerful quotation from Eric Hobsbawm: "The job of the historian is to remember what society prefers to forget."[18]

Sometimes forgetfulness just happens. Sometimes it's very premeditated and intentional. I do suspect that Covid will come to be characterized as a kind of fluky, exogenous, horrible, acute event. A lot of the things we have seen in the past twenty years that are really social crises are treated that way. For example, the 2008 financial crisis. It did not lead to a fundamental rethinking of how the economy works and how it is regulated, in the way many of us thought it would. Or the BP oil spill in the Gulf of Mexico. Not on the radar of most Americans right now even though it was one of the most catastrophic environmental disasters in recent world history. Or the Coal Ash disaster at that time in Tennessee.[19] It is still causing all kinds of damaging health effects for people who live in that area. But these events are all treated as acute episodes and not as a result of long-standing processes. We need actually to find the underlying processes and not just surface manifestations that we try to treat away.

I am encouraged—and this is sort of a generational thing—by some of the younger epidemiologists and model-builders who are trying to think through ways of doing their work in a much less unidimensional way, that takes into account the influence of social structures on who gets harmed and who doesn't in pandemics like this. There's a brilliant epidemiologist at the University of Michigan named Jon Zelner. He, other authors, and I brought out an article recently (he was definitely in the driver's seat and I was just along for the ride) about the kinds of pandemic modelling of Covid-19 we've all become very familiar with.[20] Our argument was that the metrics from many models are helpful for planning for disease burden, hospital capacity, and to inform nonpharmaceutical interventions, but they have systematically failed to account for the structural factors that lead to socioeconomic, racial, and geographic health disparities.

The various metrics coming from those models, that tell you the average spread in the neighbourhood, that there are more cases today than yesterday, the famous R_0—all the numbers we became very familiar with—can be aggregations that mask the uneven impact of something like Covid. Future models need to try not to mask that aggregation but to make it central. I see a lot of people who are really interested in this. So, I am hopeful on that front.

I do think a younger generation is asking tough questions and challenging paradigms. But, as we both know, paradigms and big science agencies are powerful. They don't like change. Will a huge event like Covid rattle them? We'll see.

MCKAY: I noted that, paradoxically, in the first year of the pandemic, there seemed to be many more people saying, "Everything has to change. We must cross this threshold and enter a new world of future possibilities. We can do things differently." Those voices quietened down over the course of the pandemic. People became less hopeful and more fatigued. These possibilities seem more and more distant. What one might call the "critical utopian energy" of the first year dissipated. Can we somehow retrieve it? Do you think that's possible?

CHOWKWANYUN: I remember something like that with the financial crisis too. The first year, some major changes were proposed, but over time, the changes were fundamentally just around the edges.

I was taken by an article by a historian named Howard Markel in *The Atlantic* recently.[21] He's a historian of epidemics. He made a lot of historians mad with it. But I thought he actually had an interesting point, which is he was not going to use the 1918 flu pandemic anymore to talk about Covid (which is what many historians, including myself, would do). He said the reason he won't is because he actually sees Covid-19 as, in some ways, largely unprecedented in terms of the scale and the people it affects and the deadliness of the virus and how contagious it is and other intrinsic properties associated with it. And he noted one thing that stuck out for me: none of the mitigation measures in the 1918 pandemic (including some of the most aggressive ones) lasted as long as the ones that have been imposed today. I think he was implying there's a human psychology to this, a kind of a frontier.

MCKAY: I think we would both hope Covid-19 leads to some profound challenges to the existing social system. And yet, I can't see who's going to mount those challenges. I just can't see the social force right now that's going to say, "This has to stop. This has to change."

CHOWKWANYUN: It takes time to recover from, you know, these kinds of events. After a recovery period, hopefully, we can all think together how to move from this without sinking into fatalism. That is the worst thing right now.

AN INTERVIEW WITH

SANJAY NEPAL

20 JULY 2022

Sanjay Nepal, who received his PhD from the University of Bern in Switzerland, is the past president of the Canadian Association of Geographers and has taught in Texas and British Columbia. He now teaches at the University of Waterloo. He is the author of four books and 132 papers, mainly focused on tourism in the modern world, with specific reference to Nepal and its environs. *Great Himalaya* (2002) examines the changing dynamics of tourism in that country, and the 2016 collection, *Political Ecology and Tourism*, coedited with Jarkko Saarinen, is highly regarded in the field. Professor Nepal has written extensively on overtourism, the cultural consequences of tourism, and on hopes that the industry can transition from being one of the planet's most conspicuous polluters to something far more sustainable.

MCKAY: Before we get to the impact of Covid-19 on the global tourism industry, can you give me a sense of how you became so fascinated by the study of tourism? My sense of your field, which has grown enormously over the past four decades—there are now more journals, articles, and books than a mere mortal could possibly read—is that it combines people who are in essence committed to developing the industry (the vast majority) with some who assess it far more critically. Throughout your writing, I sense an attempt to strike a realistic balance. The central theme might be that mass tourism will always be with us and the point is to render it environmentally sustainable and socially responsible. Over your long and distinguished career as a tourism scholar, what changes have you seen in this sphere, and are these goals becoming distant dreams, given how fast and how quickly the industry has grown since the 1980s?

NEPAL: My initial exposure to tourism was somewhat limited, in the sense that I was trained as a geographer—my master's thesis was on environmental planning. I looked at community and resource conflicts, particularly in the context of national parks and protected areas. Tourism was part of my PhD, but it was very interdisciplinary, looking at ecological and socioeconomic impacts. But then, in the end, I realized that, no matter how much you synthesize, ultimately much of it comes down to the people planning and managing tourism and whether or not they get those policies right.

To be honest with you, I think many industry leaders, including writers, would claim they are in the *business* of tourism. What that means is that tourism can only survive if it continues, continues to expand, as in any other economic sector. That's what we're seeing today. It is only as a *business* that tourism can thrive.

I am from Kathmandu. Our ancestral home was very close to what is today considered the hub of Kathmandu's tourism centre. Even as a kid growing up, on the dusty streets of Kathmandu, I was exposed to tourism and tourists, early on—when I was ten or eleven years old. Eventually my mother was forced to sell that ancestral home, partly because of issues of drinking water scarcity, and so on. So, I consider myself someone that has been displaced by tourism, or at least by the forces associated with tourism. That has been my introduction to tourism. I think it is fair to say that I look at tourism with a critical lens—acknowledging its positive influences but also its detrimental impacts on people and places.

I came to Canada to do my PhD at Western. I wound up getting my degree in Switzerland. I came to tourism with an academic background in human dimensions of wildlife conservation. And one of the things I realized was that tourism always seemed to be the go-between, linking people and wildlife. I thought: "It might be quite interesting to look at tourism."

Geographers have been in the forefront of tourism studies. In Canada, we have pioneers of tourism studies at Western and Waterloo. In geography, we tend to look at tourism issues from a very critical perspective. As you rightly pointed out, the vast majority of tourism journals are focused on how *do* tourism, how to expand tourism. Sociologists, anthropologists, and geographers tend to look at it with other questions in mind.

We're looking at some 1.5 billion plus tourists in the world in a given year. In my house, I keep a 1956 issue of *National Geographic* magazine, from the time before intercontinental travel became possible for most people. Today, if you think of 1956 in terms of a timeline, that's a very short period considering it took us centuries to get from a primarily agrarian society to a tech-dominated industry. The history of modern tourism, as we know it today, is barely sixty-five years old. In that time, we have seen tremendous growth in the tourism industry. We've also seen its tremendous negatives, in terms of its social, cultural, environmental, and economic impacts.

Tourism provides a great opportunity to look at contemporary societal issues. It's fascinating. It's mind-boggling. If you really want to understand global changes, it is very useful to look at them through the prism of tourism. Social scientists are interested in examining change in a society. Tourism as a global force has the power to accelerate the speed of change in communities around the world. It's fascinating.

MCKAY: A lot of what you're saying seems congruent with the political ecology approach of your earlier work in 2016. Tourism, you argue, warrants taking a much more holistic approach.

NEPAL: That's what's fascinating about it.

MCKAY: My second question relates to the first. In rural and peripheral areas, tourism is often the "industry of last resort," once forestry, mining, agriculture, fishing, et cetera have declined. Your (2008) study of Valemount, British Columbia, shows how one beleaguered mountain community hoped tourism development would boost the local economy.[1] Yet, that community was divided, with many with the longest and closest attachment to it being most skeptical of tourism as a panacea. Critics of the industry might suggest that, however tempting the short-term rewards from construction work and the smaller number of permanent jobs, tourism is a faulty development strategy because it plunges vulnerable communities into dependence on a global marketplace and the fickle tastes of tourists. Nothing in the world of tourism stays the same: attractions come and go, tourist markets fade, and revenues from transnational chains are swiftly repatriated to their home countries. Has tourism really paid off for such communities? Or does it mean vulnerable communities mortgage their futures to developments far beyond their control?

NEPAL: There were these two big resort developers coming into the town of Valemount, a community of fifteen hundred residents just forty-five minutes from Jasper, including a lot of transplants from Western Europe—places like Austria and Switzerland. They're drawn by the beauty of the landscape. It was a great opportunity for me to do that research. I said to the municipal staff: "I want to run a town hall meeting to discuss the pros and cons of resort tourism," and the municipal staff said to me, "Valemount people are a bit passive, you might not get many people to participate. But let's try and see what happens." So, I and some of my students went there and, lo and behold, we have thirty-five people show up at this town hall meeting. It suggested that the people there were really passionate about tourism and tourism-related opportunities, as well as the costs they entail. As you rightly point out, those who had been long-time residents were most skeptical of tourism, this resort development, and the economic spin-offs from that project. They were actually a bit territorial in the sense that some of them were saying, "We used to go on all kinds of hikes and enjoyed the recreational opportunities here. Now, if you have outside tourists come here, that small-town opportunity is not going to be there anymore."

My position at that time was, let's look at the situation of the single-industry towns. Let's look at some of the interior BC mountain towns. Many were single resource towns. Pulp mills were shutting down. The lumber industry was suffering. Gold mines had been shut down in places like Kimberley. They were all transitioning to outdoor recreation amenity tourism and that type of thing.[2]

My paper was really about options. Say the pulp mill, or the mine, shuts down: What do you do next? People are hanging onto whatever they can. They find this place worth hanging onto. In a beautiful, amenity-rich landscape, tourism naturally comes to people's minds. Those in favour of the project at Valemount were fully aware they were not going to get thirty dollars an hour, the rate in the lumber industry at that time (2007–08). You could probably get twelve dollars an hour, if you're lucky. Given the options in front of you, what do you do?

I've mostly worked in remote communities, including in Nepal. Tourism presents itself as an option. If you have a homestead and live in a beautiful landscape, a beautiful area, you could quickly turn that into a homestay, some kind of a tourist accommodation. There's an easy way into the industry for people with limited resources and opportunities.

MCKAY: To quote from your piece on political ecology and tourism: "Despite the long history of environmental degradation associated with tourism development, tourism is viewed as less destructive than other forms of resource extraction. It is argued that the benefits of tourism outweigh its costs, but the true costs have never been given a serious consideration in tourism research."[3] In situations like the one you described in Valemount, it seems like people are presented with just two options: die as a community or adopt tourism. But really, aren't there many more options than those two? And doesn't selecting tourism as the main one foreclose other things you might have done? And can't a community debate the precise form tourism is going to take?

NEPAL: Yes, exactly. The opportunity costs. And the externalities of tourism, its true costs, have not been assessed. Of course, a cynic like me would say that all industries involve externalities. Maybe there are different ways of conducting this business, right? We have never really considered the social, cultural, even environmental costs. Maybe there are different approaches to tourism. Maybe there are some approaches that have worked for remote and smaller communities. It is worth addressing how the tourism industry can consider the costs of doing business and present challenges and opportunities associated with tourism to people seeking to develop it in their community. Perhaps a different (i.e., one that considers the externalities) approach to tourism would is necessary.

MCKAY: Turning now to Nepal, one of the most famous recent photographs of Mount Everest showed a line of tourists near the summit, looking for all the world like frazzled customers at a check-out counter at Costco. "We want our moment of sublimity! We'll even climb past dead trekkers to achieve it!" Your work reveals that, for the Sherpa, Everest—or Sagarmatha—had deep spiritual significance, with the *beyul* (sacred, hidden valley) and its mountains, forests, and lakes inhabited by deities, a meaning that is slowly receding as people become more reliant on tourism and its secular ways.[4] The climbers of Everest are presumably in quest of a sublime experience (as well as bragging rights). Yet their commerce is undercutting other people's quest for a similar spiritual experience.

At least from some perspectives, this is the epitome of colonial arrogance, transforming a sacred landscape into an object of commerce and personal gratification without much consideration of the meanings it had for local people and their culture. In their quest for an escape for modernity, tourists succeed mostly in diffusing it. From my perspective, this is a perfect example of rich tourists killing the very attraction they profess to revere. And what they are establishing at Everest's base camp is a kind of hypermodernity, with all of its current environmental and social challenges. I am reminded of geographer David Harvey's comment: "To the degree that the taste for reckless and senseless over-consumption is curbed, there could be some long-term benefits. Fewer deaths on Mount Everest could be a good thing."[5] Would you agree?

NEPAL: Everest, I always say, is full of contradictions. That was my PhD field site. I offer field courses from Waterloo. I've been to the Everest base camp six times. It's full of contradictions.

Obviously that arrogance is there. And when I go to Everest, compared to the late 1990s, it's much more commercial. The spirit of adventure is not prominent. Tourists are there in pursuit of authenticity and, in the process, they are undermining the very thing they are seeking, which is a great contradiction.

But you also have to keep the local perspective in mind. If you talk to the Sherpa people there, they cannot imagine a future without tourism. "Prior to the advent of Everest tourism," they say, "we were really poor. We were one of the most backward communities in Nepal. And look what we have become!" Some of them have become immensely rich. One of the local representatives even became the Minister of Tourism, of all things.

I read one article in a national daily in Kathmandu in which a different point of view about crowding on Mount Everest was presented. I think it was one of the Sherpa guides from the Everest region who suggested that the photo of three hundred people lining up to climb Mount Everest was just the consequence of the narrowness of the window of opportunity in a short season. And he showed an alternative photo, with one climber from Germany, who climbed in late June (I think) and was the only climber. Then he said: "You'll always publicize the first photo and you don't notice this one." There's some truth to that.

Overall, I personally do not like the direction tourism is moving in Everest. But, having said that, I also like to consider the counterargument, that Everest is also one of the best examples of locally controlled tourism. The Sherpas have been able to determine the type of tourism and the speed of development and change they want to have. The Nepali government has very little to say about Everest tourism, other than determining who gets to climb the mountains and collecting climbing and trekking fees. Local control of tourism has been a success story, even though the success has not been without the costs associated with tourism development. Many of the major players in Everest are very probusiness. If you talk to them, their response will be: "The more, the merrier."

In tourism you often find contradictory experiences. The sacred and the profane at the same time and in the same place. Many of those three hundred tourists climbing Everest are doing it for reasons that are BS, but there are some who will tell you, "I really find Everest to be a deeply spiritual journey for me." Tourism experiences are personal and also time- and context-specific. One of the reasons I was really drawn to the study of tourism is that it confronts us with an intractable problem. Its good side and its bad side are not neatly distinguishable.

MCKAY: Nepal, you write, planned a bumper tourism year in 2020, anticipating perhaps two million tourists, a goal you characterized as "crazy." The prepandemic tourism economy provided jobs but produced many other problems. "Roads that have been haphazardly dug out in the mountains have not only increased the frequency and intensity of landslides, they have simply ruined the aesthetic appeal of the mountains," you write. "Annapurna is no longer a classic trekking destination, its mountains that evoke a sense of adventure have been crisscrossed by hazard-prone and hazard-inducing roads. Khumbu (Everest) has become overly commercial, people trying to cash out tourism as if there is no tomorrow."[6]

Then came the pandemic, plunging the country and the tourism economy into crisis. How is Nepal regarding tourism now? Is it still going to pursue mass tourism with the same almost "crazy" energy? Are Nepalese themselves critical of the environmental damage of the industry, as demonstrated by the renowned garbage dumps littered with debris in Everest's base camps? How are the Nepalese thinking about postpandemic tourism?

NEPAL: Here's the spoiler for you. It's business as usual.

Having said that, a few things did happen in the course of the pandemic. If you look at tourism from the perspective of communities, and you know communities that are trying to gain some footing in the tourism industry, whether it's in the Everest region or in the places that I just returned from, they see tourism as a good thing.

But they are also very clear on what type of tourism they want. They are not thinking of this industrial style of mass tourism. They are not thinking of the tourists who crowd Kathmandu. They are not thinking of tourism as just a business. (You know, there was a time when there was a proposal for a gondola going to the tourist hub in Everest!) There are all kinds of tourism investments being proposed. That's one side of it. It's business as usual.

On the other side, there was an uptick in domestic tourism during the pandemic. People would say: "We didn't realize there are so many domestic tourists. There are many Nepalese who want to explore Nepal in the absence of global tourists." They suddenly realized that there is this untapped market within Nepal. So, many communities started providing services to Nepalese trekkers. I am a bit wary of this growth of domestic tourism, partly because you're basically adding to the mix. You're actually looking at an expansion of tourist numbers.

You have to look at it from both perspectives. People in the remote rural community to which I just travelled look at tourism not as the main economic activity but as a supplemental activity. They might have a few animals and a piece of land and could use cash income. Tourism is part of that mix. And I think if you do that, if you consider tourism as one of the diverse economic strategies, then it might do some good. If you look at tourism as the sole provider of your economic prosperity, then it's not a good way to look at it.

MCKAY: Some people would say the Nepalese case illustrates the problem of gross dependency on tourism. Among the Sherpas, the two-year interruption must have caused acute suffering.

NEPAL: On almost every visit to Nepal, I used to buy handmade woollen carpets in Kathmandu. I told my student, who was with me in Kathmandu this year, that carpets are good souvenirs to bring back home. I wanted to show her the shop in Thamel where I bought the carpets. It turned out the shop was closed. I learned later they had moved elsewhere where the rent was cheaper. It's the pandemic effect. Not only that shop had to relocate to a cheaper place—countless hotels, restaurants, jobs disappeared in the absence of tourists. There was an almost 83 percent downturn in tourist numbers. That was a bit scary. That should offer a big lesson to tourism's advocates. You cannot put all your eggs in one basket.

MCKAY: Yet it seems that's what they're intent on doing, once again.

NEPAL: I'm Nepali. The mindset seems to be, if I understand my country, that as long as Nepal remains beautiful, with its majestic mountains and so on, tourists will always come back. As long as Mount Everest is there, we're not going to be short on tourists. I think this is common thinking among tourism entrepreneurs in Nepal. I sit on the fence. Tourism is good, tourism is bad. OK, how do you maximize the first and minimize the second?

Those involved in the tourism industry don't see it that way. And, I have to say, *Lonely Planet* does not help. *Lonely Planet* came up with a list of top ten countries to visit in 2022. I think Nepal was number eight on their list. The tourism industry in Nepal was euphoric about the *Lonely Planet* ranking.

MCKAY: You write: "Certain areas need to be totally off-limits to tourism development, while some areas should limit developments to maintain as highly attractive high-value tourism destinations. Tourism need not be developed everywhere!"[7] Yet, given tourism's transnational and amorphous character, with a million moving parts, who could rule out areas tourists want to see? If tourism is a human right (a suggestion broached in September 2017 in the *Framework*

Convention on Tourism Ethics from the United Nations World Tourism Organization [UNWTO]),[8] won't any limitation on tourists' freedom, even in the name of the survival of the planet, spark intense resistance?

And *is* tourism such a right? Do we have a human right to be tourists? Do I have a human *right* to climb Mount Everest? Don't we also have the collective *right* to set limits to tourism?

NEPAL: When I wrote that, I was thinking of some remote, pristine places that are still unexplored. There are many places around the world like that, including in Nepal, which I usually write about. These are fragile areas and need to be protected. We don't want tourists there. Having said that, it's really difficult for the government. I'm not a politician. I don't want to work for the government, and I sometimes pity the government bureaucrats because we always gang up on them. "You could have enacted this policy or that policy!" I do think there should be places where tourism development should be prohibited.

With regard to the UNWTO declaration on tourism as a human right, it's a ridiculous statement to make. It would basically mean 7.5 billion tourists on the planet. UNWTO is in the business of expanding tourism as a growth opportunity. That's their bottom line. And—here's the cynic in me—all this talk about climate change and tourism and protecting traditional peoples—I don't want to say they're not genuine. But it's often, to me, like a big greenwash. The bottom line of the tourism industry is profit, and in the main, the way to reap profits is to maximize your numbers of tourists. You maximize your numbers by marketing: "Remote. Pristine. An Exclusive Product." Come to Churchill, Manitoba, and see the polar bears before they're gone.[9] On the one hand, we seem to be saying: "Polar bears are important, let's protect them." At the same time, you're creating a situation likely to further jeopardize that protection.

MCKAY: Your work on the political ecology of tourism suggests the significance of David Harvey's theme of accumulation by dispossession. Isn't that happening all around the world, people speak of "conserving" and "protecting nature"—when often what that entails is dispossessing small producers, disestablishing entire populations from areas in which they had previously flourished, and removing poverty from the tourists' sight-lines (since acute poverty is rarely picturesque). There is a real class dynamic to this phenomenon, is there not?

NEPAL: Isn't it ironic that so many of the world's most beautiful places are also the poorest? Yet, I see tourism as a potential solution—not *the* solution, *one* of the possible solutions—to address issues of poverty, community empowerment, and so on. If you look at Sherpa women, all of a sudden they have been greatly empowered. They have cash. Who are we to say that's not good? We tend to look at these issues as outsiders looking in. Why don't we let them look too? Why don't we let the communities decide how they want to proceed?

Some of the remote communities I studied in Nepal were rich seven hundred years ago. Prior to colonialism, prior to the spread of globalization, there were prosperous communities in places such as Dolpo (where I am currently conducting research). The communities there built magnificent cultural monuments (e.g., Buddhist monasteries) that tourists today can visit and see for themselves. Dolpo might be considered a primitive place from a western perspective, but its rich cultural history also provides a counternarrative to that perspective. Today, perhaps they once again will have the capacity to determine their own future. We need policies that facilitate community empowerment and control, not politicians and government bureaucrats who dictate what kinds of development for whom, how, and when. The tourism industry needs to be cognizant of the historical significance of places and communities that have not only survived but thrived for generations. They need to be mindful of local aspirations and capacities, traditions and sensitivities, and use that to develop and promote a type of tourism that could be a win-win for all.

MCKAY: So much comes down to local control, doesn't it? Yet as your research points out, communities are always divided, with some seeing in tourism a way to achieve their own interests and others far more skeptical. So much of what you're recommending comes down to the rigorous defence of local control. The various parts of the community have to have a considered strategy and stick to it for years—and not be swayed by the people who want the sector to grow and grow and grow at any price.

NEPAL: Right. So much of it comes down to local control. I'll give you an example. I spent thirty-five days on foot in Dolpo with my graduate student during the summer of 2022. We trekked and rode horses to talk to people in remote villages. We even reached some villages that were within four to six hours of the Nepal/Tibet border. They would really welcome economic opportunities. This is a place the Nepalese government in Kathmandu has neglected for decades. While tourism is seen as an opportunity to improve their livelihood and change their lives, local people were also saying: "We want tourists on *our* terms, not on the terms of the government or of the tourists."

MCKAY: You recently coauthored an important piece on overtourism with a focus on France, the US, China, Spain, and Italy. Antagonistic relations between tourists and the toured-upon have been noted since the 1970s, yet of late, the tensions have become explosive, with some even speaking of "tourismphobia." In Barcelona, a 2017 poll suggested tourism was the residents' number one problem, and youths spray-painted tourists' vehicles with sayings such as "tourism kills neighbourhoods" and "tourist go home, refugees welcome." Similar protests took place in Madrid, Ibiza, Venice, Mallorca, and elsewhere. You ponder the appropriateness and efficiency of corrective taxes and fees, all designed to cure the problem, yet sometimes doing so without really pricing the industry's externalities and the new models of accommodation.

Don't all such measures defy the neoliberal master-logic of our time, making them unlikely to succeed? Taking your point that "it is important that tourism management policies are not implemented within a neoliberalism framework which only promotes capital accumulation but the distribution of wealth remaining uneven,"[10] if we really want to save Venice from the "golden hordes," aren't stronger counter-neoliberal measures, aimed at limiting tourist flows, warranted? If I want to visit Venice, and add myself to the city's 1.3 million or so other tourists in a given year, should I be free to do so, provided only that I can pay for it? Or don't I need to reflect on what it is I hope to find in Venice and perhaps enter a vetting process with a worked-out defence of what I hope to discover there?

In this piece on overtourism, you get into the nuts and bolts of policies that might make a difference to the most affected cities—the sorts of taxes and fees that could respond to the assault on them by Air BnB.

NEPAL: I might have been influenced by my coauthor, who is a trained economist. I think one can imagine a mix of incentives and disincentives to influence tourism flows. For example, in many places, there's no such thing as an entrance fee. In Dolpo, you do have to pay because this is a restricted area close to Tibet. (I think the Nepalese government is sensitive with respect to China.) This policy of limiting access to foreigners in border regions goes back to the 1950s. If you want to visit Upper Dolpo, you have to pay a minimum of five hundred dollars for a ten-day trip. So, that's fifty dollars a day. So, in a sense, this is example of an exclusive form of tourism. Most of the people I met there have the means to pay that much money. Putting a premium price on the experience is, I think, definitely a possible option. You're filtering out the tourists. A not-so-good thing about this tourism policy in Dolpo is that it gives immense power to the central government and resources (in the form of tourism revenues) to exercise that power. What do the local communities get in return? Almost nothing. Paying that premium price for the exclusive trekking experience in Dolpo would be alright, I think, if that revenue was used to improve the lives of the people living there. But that is not what is happening today. This must change. Otherwise, a day will come when people will say no to tourists, just like the backlash we have seen against tourists in other parts of the world.

And you speak of Spain. Barcelona is a primary tourism destination. In Spain, tourism contributes about 12 percent to the GDP. Now, if you don't have tourism, imagine what would happen? You need well-considered incentives and disincentives. You can have all this antitourism backlash. I always begin my classes by saying that people hate tourists. People in Barcelona, people in Venice—they hate tourists, but they love tourism.

MCKAY: We come back to your theme of contradictions.

NEPAL: Tourism is embedded in the modern economy. Addressing those contradictions is quite critical to understanding the nuances of tourism.

MCKAY: If the pandemic has been tragic for many and troublesome for most, academics who study tourism might at least derive some satisfaction out of their field's new prominence. The topic of tourism is generally not taken very seriously in academic settings. Suddenly it seems much more important, because the pandemic has been brought to the planet, in large measure, thanks to mass tourism, an unrivalled mechanism for spreading viruses. Mass tourism has been revealed to be a kind of weapon of mass destruction. It's quite dangerous. It's spreading disease much faster than the Mongol armies of the fourteenth century.

If the majority of tourism-related academics feel a responsibility to help the industry grow, a growing minority now want to rethink its very fundamentals. Do you think the pandemic will change how academics, and the public at large, look at tourism? Might its glory days be coming to an end, in an era of pandemics?

NEPAL: You are going to see these problems with business-as-usual tourism. The pandemic sent us a clear signal. It made very clear that the externalities of tourism, along with other industries, need to be built into our sense of the true cost of doing business.

You could, when I was a child, go to a mountain top, or even onto the rooftop of our house, and you could see the chain of snow-capped mountains very clearly. There was one place where you could look east and see the summit of Mount Everest on a clear day. Then that became no longer possible. But, in the pandemic, it became possible again. It is a good illustration of what we have lost in this maddening rush for economic prosperity.

We're also dealing with global climate change, natural disasters, some of which are climate-induced. There are reports of receding glaciers in the Himalayas and snow not staying on the ground for long. Climate change and natural disasters are going to change the dynamics of tourism. If you don't have snow, will the Himalayas still be aesthetically pleasing and therefore attractive for tourism development? This is a good question to consider.

The Economist and the *Globe and Mail* have been talking about "mindful tourism."[11] The *New York Times* ran an article on "regenerative tourism."[12] The idea is that we cannot continue to practise tourism the way we practise it today.

So, we need to change. Tourists could work to become educated on the cultures they visit and the environments they're visiting. Similarly, local communities could learn about foreign cultures from the tourists. There is great opportunities for meaningful cultural exchanges—that is the positive strength of tourism that needs to be harnessed.

Let me give you a micro-example of a resource-intensive practice we could change. Many tourists want French fries. Get French fries, you're happy. But, French fries are the most resource-intensive food because you have to heat the oil, which can be problematic in high mountains. For some reason, the local Sherpas thought, "If we feed the tourists with resource-intensive food, like French fries, they will be happy and we'll have repeat customers." Even smaller things like that can change. The tourists needed to be more mindful of their resource consumption habits too and not just engage in relentless pursuit of leisure, no matter what.

This idea of regenerative, mindful tourism is going to stay with us for some time. I hope policymakers are cognizant of this new trend. And that they realize a "Small is Beautiful" approach to tourism is preferable to mass tourism, both for tourists and the people they visit.

Tourism is here to stay. Travel is driven by curiosity. As long as people remain curious about the world and its people, including the distant and remote corners of the world, tourism will continue. Tourism itself is not necessarily evil, as some say it is. It is the practice of tourism that needs a thorough reconsideration in light of the challenges—global warming, natural and human-made disasters, war—that lie ahead.

PART THREE
CHOPPY WATERS AHEAD

PART THREE

CHOPPY WATERS AHEAD

AN INTERVIEW WITH
J. MICHAEL RYAN
10 JUNE 2022

J. Michael Ryan is associate professor of sociology at Nazarbayev University, Kazakhstan. He served as a researcher for the TRANSRIGHTS project at the University of Lisbon and has taught courses at the American University in Cairo and in Ecuador and at the University of Maryland. He also worked as a research methodologist at the National Center for Health Statistics in Washington, DC. He has brought out more than a dozen books, including *Core Concepts in Sociology* in 2019 and *Trans Rights in a Globalizing World* in 2020.

During the pandemic, Professor Ryan has not only given us *COVID-19: Social Inequalities and Human Possibilities* (2022, coauthored with Serena Nanda) but also a two-volume collection of general essays: *COVID-19: Global Pandemic, Societal Responses, Ideological Solutions* (2021) and *COVID-19: Social Consequences and Cultural Adaptations* (2021). The Routledge Covid-19 Pandemic Series, which Professor Ryan edits, lists nearly a dozen additional volumes, with many more doubtless to follow, making it one to watch for those of us trying to keep track of the impact of the pandemic.

RYAN: I might also mention that I have personally edited four more volumes, and I just found out yesterday that those just went into production. There are more volumes coming out soon. My mind, thankfully not my body, has been full of Covid.

MCKAY: A productivity level that puts the rest of us to shame. My first question relates to this term "syndemic," a neologism coined in the 1990s by anthropologist Merrill Singer, a student of HIV/AIDS, that we have used for our magazine, and which has clearly also influenced your work. Could you give people unfamiliar with this term an insight into why this concept matters to you? And would you be open to the argument that only a radically integral analysis can offer us realistic readings of the underlying *causal* forces whose dynamic interactions make such diseases possible—an "upstream" as opposed to a "downstream" analysis, so to speak?

RYAN: The concept has been very influential in my work—not just the term but the concept. To be honest, it was not something I'd thought about before coming to work on Covid-19 issues. But since I did, I wish I would have been thinking that way a long time ago. The concept matters because diseases don't exist in isolation. They share the world with us, and we need to understand the world they live in, which is the world we live in too, if we're to understand them. In a way, just as human beings are socialized by their environments, so are diseases. We view these agents as diseases, whereas we are hosts to them. We're also reliant on bacteria and viruses for our survival. Up to 8 percent of human DNA is actually in part made up of ancient viruses.

I do also think we need to have an upstream analysis, though this gets complicated in the same ways that I think intersectionality is often difficult and complicated. It's difficult to include everything and difficult to think about blended interactions, rather than just being additive, which is maybe the problem you're signalling with a downstream analysis. We need to think about the conceptual limits so we don't pare everything down to a level that would not be useful for a broader social analysis. We're all unique individuals with unique experiences, and those are all important to recognize. But also, we need social concepts.

When I first set about doing this, I initially, narrowly thinking just about sociology, issued a call for contributions for what was supposed to be a single volume on the sociological perspective. I realized really quickly that that was wrong and very short-sighted. I ended up with over a hundred proposals. That's how the first volume morphed into two and from just sociologists to a wide range of social scientists. It got me thinking: we really need to put this work in broader conversations. It's not just about sociology.

As you've noted, and as I try to argue in my work, we need this broader social scientific perspective as a corollary to (or companion of) the medical perspective. I often distinguish between the virus (which I see as the more medical) and the pandemic (which I see as more social). But I really don't do that to draw boundaries but to show

how the two are already joined together in a syndemic. These things are all inherently social. How do we classify what a virus is? What constitutes a pandemic? What does it mean to have a lockdown? What are the policy issues? I agree that things need to be more holistic. Our analyses need to be more syndemic across the board. We need to take up these broader or more integrated perspectives.

MCKAY: The thesis sustained by an emergent school of epidemiologists, biologists, social scientists, and other scholars is that things like Covid-19 (and global climate change more generally) are complexly interwoven phenomena whose origins lie in fossil capitalism launched over two centuries ago, along with the massive deforestation and industrial agricultural practices such capitalism has more recently entailed. In their holistic interpretation, a "metabolic rift" has opened up between the socioeconomic systems upon which humans materially rely and the intricate evolutionary processes of the nonhuman natural world.

Capitalism is certainly present in your book as an object of critique—"medicine must be removed from the jaws of capitalism," you and Serena Nanda write[1]—and one is rarely in doubt about your sympathy with the exploited and oppressed. Yet, I was wondering, would it be fair to say that capitalism is still a fairly peripheral concept for you?

RYAN: I would agree that capitalism could be considered a fairly peripheral *term* in my work. But I would argue that it is a, or probably the, central *concept* driving my work. I deal mostly with the epiphenomena of capitalism rather than analyzing the system itself. I think it's important to do both. That's why I appreciate the work of people who are taking the system to task. But, I also think it's important to deal with the effects as well as the causes. I certainly see capitalism as the spectre haunting everything.

I also focus more on the pandemic itself. So for me, the pandemic is the focus, even if it's undergirded by capitalism and by other humanly created social systems—race, gender, national borders. Mine is not a critique of capitalism through the lens of Covid. It's an understanding of Covid in the era of capitalism.

MCKAY: I noticed in particular the influence of Karl Polanyi and thought to myself your perspective was Polanyian. In one place, you draw on Polanyi specifically, but I sensed he was important to you more generally as well.

RYAN: I happen to be a big fan. I'm glad that came through. In an earlier life, I was interested in the relationship between populism and inequality in Latin America, and I was very focused on using Polanyi, especially to understand Bolivarian socialism in Venezuela. He's too often overlooked.

MCKAY: He creates a vivid sense of the immense social dangers of a totally marketized society. His general insight was, you can only commodify things so far and then there will be a general recoil against total commodification. Contrary to neoliberalism, it's just not tenable to render Polanyi's "fictional commodities"—land, labour, et cetera—as straightforward commodities without incurring massive social costs and risking general social upheaval. That's a message that surely resonates in 2022.

RYAN: I hope you're right. Just when I think capitalism can't surprise me anymore, it does. I would not be surprised if a lot more things become commodified. Water is more and more becoming a commodity. I'm told air is becoming a commodity in China. I do think the capitalist system needs to be the main target. But it shouldn't be the only one. Sometimes using that term covers up individual responsibility. There are people, individuals, making choices. Not engaging with that level sometimes eliminates some possibilities for hope—and we could all use more possibilities for hope right now.

There's been a lot of discussion about this being a zoonotic disease—where did it come from? Bats, pangolins, foxes, we don't seem to know. I also think that we often conveniently forget we give diseases to other animals as well, including Covid-19. They give them to us, and we give them right back, especially in zoos and other places where animals are constrained.

While the viral jump might be related to environmental forces, the spread of the virus is much more closely related to human, social, and political structures. I guess we could put capitalism at the root of all of that. I do think it's important to recognize capitalism when we're talking the pandemic. Where do we put the blame? It surely doesn't belong on a bat in China. It probably didn't want to get eaten in the first place.

MCKAY: A lot of the scholars who influence me, like Andreas Malm, work very hard to establish a contextualized and nuanced and specific interpretation—not just to go back to a knee-jerk, reflexive turn to "capitalism" as our obligatory term. Others, of course, take a more mechanical approach.

RYAN: We need to ask, what aspect of capitalism, which form of capitalism, whose capitalism, right? The form of capitalism in China is not the same as in the US. It has to become more nuanced. Capitalism is often used as a sort of catch-all.

MCKAY: Throughout *COVID-19: Social Inequalities and Human Possibilities*, we find an extraordinary wealth of examples from around the world, and one of its great merits is its breadth of coverage: from Kazakhstan to Kenya, we engage with people and countries struggling with many of the same problems. An extraordinary wealth of examples. I think you can't really engage with Covid-19 today without engaging with your impressive work.

At the same time, more critically, I was struck by the survival in the text of common-sense Cold War sign-posting. In your treatment of geopolitics in your monograph, for example, we encounter the "democratic state of Israel" (70), the "autocratic state of Russia" (70), the "totalitarian nation of China" (77). We also meet up with "The West" (75), contrasted with the "world's poor nations" (145). There are, it seems, primarily, two regime types: "democratic governments vs. authoritarian governments" (119). I don't have a fixed and firm alternative to these terms, but coming from a Marxist framework, they do strike me as rather static. There are many alternative rubrics, such as "empires" and "imperialism" and "colonialism," that are not front-and-centre here.

Is there a case for retaining and developing, above and beyond your primarily ideal-typical description of regimes, an analysis of systems of accumulation and political power that assigns each regime its role in the world order? And, under conditions of capitalist globalization, might not the neoliberal transformation of those systems over the past four decades have placed all scholars under a new obligation to reinterpret a world that is both similar to and radically different from the one analyzed by twentieth-century sociologists? The boundaries of nation-states don't mean the same things anymore. You've got global processes of accumulation that mean we're in a radically different world than the one that preoccupied twentieth-century sociologists. What would you say to that?

RYAN: I think I agree with you in that a lot of that terminology is problematic. Part of that arises, no doubt, from my disciplinary training.

I've struggled quite a bit myself to come up with better terms. I'm never quite sure what to say in a way that can be conveyed in an easy-to-understand concept. "The West" is flawed. "Poor countries" is flawed (I like to think of them more as "impoverished" countries). They're all flawed. How do we deal with that? I think it speaks to broader issues of using commonly understood vernacular terms while also trying to work within the framework of intersectional analysis. This problem has only been exacerbated during the pandemic. It is definitely worthwhile coming up with better terms. I'm just not quite sure what they are or how to do that.

You also raise the question of boundaries not meaning the same thing anymore. I find that really interesting. A lot of my work has been around issues of globalization. Many political scientists debate whether states matter anymore. I think Covid *should* change a lot of those conversations—or have a lot to add to a lot of those conversations.

While it's true that maybe boundaries and borders are mattering less, I think we can see, with Covid, that they still very much matter. When people went into lockdowns, it was all about borders. Your passport absolutely mattered. We saw a resurgence and importance of physical territoriality, especially for those of us who are not members of the elite. Clearly money was able to flow quite easily, as it always does, but I think human beings took a step backwards.

MCKAY: And I suppose one could reference the rise of nationalism, which is also all about borders. Many in the 1990s declared nationalism dead and gone as an atavism that no longer corresponded to economic realities. I don't think many people in 2022 would say that nationalism is kaput.

RYAN: It's very much alive and well. One could even say that Covid might have helped nationalism because, in places like the US, we had not had such a clear enemy since Iraq or Afghanistan. All of a sudden, it was China. Now we could definitely blame Covid on them. And why did the Chinese do this? All such arguments were inaccurate and nationalistic but often effective. Covid seems to have added fuel to this conservative fire.

MCKAY: Neoliberalism haunts your book, with one core argument being that the pandemic, far from constituting a crisis of neoliberal order, is actually a kind of "blessing" for it, along with nationalism and neoconservatism. The "problems of the rich" will continue to be presented as "perils for all of us," while "their gains, and our miseries, are seen as something individually earned," you write.[2] Can you provide us with a summary statement of your position on the socioeconomic origins and ideological framings of the crisis?

RYAN: I go back to a term we already talked about: capitalism. In various forms of inequalities—in racism, in sexism, in heterosexism, completely arbitrary national borders, hierarchical global citizenship schemes. All the inequalities and inequities that were already haunting our contemporary world became more visible.

MCKAY: Some of us might think that the neoliberal reactions to Covid-19 have offered a classic example of McDonaldization as analyzed by George Ritzer, a contributor to one of your collections.[3] In what ways has Covid-19 served as a "blessing" for it? Some of us might view Covid-19 as the ultimate indictment of a capitalist system and the neoliberal ideological framework established to defend it. Just-in-time production and distribution, the paring down of the social welfare state—these are not well-suited to health systems in crisis. We really needed, rather, a just-in-case strategy. One could say Covid-19 has not been a blessing for neoliberalism because people will come to see just how deficient these hegemonic models are. You can't rely on them. And neoliberalism as a form of "hyperindividualism" has been shown to be highly destructive. So, in what sense is Covid-19 a *blessing* for neoliberalism?

RYAN: Just last night, Ritzer and I gave a talk on Covid and McDonaldization. One of the things we talked about was this: the just-in-time versus just-in-case argument. The pandemic revealed that just-in-time wasn't working in public health. Or rather, it works well until it doesn't. And, today, we don't need just-in-case for *what* might happen but rather for *when* the next case arrives.

If we're thinking about pandemic issues, there will be another pandemic. I hope the lesson we'll draw from this one is that just-in-time doesn't work. We need to be thinking more in terms of just-in-case, a flawed term in this case because the question isn't really about if, but when.

In terms of the broader arguments about neoliberalism and hyperindividualism, I agree with some of what you're saying. But I'm wondering: Who is seeing these results? Perhaps we are because it's the kind of thing we think about. I don't think most voters are seeing the same thing. I don't think most politicians are. It was very clear for many of us before the pandemic that hyperindividualism was not sustainable. It is destructive. But, I think the pandemic, for many people, has made them into bigger supporters of hyperindividualism than before. I think we're seeing reasoning like this: "I don't care if you have vaccines, as long as I have mine, and I know there's more, at least for me, somewhere."

Vaccines are a very interesting case. We really have been talking about a just-in-case approach on the part of wealthy countries—those in a position to hoard. Canada, I hate to say, has been one of the worst offenders. At one point, Canada had six times the number of vaccine doses it could use. The US had about five. When you're beating the US on something like this—there's an issue there, right?

Hyperindividualism has been given a boost. We're seeing the flourishing of neoconservative politicians who have really benefited from the pandemic. They got a big boost. It allowed them to push through neoliberal policies, neoconservative policies, and you weren't paying attention because you're too busy looking over here at the shiny ball to notice what's happening during the pandemic:

"I can distract you with that. You don't know what I'm doing under the table."

In that sense, I think they've actually been strengthened by the pandemic. I hope I'm wrong about that. I think we're seeing all signs pointing to things getting worse, unfortunately.

MCKAY: As a scholar of sexual minorities, with specific reference to the struggles of trans people, you are really distinguished in the burgeoning field of pandemic studies for your consistent focus on the LGBTQ+ community, not only in your coauthored book but in your collections of essays.

I'd like to ask two related questions about this. First, related to the questions we've already touched on, do you think the pandemic signals a paradigm shift in the way such minorities are conceptualized—that we, in essence, have moved from being rights-bearing individuals free to make most of our own decisions about how we manage our sexualities to being vectors of disease posing a menace as "foreigners" to the societies in which we live? Can this not be seen as a major opportunity for people who want to push back on the rights of LGBTQ+ people?

And second, have you noticed how thoroughly the HIV/AIDS epidemic has been shunted to one side in historical assessments of Covid-19? I keep noticing, in summary histories of pandemics past, everyone goes back to 1918–20. Again and again, one reads: "This is the most dire pandemic since the Spanish Flu." The last big pandemic. Never anything like it since. A "Black Swan" event. Doesn't one just have to say to these folks: "Sorry, but you're just wrong"? HIV/AIDS, with an estimated death toll of around thirty-three million globally, still far outranks Covid-19 (estimated death toll, from the latest statistics, of fifteen million) in terms of its tragic consequences. So, much that we've been told about this being an unprecedented pandemic is, in a straightforward way, incorrect.

The excision of HIV/AIDS (along with the many other spill-over diseases from the 1970s on) could suggest an almost wilful blindness to one of the more damaging implications of capitalism as a way of life—that is, its unplanned, chaotic but pervasive and dangerous intensification of human interconnectedness—and to the fact that we have been living for four decades in what some call the "Pandemicine."

Zoonotic overspills have become quite normal, and pandemics are likely to arise from them. Would you agree?

RYAN: On the first part of your question, I don't think there's been a transition from being rights-bearing individuals free to make most of our decisions about how we manage our sexualities because I don't think most of us have ever known that privilege, to have it as a point to transition from. Certainly not most people in the world. Even in places where that might be the case for the privileged, it's still something relatively new. So, I'm not sure there's been a transition because I'm not sure we were ever at that starting point. Certainly not everyone.

You know, I identify as a gay man. I'm married. I have a husband, not a wife. So, I've had some of this personal experience moving around the world, and in many places I've lived which would generally be seen as fairly homophobic, I've fared much better [there] than when I go back to my small town in Indiana. I'm from a small town of about five hundred people in the rural corn fields. Trump belt. Mike Pence was governor. He put Indiana on the map for the anti-LGBT laws he was passing.

It gets quite complicated in that sense. I think our ability to manage our sexualities is also something we have to look at more intersectionally. I have more privilege to manage mine, in lots of cases, because I'm from the US. As I live abroad, I'm often seen as a foreigner first, right? So who cares what I do? I'm also often seen as wealthy in the countries I live in, so that brings advantage. I'm a college professor, so that brings some advantage. I certainly have a much easier time of it than my LGBT+ students here in Kazakhstan.

It's complex for LGBT+ people who have become a target. There have been some documented instances of this. In South Korea, for example, there was a huge backlash when an outbreak there was traced to a gay night club. There has been the passage of homophobic and transphobic bills in a number of countries. Being a member of a sexual minority also puts you in a more precarious position during a pandemic because of pre-existing issues for a lot of people. The ability to access medical care. Housing discrimination. Lack of support for those in same-sex relationships. Not getting the same bail-outs for your families because our families are not recognized.

As for the second part of your question, you know I'd actually be a little reluctant to draw many parallels between HIV/AIDS and Covid-19. I think we can draw some, but I'd be against many comparisons for a couple of reasons. They're very different diseases—different types of diseases. They spread in very different ways. I think we could draw useful parallels between other diseases in general that have been sidelined, such as malaria, tuberculosis.

Take hydroxychloroquine, commonly used to treat malaria. Suddenly, they ramp up production of it. Now it's being stored in warehouses all over the place because they ended up not using it. I was scratching my head about it. Where has this been? Millions of people are dying every year of malaria. Why are you doing this? Why are you now letting it sit in a warehouse when you could be wiping out malaria?

Well, the answer is (and this also applies to HIV/AIDS): we don't care, right? It's not something that's probably ever to kill me or kill you, or kill most people with economic resources. I've lived in many malaria zones, and I just take a pill, right? I have access to the pill, I am able to pay for the pill. When it's not a threat to people like me, it gets ignored. When it's not a threat to those in power, we sweep it under the rug.

The same thing applies to HIV/AIDS (which was first called GRID, gay-related immunological deficiency). It was completely swept under the table because it affects people who didn't matter in most eyes. It was men having sex with men, drug users, sex workers, people that society doesn't really care about—this was the perception, even if it was completely wrong. A number of countries have downgraded it, in fact, from a deadly disease to a chronic condition akin to diabetes—something to manage. Now, it's just killing people in Africa, not so many Europeans, so we allow ourselves to forget about it.

I also think the impact of Covid has been different. HIV/AIDS has killed thirty-three million people, but that has been over four decades. Meanwhile, Covid-19 has killed about fifteen million, we think, in about two years. How many people will it kill over four decades? And Covid-19 is also getting more attention because of the kinds of people Covid is killing. Now, it's killing international jet-setting folks from more privileged locations. That's different. *Now*, it's a global crisis, *now* it's an epidemic.

MCKAY: Taking all your really good points—that HIV/AIDS and Covid-19 are really different diseases and their social and medical trajectories have been quite dissimilar—they are still comparable in another sense: that they're zoonotic diseases, reaching humans from other animals, likely as a consequence of the development of hitherto unexploited terrains in the Global South. They both testify to the challenges of human connectivity. They would both be unthinkable without the radical new forms of human interconnectedness that emerged in the 1970s–80s.

For all the benefits of that global interconnectedness, in its unregulated, capitalist form, it has turned out to be one of the most dangerous weapons pointed at ourselves, ironically, through the human experiences and linkages many of us treasure. Through mass tourism, because of insanely accelerated levels of accumulation and just-in-time processes of production and distribution—we're all in harm's way. We're all in each other's neighbourhoods all the time. This is in some ways a very good thing, but it can also be a very dangerous thing, if it's unregulated, if it's driven by purely capitalist motives.

The very global interconnectedness that is so valuable in sharing ideas and crafting movements is also really a dangerous phenomenon when it takes an unregulated, hypercapitalist form. That would the basis of the comparison. They are both zoonoses that became pandemics through the instrumentality of global capitalism.

RYAN: Yes, I can see that connection. I think again I would probably broaden it out to other zoonotic, and non-zoonotic, diseases. The issue of interconnectedness is something we've all thought about during the pandemic, both on the physical and social levels. I've thought about it quite a bit. I've had some unique experiences over the last couple of years.

From March to November 2020, I was here in Kazakhstan, at the university. I actually live on campus; we're in a gated compound right on the edge of the city. When I look out my window right now, it overlooks the vast steppes of southern Siberia. This is an area I might not normally want to be in. But during a global pandemic, it was kind of nice. There aren't many tourists. I'm on the edge of the city. I'm very isolated. So, in that sense, I felt much better than if I were living in Manhattan.

I left here then, and my husband and I went to the Canary Islands where I'm undertaking research to study the impact of the pandemic on tourism there. We ended up staying there for seven months. It was interesting to see the impact of Covid-19 on the locals, because about two million people live there, but fourteen million people arrive every year for tourism. This is a place that runs on that. We stayed in very remote houses, very isolated, but we would on occasion drop in on tourist centres. There weren't many tourists, but you could quickly recognize them. Because they were the ones who weren't wearing masks. They were not acting responsibly.

Then I went to my small town in Indiana, a small, isolated community. No one was following health protocols. Nobody's wearing a mask. There's a big push-back against vaccines. It was frightening—there, more than anywhere, I felt isolated. Yet, it's the place where I had the most people physically around me. I just wanted to be away from them.

Throughout the pandemic, we have had to recognize the difference between "physical connectedness" and "social connectedness." A lot in this pandemic has come down to the idea of "social distancing"—one of my pet peeves. I correct it every time I hear it: "No, no, no, physical distancing." I think conflating those two terms is inaccurate, and scary, in lots of ways. Health measures don't rely on being socially distanced, they rely on being physically distanced.

MCKAY: I know a lot of South Asian scholars have also queried the term ["social distancing"], since it's redolent of many of the worst aspects of the caste system and its destructive consequences for those occupying the lower rungs of it.

RYAN: Yes, in one of our forthcoming books, we have a chapter looking exactly at that—at Covid as a new form of untouchability.

MCKAY: In North America, there has been much polarized discussion about lockdowns, with schools in particular attracting a vast amount of commentary. I found your book really refreshing in its willingness to give some time to critics of lockdowns, especially in the Global South, where masses of people risked starvation as well as further sickness as a consequence of them. So, is this one lesson to be learned from Covid-19—that comprehensive testing and tracing (on, say, the Japanese or Vietnamese models) is to be preferred to comprehensive lockdowns? Over the past two years, have we discovered both the strengths but also the limitations of lockdowns as ways of handling pandemics?

RYAN: I am not such a fan of testing and tracing, I have to say. It's expensive. There's a lot of environmental waste. There are a lot of flaws. It's good—I'm not saying stop testing and tracing—but there are better ways. And practically speaking, once I'm tested, I can contract Covid-19 again. I think there are better ways. And one of them is lockdowns. I think the problem with them was often the way they were enforced and who they were implemented to benefit. You know, globally, if we had been able to tell everyone, "Go home and don't leave your house for two weeks" at the very start of the pandemic, it might have been over in two weeks. It's idealistic, of course, to think we had the capability to do that. Still, it could have happened, had we dedicated our resources to it.

So I think the problems have arisen from the way they were handled. Lockdowns were carried out in a very patchwork manner. That made them inefficient. It's not effective if I'm locked down and my neighbour doesn't obey the rules. Why am I locking down, doing my part, and they're not?

The push-back against lockdowns got overblown in a lot of ways. We were clearly not locking down those protesting against lockdowns, so it was a little hard to see what they were protesting against. Same thing with the antimask demonstrations. A lot of people weren't masking in the first place. It's not that we used lockdowns, but that we didn't use them correctly.

MCKAY: A historian might make the point too about how meaningless it is to talk about lockdowns in the abstract, if you're not talking about *when* they were imposed, without any sense of their context or timing. In the US, for example, lockdowns happened after the virus had been allowed to circulate for months. Critics of lockdowns were, in a sense, right, in that they said, "Imposing this now is not going to change the situation." When you're three or four months into the pandemic, the horses are out of the barn, to use a colloquial expression.

Whereas, if you locked down quickly, right away, and rigorously, you might achieve a very different result. Yes, you are going to make some false calls—as the WHO has done in past years. But one lesson of Covid-19 would seem to be: act fast and demand a high level of adherence to what you've decided to do for a short period of time—three weeks, perhaps, but not two years. These are surely questions to be asked about lockdowns: when? where? for how long?

RYAN: Lockdowns can't keep going on forever, right? But that was never the intention. They should have been very short and, if everyone would have adhered to them, we would have forgotten about Covid a long time ago.

And yes, we did it too late. And the people driving the policy themselves didn't adhere to it. I really have no problem pointing the finger at them, the people who violated health protocols. I don't have much tolerance for that sort of thing. They're often the ones protesting. I'm not afraid to go up to them and say something. It can be exhausting, but it needs to be done.

It's maybe a case where language matters quite a bit. "Lockdowns" sounds like being in a prison. Perhaps "shutdowns"? Or "pauses"? Or "stay-at-home social responsibility?" Or even a "staycation"? It could have been framed that way instead of having this penal connotation. And we *might* have then found greater compliance.

MCKAY: One of the great aims of your book is to "add the social voice to the medical conversation."[4] In the two-volume set of primarily sociological/anthropological interpretations of Covid-19, we encounter myriad different schools, the result, one imagines, of the transformation of these disciplines in the wake of poststructuralist and postmodern influences hegemonic over the past four decades.

But, might it be a time for sociologists to supplement their often very sensitive and stimulating sense of the power of political and economic ideas with a sharper appreciation of the class realities underlying them—to trade in, so to speak, some of their volumes of Derrida, Foucault, Latour, and Butler for the older works of Polanyi, Tawney, and Macpherson—or maybe even Marx, Engels, and Gramsci? If the pandemic has constituted, as you write, the "working-class crisis,"[5] does this not suggest that some of the themes of contemporary sociology need to be revisited, given how many sociologists since the 1970s have bid a dry-eyed farewell to the "working class"? I don't get the feeling they were too choked up about saying goodbye to the working class—they seemed anxious to move on to sexier topics.

RYAN: I think what sociologists focus on depends a lot on where they've trained. There's quite a difference between the sociological training you'll get in Europe, for example, versus the US. The "post" influences you talk about were very popular in Europe. They were more short-lived in the US. I didn't read a lot of them for my graduate classes, though I have read many of them since. I'm not sure I ever read Derrida as a student.

I'm not really a fan of those "post" works myself. In the context of the pandemic, they often don't push for change. They're not political enough for my taste. I think they're politicized, but a lot of them actually advocate against radical changes—and leave one just sitting back and enjoying the problems they reveal. And they're often written in intentionally very complicated terms. Sometimes they're purposefully written to be impossible to understand. I don't find that useful. I think the role of academics, sociologists included, should be to write in a way that people can understand it. Many academics write mainly for each other, and that's about it. We write to get published, not to make social change. I think that's really problematic.

There's been a marked shift in social sciences away from the humanistic principles we might find in Marx and others. Ideas of helping society have taken a back seat to professionalization—publishing articles, generating citations. I think academics are turning into assembly-line workers instead of thinkers. Students are turning into customers. And universities are turning into corporations. So, there's less room to be critical of the class system if that system is supporting your institutions. When you do that, you're at risk of losing your job, and if you don't work, you don't eat. These topics have become too professionally risky.

I also think there's been a distortion that has fuelled all of this; that is, the way we view experts. Who is an expert? That's been really key during the pandemic. If we're looking at Trump or Cardi B or these people posting conspiracy theories on Twitter—more people are getting their medical news from those sources than from medical professionals.

MCKAY: I'm really struck by the way that people seem to want science to deliver certainties. They will rake someone like Dr. Fauci over the coals because he changed his mind on this or that issue. I'm not saying he should be beyond criticism, that he shouldn't be challenged in the public sphere, but to hope that science will give you certainties is to fundamentally misunderstand the scientific enterprise. It is not going to give you certainties. It's going to give you a range of probabilities and useful concepts and techniques for reading the available evidence, all subject to future revision and further development. Many people do not want that. They are in search of something that looks quite a lot like a secular religion. They want inerrant truths.

RYAN: This was the first time many people were exposed to how science works, and especially how vaccines are developed. There are, inevitably, errors. There are lots of mistakes. There are people who get sick during trials. Normally, we don't know that—it all happens behind closed doors, over a decade. Suddenly, it was in the spotlight. When someone like Fauci, or whoever, shifted their best advice, many people became unglued. "You said this! Then you said that!" Well, that might have been correct at the time, but it isn't now.

Science has changed. The empirical evidence has changed. A lot of people don't understand that. In some ways, the pandemic was a missed opportunity to educate people in how science works. We call them "clinical trials" for a reason. This was a new disease we didn't know too much about. We still don't know as much as we need to know. But people want certainty. They don't want you to change your mind based on the best available evidence at the moment. Or at least it's been politicized that way.

I'm not sure the average person minds that much on other issues. They don't seem to mind when that happens with other issues, like advice about smoking (although former vice president Mike Pence said there's no evidence that smoking kills people, but he's a little behind on most things). When that sort of evidence changes, most people seem open to that. But I think when they came to Covid-19, they could be very close-minded. I think the analogy to religion is a good one. They wanted a solid answer. You better not change your mind. But it's just not good science to stop asking questions.

MCKAY: "Memories will fade," you write[6]—and one senses they are already fading. Without decisive battles, valiant heroes, sneering villains, clear-cut turning points, or conclusive armistice agreements, the pandemic is very unevenly drawing to a close—or perhaps we're just entering a new phase with new variants. It lacks the narrative shape of a war. Not even close.

If some of the problem of fading memories and inaccurate representations lies in the self-interest of those with every reason to forget how they mismanaged the situation—"that was then, this is now, let's forget all about partygate"—could a cultural theorist also make the argument that an additional reason why Covid-19 will likely fade in memory is that our militaristic metaphors fail to capture an event that fails to conform to our narrative expectations? I don't think the pandemic is ever going to yield a narrative with a clear-cut beginning, middle, and end. Would you agree that, for all the militaristic metaphors people have thrown at the pandemic—your books are great on this—Covid-19 really has not conformed to our narrative expectations?

RYAN: Let me start by saying that I think a lot of those contrasts between strong men and sneering villains and valiant heroes are not clear-cut. It depends on who you are and what your perspective is. A hero in my eyes might be a sneering villain in somebody else's. Also, a lot of people are not trying to turn the page to hide their mismanagement because I think a lot of them would say they managed it very well.

Science doesn't sustain that conclusion, nor do the facts—but these folks tend to be people who weren't really concerned about facts, anyway. Trump, for example, remains convinced he handled Covid-19 really well. I don't think they want to turn the page because I think they think they did a great job. Unfortunately, at least in the US, since Trump, we're living in this universe of alternative facts. I think that makes analysis difficult. I think it makes understanding these populations difficult.

In terms of using metaphors, I think they are both problematic *and* useful. They're problematic in that they're not precise enough. They're useful because they can help us understand what's going on, especially for people who aren't experts. I'm really interested in astrophysics, I find it fascinating, and Neil Degrasse Tyson can tell me a lot about the subject through metaphors. I'd never be able to understand it otherwise. Metaphors can be very useful.

I definitely don't think the pandemic is drawing to a close. I think you're right that people want to turn the page. I get a little nauseous every time I hear someone say, "Living with Covid." It makes me nervous and upset.

MCKAY: That was actually even the title of an official British policy paper, released when Boris Johnson suspended a lot of the precautionary practices associated with Covid-19 in February 2022.

RYAN: It makes me nervous, for several reasons. One, we don't have to be *living* with Covid when we have the tools to wipe it out. We could enforce them. So, that's frustrating.

Second, we're still very much in the throes of this pandemic. The kinds of numbers we're seeing from some countries are way above what they were in 2020, right? Globally, we're still averaging around a half-million cases per day. It's actually just falling a little bit under that. When it first hit half a million cases per day, everyone became unhinged: "What a catastrophe!" Now, nobody cares, and the situation has actually got worse. So, we're not past it.

I think we've subordinated our social awareness of the pandemic. Not just about things like masks and lockdowns. A lot of people don't think twice about going to a crowded bar or a big birthday party.

It was graduation on campus here today. My apartment window overlooks the main part of campus. I didn't see a single mask. Covid-19 is largely under control in Kazakhstan, but we're not that distant from it. I think we need to challenge the mentality of people who think we're past the worst of the pandemic. That mentality needs to be reframed. Another one is coming.

I get a lot of proposals from scholars who want to study the postpandemic world. I largely reject those. I think we can speculate, perhaps make recommendations, but we can't analyse a period that we're not living in yet.

Why do we forget? There are historical events that are historically highlighted, that we will never forget—one thinks of 9/11 in the US. Or something like "Remember the Alamo." I don't think most people know *why* we're supposed to remember the Alamo or really know where or what the Alamo was. But they do know this slogan. I think, similarly, that we are already forgetting the pandemic. Already, and too soon.

I don't think we're going to build museums to the pandemic, along the lines of the ones we constructed for 9/11 or the Alamo. I think we're going to sweep it under the rug because it has unveiled the weaknesses of capitalism (to come back to that word and tie together a lot of our discussion). It's fuelled inequalities. It's also put them in our face in ways that are much more difficult to ignore. We just want to ignore them. We want to take the pill and go back into the Matrix. That, of course, is very dangerous because when we go back in, it's going to grow even worse, in the future. The fact that we kept ourselves in the Matrix, to continue with that analogy, is a lot of the reason Covid-19 has had the devastating impact it has had.

I've had a lot of people ask me what surprised me about the pandemic. My answer is: not much. I was not surprised that it affected people unequally, based on sex and gender and sexuality and economic standing. I don't think most people were surprised. That might prevent us from being able to move forward in a constructive way. We *should* have been surprised the pandemic would have such a socially unequal impact. The virus doesn't discriminate. Human systems, human beings, discriminate. We've grown accustomed to these sorts of inequalities, perhaps we're not even looking to change them.

MCKAY: Which means, perhaps, that Covid-19 has not constituted the cultural turning point some of us hoped it would be?

RYAN: In the early days, I was much more optimistic that the pandemic could be a turning point. Time wears on. I'm less convinced of that. People are so eager to forget, they're so eager to move past the pandemic. It rarely makes the headlines in the US. Take the one-million-death point: I could not easily find it in the media. You had to dig for it. It should have been a "Boom" moment, right? But it wasn't. I'm not sure we're going to take lessons from this.

The pandemic is fuelling inequalities. People who already pulled the wool over our collective eyes now have more money. It's well worth noting that the pandemic was not economically devastating for everyone. We are now witnessing a race between Bezos and Musk to determine who is the richest man in the world. And "man" is an important word there. That's making more headlines than the numbers of people pushed into poverty.

The pandemic has fuelled a lot of arguments against science, against education. The antivax movement wasn't so very big, but it has become very vocal. It's a small group—they're just very loud. I think that group is going to grow bigger.

Unfortunately, I think the pandemic might be fuel for an even more unequal and unjust world. It's not a very happy note. I'm a sociologist. I'm trained to be depressing. I honestly hope I'm wrong.

A big part of what motivates me to do all this work on Covid-19 is the way it is shaping up in memory and culture. I'm frequently asked: "When do you sleep?" I have put out a lot of material. It's really overtaken my life, purposefully. I see it as activism, in a sense, because I want this information to get out there. I want to push and promote understandings of what's going. I want it to stay in our social and cultural consciousness. I am not a medical doctor—I can't help out in a hospital. I am a social scientist and, hopefully, I can help out with these understandings. That's what's been driving me. The push to make myself wrong—this analysis that things are going to get worse. I really want to be wrong about that.

MCKAY: It's almost an intellectual duty to rise to this occasion?

RYAN: Yes. I also hope that Covid-19 doesn't become another fad. Studying Covid became sort of a bandwagon thing, right? Everybody suddenly hopped on board. I think people are now hopping off board rather quickly. Some people are weary of it. It can be exhausting to think about. I hope it doesn't just seen as something that's segmented, isolated, because we've seen the possibility it has to be this turning point.

It is going to change society. It has already changed the direction of society. We just have to decide how. Are we angling further down or angling further up? Further down, I suspect, but I'm going to keep working late nights until I can help us be turned back up again.

AN INTERVIEW WITH

LAURA SPINNEY

15 APRIL 2021

Laura Spinney is a science journalist and has written for many of the influential journals, such as *Nature*, *National Geographic*, *New Scientist*, and *The Economist*. She is the author of five books, both fiction and nonfiction, including the acclaimed *Pale Rider: The Spanish Flu Of 1918 and How It Changed the World* (2018), which is a spellbinding history of a past pandemic whose long shadows have been cast over the present pandemic.

MCKAY: Laura, as the author of *Pale Rider*, you have argued (drawing in part upon the works of evolutionary pathologists) that the influenza epidemic of 1918 spread around the world largely because of the unprecedented mingling of people on the Western Front in the First World War. (There are three possible candidates for the location of the first outbreak.) That suggested to me something of the *active* role humans can play, sometimes unwittingly, in the spread of diseases. I really love this passage in a recent piece you wrote in *The Guardian*, which says, "The key thing to understand is that we are not passive bystanders, we form the virus just as it forms us."[1] Can you connect this observation to your classic study and then say a bit about what lesson it might suggest to us about passivity and activism in the 2020s?

SPINNEY: Thanks for a great question. For a long time, throughout the Middle Ages and after, people thought of epidemics and pandemics as acts of God. They were very fatalistic about them. They were just things that struck. You probably deserved illness, somehow. There was certainly nothing you could do about it—you just had to endure it. Beginning with germ theory in the middle of the nineteenth century and a better understanding of hygiene and infection control, we started to realize that that wasn't quite true. You could have an impact on infection. You could control it. And then science evolved.

Now, we understand that, in fact, we shape epidemics and pandemics in a much more fundamental way. We talk about spillover events, zoonotic diseases that move from animals into humans. We shape the whole ecosystem that makes that possible through our use of the environment, through farming, through wildlife trade, and so on. We no longer can think of ourselves as passive bystanders. Once the pandemic is upon us, we understand that we can also shape the virus in terms of how it mutates, how it evolves, how infectious it is, and how severe the infection is.

One evolutionary biologist maintains that the reason the 1918 flu was so lethal (it's estimated to have been at least twenty-five times more lethal than any other pandemic flu we know about in history) is because of the exceptional conditions that prevailed in the world at that time. You had, on the Western Front, millions of young men packed into the trenches for shorter or longer periods of time, already not in a very good state, stressed, hungry, tired, suffering from other infections, injuries. Notably, their lungs were often gassed. So, they were very vulnerable to a new infection.

When a new pathogen emerges over time, it should moderate its virulence in order to achieve a more benign equilibrium with its host—us. This didn't need to happen in the trenches in 1918. There was literally no price to it racing through this population of young men, since they were going to die anyway, and it could just easily transmit to the next one. So, the idea is that, because of these conditions, it stayed virulent far longer than it would have done and still highly contagious and spread around the world, helped again by the movements of troops and civilians at that time.

We shape the evolution of the virus. Vaccines put enormous selective pressure on the virus. The uneven rollout of the vaccines across the world that we're seeing at the moment is another way we're shaping its evolution, because the pressure will be on it to escape.

MCKAY: Sticking with this memory of 1918, one of the big themes in the British discussion, especially, has been what some would call the misuse of the memory of 1918. Devi Sridhar of the University of Edinburgh and others have been saying that, really, British planners were fixated on 1918 as *the* pandemic.[2] That led to fatal policy errors. They made the mistake of treating coronavirus like the flu and left it too late to lock it down, going for a strategy of mitigation rather than elimination. Richard Horton, editor of *The Lancet*, says that "imagining Covid-19 as a rerun of the flu led to the greatest science policy failure in a generation."[3] Did the heavy, heavy shadow of 1918 have policy effects in 2020? And, more broadly, do historians have a professional obligation to make themselves unpopular by saying, "No, you're getting history wrong"?

SPINNEY: There's a certain irony in this conversation. I wrote my book because *nobody* was talking about 1918. We were approaching its centenary, and nobody was talking about it. Only a year ago, public health experts were wringing their hands over the fact that we never remember pandemic lessons. We go through this cycle of panic and complacency. We panic when the new pandemic emerges and then we forget it immediately. We don't learn the lessons, and voilà, the pattern continues. So, I think it has to be a question of *which* lessons to take from history. And that, of course, is the nub of it. That's where all the difficulty lies.

Flu and Covid-19 are fundamentally different diseases. They're both respiratory diseases, they have some things in common, but the pathogens belong to different families. They behave differently. I think that is what is preoccupying the experts you talked about, and with good reason.

So, for example (and they've acknowledged this), the consensus on flu is that it cannot be eliminated. It spreads through a population too evenly and too rapidly, so the best you can hope to do is to mitigate it, suppress it. You can't eliminate it. And that was the assumption of many countries at the beginning of this pandemic. But Covid-19 doesn't spread in the same way. It has a different profile in terms of infectiousness, in terms of severity, in terms of the time it takes to move from one person to the next, its incubation period. All these things are very different.

Even though the 1918 pandemic was caused by flu (which, as I've said, behaved differently), there are practical lessons to be learned from it. There are quite recent studies that have looked back at the historical data and have shown, for example in the United States (where often the data are best on 1918), that cities or regions that locked down hard and early saved more lives than similar regions or cities that took their time or were less determined about it— in terms of saving lives, but also in terms of the rapidity of the recovery of their economies. So, the overall lesson is sort of the same. I think perhaps our tendency to want to compromise all the time—between saving the economy and saving lives—has led us astray.

There are general lessons that we should learn from pandemics—and that we should be tackling between pandemics rather than waiting to be reminded by them. So, for example, in 1918, as in every pandemic since and again in this one, health inequalities in society are highlighted. These inequalities offer the virus a way into our societies. They gain a foothold in a population through the most vulnerable. There's nothing stopping us, if we wish to, from tackling those problems outside the pandemic and reducing health inequalities, making our health systems more inclusive, and so on.

I think the good news is that we *do* seem to learn lessons that we can take away in a general sense, and our response to this one has been wildly better than our response to 1918 in all sorts of ways. The obvious example is the rapidity with which we've developed vaccines—but also, the rapidity with which we detected this novel infection right at the beginning.

MCKAY: It reminds me of your point that humanity seems to suffer three pandemics every century, if you're looking back over the last five hundred years. If we regard this as kind of a "starter pandemic" of the twenty-first century,[4] in the next pandemic, we should keep elimination on the table as well as mitigation. The one lesson we can draw from this is that elimination should not be removed from policy discussions at the outset. I think the great challenge is how fast people have had to think about this—they had to make decisions about it basically by the middle of January at the latest, before things got out of control. Keep elimination on the table and not exclude it—that might be one verdict on the British experience.

SPINNEY: Well, I think that the more general lesson is: keep your mind and your eyes open. I was speaking the other day to Michael Baker, who is one of the New Zealand epidemiologists who shaped their response.[5] He was really interesting. He's a vocal proponent of "No Covid." Elimination. He thinks it's still possible, at this late stage.

He says that, back in January, he looked at what was happening in Wuhan, a city of eleven million people, and he saw that they'd been able to contain the disease. He thought, if they can do it, then we can do it. He was absolutely flabbergasted when the WHO released its first report back then, which said mitigation and suppression are the way forward (corresponding to the strategies that are normally put in place for flu) and was not even considering elimination.

It's not that, after the end of January, it would have been too late. It's just that it gets harder and harder because you get an exponential growth of outbreaks. So, the earlier you act, the better, and also the earlier you act, the easier it is, because the smaller the problem you have to contain.

In my writing, I was trying to look forward and say that, next time—because there will be a next time; it's three pandemics per century on average over the last five hundred years—but I was just trying to say, let's consider it. Let's remember that, at the beginning of the next pandemic, we'll probably know as little about it as we did about this disease. So, why rule out elimination when you are still in a period of maximum uncertainty? Why not consider all the options at that point? What, effectively, is there to lose? Because you can talk about that much stricter lockdown and the impact it has, but if you look at how much suffering has been entailed by the sort of half-hearted lockdowns we keep going into and out of, a small, contained, hard lockdown at the beginning might have been much less painful in the long run.

MCKAY: Compare that with what you see in the many Asian Pacific countries with various political systems: Taiwan, New Zealand, but also China and Vietnam. They were, perhaps, in some cases, influenced by different attitudes toward the state and the individual and the state's obligation to direct society (as maintained by proponents of the "Confucianism" hypothesis). But, one might also underscore their recent vivid memories of SARS in 2003. So, I think maybe when historians look at this over time, they'll say there was a striking difference between how countries responded, and one of the fissures they might trace is one between Asia-Pacific countries and Anglo-American ones, which have tended to follow a laissez-faire pattern. Would you agree with that?

SPINNEY: I would, absolutely. We sat and twiddled our thumbs for ages. There was a sinister dimension to that: "This is a Chinese problem, it's not our problem"—as if it was going to stay within China's borders.

The countries that have thus far done well are of very different political stripes. The only thing they have in common, really, is that they learned from recent pandemics or epidemics. Memories of SARS are very vivid still in China. It was very frightening. It had a much higher mortality rate than Covid, and most of the fatalities occurred on the Chinese mainland. Taiwan also learned, Vietnam also learned, South Korea learned. They all learned the need for certain things— for example, the need to be able to connect information sources in the interest of test-and-trace, to be able to track infection, to identify it early on, and contain it. That's even been possible in democratic countries.

So, it's not that it's impossible in a democratic system. They've proved that. I think what it shows is that experience of previous pandemics is a learning experience for both governments and people. Governments learn, "Okay, we need these tools for when the moment arrives." People need to realize that there's a need to give them those tools. There's a need for compliance. Solidarity is part of the response. Community compliance is a part of the response. You can see all of that in those countries.

MCKAY: I've been really struck by how much people use war metaphors in talking about the pandemic. You yourself talk about a "biological arms race" between a pathogen and its host.

SPINNEY: It's true.

MCKAY: I've noticed that many in Anglo-America and Canada used the analogy of the struggle against Nazi Germany. I wonder if there's a risk of such martial language? Or two risks? One is that it encourages us to think still that we're at war with nature, we're at war with a virus, when in fact we have coevolved with the virus, we're part of nature, and it should really be a question of managing our metabolism with nature in a more rational way rather than being at war with it. The other risk I see is a transition to martial language in general: we slip into a Cold War way of thinking about attributing this to a malign and malicious Other, desperately trying to undermine our state's power. We're really back to the 1950s in terms of a very polarized world.

SPINNEY: I am guilty of using these metaphors, although I try to avoid them as much as possible. My thinking on this has evolved over the last two years or so. I think there's a few things going on. First of all, I understand why Joe Biden and others use this kind of language. They want to help people get over a kind of natural passivity. They want to persuade them to act. Second, I also think it reflects the changing understanding of pandemics that we were talking about earlier. The fact that we aren't passive and that we do shape them. And so there's a certain justification for talking about it as an enemy that is trying to outwit us. There is a sense in which we *do* need to outwit it.

The third thing: pandemics, whether we like it or not, are fundamentally political. There's no better example of that than the naming of the 1918 flu—the "Spanish flu"—when there was nothing particularly Spanish about it. It was called that because Spain, being neutral in the war, did not censor its press, and so when the first cases of the flu erupted in Madrid in the late spring of 1918, they were reported in the newspapers. The patients included the King of Spain, Alfonso the thirteenth, so it became very visible very quickly. In the belligerent countries, they censored their press because, supposedly, they didn't want to lower the morale of their populations.

In our time, Covid-19 is taking place in the context of, among other things, a trade war between the US and China. If you look back over the last year, we've all seen how the WHO has been used and abused by those two powers. Sometimes it seemed like it was just an arena for their continuing trade war to be fought out in. That, maybe, is one of the problems we'll need to address after this pandemic: to create a stronger global health organization that has more teeth.

I think it's probably not so damaging for us to use that kind of warlike language if we understand that the enemy is a virus—our enemy is the virus—but, if we think our enemy is China, then it's not very helpful. Those two understandings will fuel different courses of action.

MCKAY: I've also noticed how we're just besieged with a tsunami of numbers. In me, they encourage a doubting outlook: "Hey, I don't really trust all the numbers very much because they seem like descriptive statistics that cannot actually be totally reliable from some of the countries reporting them." And secondly, they misrepresent the pandemic as a purely natural phenomenon, like a wave in the water. We keep on talking about "waves" of numbers and "flattening the curves." Would you agree that people have been fighting about the numbers in a way that undermines the credibility of the very important enterprise of epidemiology?

SPINNEY: We are not very good at relating to large-scale death, whatever the cause of it. I tried to explore this a little bit in my book. I was trying at the time to explain to myself, as much as to anyone else, why our memory for pandemics is less good than our memory for wars. We forgot this terrible catastrophe that killed more than any other disaster in the twentieth century and maybe in any other century.

In 1918, there was no such thing as a lab-confirmed diagnosis of that disease. Today, lots of people are asymptomatic. People may experience mild symptoms at home, never see their doctor, but go on to have Long Covid later. There are always all these problems.

The chances are that the figures we're working with today for Covid-19 are underestimates, but we don't know. It's easier to count the death toll of a war (at least it was in the days when soldiers wore uniforms and they all fought on battlefields in the same place). The data are more accessible. It's easier to build a picture of that disaster and get a sense of the scale of it. In a pandemic, on the other hand, I think the overall picture takes time to develop as we draw in the data and as we build on them. We document these kinds of disasters in a very different way, and because of that, we remember them differently.

MCKAY: In your book and your journalism, you pose the question about how we remember pandemics. As I read your book, you're saying, "Well, one of the problems of public memory here is that the pandemic didn't have the right shape. It doesn't conform to the beginning, middle, and end of a classic narrative structure." It's very hard to tell when a pandemic is over. We would like a pandemic to conform to our schemas. We think, for example, it should feature a third and final act. Unfortunately, pandemics don't conform to our conventional understanding of what a story should look like—with a precise beginning and also with heroes and villains. The heroes and villains are going to be hard to discern in this one. And, in 2023, what act are we in? In *Pale Rider,* you tell us memory is always a work in progress, and you write in your journalism of plans to commemorate the virus by monuments in London and in Montevideo, Uruguay (where there's an interesting project in the works).[6] How do you think we'll commemorate this pandemic so it might be remembered by future generations?

SPINNEY: Here's a shocking statistic. I live in France, and here in the 1920s and '30s, there was a kind of a rash of building of monuments to the First World War, about 170,000 of them in all, most of which are still standing. I don't know of a single monument in this country to the 1918 flu. The closest I've come: I found a simple stone cross on the Swiss side of the border in the Jura Mountains. What's interesting about that cross is that it's to the soldiers who died of the flu. And so, even in that one monument, there's a sort of confounding of the two disasters. Again, the war continues to overshadow the pandemic. And yet, we know the flu killed many more people than the war did. It is quite extraordinary, I think, the overshadowing and the forgetting of the pandemic.

There's a debate going on now among memory experts as to whether this one will buck the trend. The thinking is that this is the first major pandemic in human history to have been digitally witnessed (apart from 2009, which was rather anticlimactic because it didn't kill more than a normal flu season in the end).

That means that anyone in the world who has access to the Internet could have, if they wanted, from the beginning of this pandemic, tracked infection rates and mortality rates in (almost) real time. They could have had a general overview of the whole global phenomenon.

That wasn't the case in 1918, far from it. It took a very long time for people in the world to realize they were looking at one pandemic rather than lots of local outbreaks of disease (the naming reflects that, in fact). Initially, the flu was given many names, and it was only later they realized they were dealing with one thing, and it attracted this unfair name, the Spanish Flu.

Today, there are a lot more data on servers all over the place, as well as in people's private archives. There's a huge collecting effort going on, all around the world, of objects, physical objects, diaries, letters, but also digital content. So, if we are better at documenting this one, does that mean we'll remember it better? And if we remember it better, does that mean we're more likely to take lessons from it when future pandemics arise? I think that whole debate is really interesting.

The memorials have already started to be built. The ones that I've been looking at have mainly been quite ephemeral. I think that's partly a sign of the times. The *New York Times* filled its front page with the names of the dead, trying to capture the humanity of this tragedy. I think that's really important, because there is something ephemeral about a pandemic. It rushes through and then it's gone. (Of course, the loss of individual people is not ephemeral.) You need another dimension as well, something that reminds us of the *permanency* of pandemics. The fact that they are a feature of humanity and have been for thousands of years. There will be others—they're not infrequent.

Montevideo provides a really interesting example. As I understand it from the pictures and the drawings I've seen, it's going to be a bowl in steel and concrete, forty metres across. You will walk out to it along a platform from an urban beachfront in Montevideo. It's suspended over the South Atlantic, and it's got a hole in the middle. It's slightly concave, so it amplifies the sound of the waves, which comes up through the hole and you can look down into the roiling sea.

When you look out from the beach—from civilization, so to speak—the monument can be hidden in the weather. And it will weather over time. The message might be: we are not the centre of everything; we are subordinate to nature, and this threat is always there.

MCKAY: There's an optimistic sensibility that some historians bring to this discussion. Okay, pandemics are part of the human experience; yet, you cite statistics from France, Britain, Italy, and the United States suggesting that majorities now believe our civilization is entering a period of general collapse. The French have coined the phrase "collapsologie" (collapsology in English), which they started off as a joke but actually is now in the *Petite Robert*—it's becoming a real word. In some instances, it seems suffused with right-wing Malthusian ideas about having to control population. But other elements are feeding into it, such as concern over global climate change. So, I'm just wondering if historians can provide human beings with a more balanced, somewhat more realistic, even optimistic sense of the future based on their research? Would you like to comment on that?

SPINNEY: I, like you, love this idea of collapsology.[7] Not that I love the idea of the world collapsing or societies collapsing, but I think it's fascinating. We go through these periods when we think the world is going to end and societies are going to collapse. I think historians would probably agree that a given society is healthier at some points than others, even if they don't go through the classic cycle of decline-and-fall that nineteenth-century historians talked about.

When I was writing about collapsology, I was writing about the sort of French version of the phenomenon where people are wanting to go back to nature. That's not the first time in history that's happened either. And in the French version it's not just climate change they're worried about—although that is a major part of it—but also the sickness of society, the fact that there seems to be these huge and very profound divisions in French society. I think it's trying to be scientific and to some extent it achieves it. Maybe in itself, it's a spur to action. Maybe you need to feel that things have got so bad that now, finally, it's time we have to act.

The problem with a lot of the collapsologists' thinking, though, is that it is quite fatalistic. Some of them will tell you the world is going to end in 2030. And if you hear that, one response might well be: "Well, I'll go and have a drink, then. There's nothing I can do." It's important we have a sense that there are solutions, and I think historians come in there. They can show us how societies passed through these moments previously.

It is true that we are facing unprecedented challenges, notably climate change. But, I think there's a balance to be struck. People need to feel they can do something, that they can act to change the situation. Maybe they also need to be a little bit frightened or shaken before they start thinking that way. We need to talk up the positives in the world, and the fact that we do change, and we do learn, and we do adapt, and that Malthus has been wrong, so far. We do tend to muddle through and find ways to produce more food for ourselves, for example.

I read, for example, a piece the other day by Stephen Buranyi in *The Guardian*, saying the vaccines are working.[8] The good news is, the vaccines are working. Let's hang on to that. I think it's important to talk up the positives.

MCKAY: You could say, optimistically, that the pandemic has knit us together far more profoundly as one humanity. In many ways, western hubris—our sense of being so much better than everybody else—has been sort of knocked down several pegs. We have enormous lessons to learn from the rest of the world.

SPINNEY: Then there's a bit of good news buried in that as well. Now we have been through Covid, the next generations will have a chance of facing the next pandemic better in our countries because they've been through this one. So, I'm not saying it's good we had a pandemic, but I am saying there is a silver lining.

AN INTERVIEW WITH
NAOMI KLEIN
17 FEBRUARY 2022

Since *No Logo* in 1999, Naomi Klein has been a must-read for everybody interested in how our planet and its peoples have been transformed by neoliberal capitalism. *The Shock Doctrine* (2007) focused on how, in conditions of socioeconomic turmoil, elites are able to implement far-reaching plans that *seem* to be responses to crisis but in fact work to secure their own narrow interests. *This Changes Everything: Capitalism Versus the Climate* (2014) picked up this theme, emphasizing how a neoliberal order was, in effect, "now at war with many forms of life on earth, including human life."[1] This theme is also echoed by Pope Francis in his most recent writings,[2] which is indicative of Naomi's global reach. *No Is Not Enough: Resisting the New Shock Politics and Winning the World We Need* (2017) emphasizes the need for progressives to break free from the forces that lock them into the reigning economic paradigm but also to enunciate a positive vision of the world we might create. Naomi has recently brought out a book aimed at a younger audience, *How to Change Everything: The Young Human's Guide to Protecting the Planet And Each Other* (2021). *On Fire: The Burning Case for A Green New Deal* (2020), her seventh major book, focuses closely on climate change as a "civilizational crisis"—one that calls into question humankind's commitment to growth-at-any-price.

MCKAY: I recently reread many of my voluminous notes on your work and was struck by both the continuities and changes within it. To what extent, your conservative critics ask, is your entire movement simply a "green Trojan Horse" whose belly is full of "red Marxist socioeconomic doctrine"? "Green is the new red," complains one of Margaret Thatcher's closest collaborators, Nigel Lawson.[3] Do these critics have a point? Would it be accurate to discern in your work a growing emphasis on critiquing capitalism as an economic system?

Can you offer us your own description of your intellectual journey from *No Logo* to *How to Change Everything*?

KLEIN: Well, I can try. I definitely see continuities between my books, in the sense that I try to follow my research where it leads me. Each book ends with me at a certain place and then it becomes a little bit unsatisfying. I end up trying to resolve the contradictions of the last book in the next one.

I think you can see that most clearly in the relationship between *The Shock Doctrine* and *This Changes Everything*, in the sense that *The Shock Doctrine* is about a right-wing strategy of exploiting states of shock as an antidemocratic tool. When I released *The Shock Doctrine* in 2007, we had a little film that went with it. The slogan of that film was: "Information is shock resistance, arm yourselves." I think I had this sort of arrogant idea that if we understood that these very unpopular policies get smuggled in under cover of crisis—then just knowing that would be armour against this cynical tactic. As I said, that was 2007. In 2008, the financial crisis happened. A lot of people understood that that crisis was being exploited in order to further enrich elites and to push through privatization and deregulation. The slogan on the streets of Europe was, "We will not pay for your crisis." But—they *did* pay for the crisis of the bankers.

I think puzzling through why that was is what made me start thinking about—well, as the title of another of my books says, *No Is Not Enough*. It's not enough just to say no to their bad ideas. We need our own crisis strategies. We need our own solutions to crisis. So, that's what set me off on the journey to write *This Changes Everything*.

We need solutions on the scale of the crises. And that is what I think a Green New Deal is. That is what I think a systemic response to the climate crisis is. And so, that's the argument I made in *This Changes Everything*.

I think there's another way of seeing how my ideas progressed. The first few books I wrote were really critiques of neoliberal capitalism. *No Logo* was. And *The Shock Doctrine* was an alternative history of how we ended up with neoliberalism around the world—this extreme form of capitalism. It's gone by many names, and I make an argument that shocks and crises played a role in advancing the neoliberal revolution.

When I set off to write *This Changes Everything*, I thought it was also going to be a book about neoliberalism and capitalism, but as you quoted in your very kind introduction, Ian, the book doesn't only talk about the neoliberal stage of capitalism and how it is at war with life on earth. It talks about the growth imperative at the heart of capitalism, neoliberal or Keynesian (although Keynes argued for a steady state). In following my research, it became clear to me that this was not just a clash about neoliberalism but the growth imperative itself.

Another aspect is that in state-centralized "socialisms"—socialism in quotes, because I think there's definitely a strong argument to be had about whether or not there really was socialism in the Soviet Union—we also find a war with life on earth, and I think that's important to acknowledge as well.

MCKAY: What would you say to the "Trojan Horse" charge?

KLEIN: That we're green on the outside and red on the inside? We're all red on the inside!

What I would say is that the research I did that led to the writing of *No Logo* was about the ways capitalism sacrifices both workers and ecologies to pursue short-term growth. A few of its examples were the sweatshops producing our disposable consumer goods, but also the Niger Delta and what Shell had done there. It wasn't a book that was engaging with climate change specifically, but it was engaging with localized ecological "sacrifice zones."

The argument at the time that you would hear from boosters of neoliberalism in the 1990s was: "Okay, yes, these places are being polluted and these people are working under terrible conditions, but eventually it's going to lead to so much growth and so much prosperity that the benefits are just going to trickle down and benefit everybody. A rising tide will lift all boats." In fact, what has happened is that the sacrifice zones of the capitalist project have expanded from those localized impacts on those places to the planet itself.

I'm not trying to hide anything. I really have a critique of capitalism that extends from the local to the global. Think of that quote from Thatcher's former chancellor, Nigel Lawson. It's not coincidental that it comes from the man who shepherded in the idea that "there is no alternative to privatization and deregulation." He is the one who has an ideology that is incapable of squaring with the reality of what is happening with our planet. He has become one of the major climate change deniers in the world. You can't believe in privatization and deregulation and growth at all costs and also acknowledge what is happening with our planet's life-support systems.

MCKAY: Along with Andreas Malm, you enunciate what you call an "inconvenient truth"—that is, there is no time for gradualism. As you write, "when you have gone as badly off course as we have, moderate actions don't lead to moderate outcomes, they lead to dangerously radical ones."[4] Do you agree with Malm that, as COP26 seemingly illustrated in late 2021, the many international conferences on climate change have essentially failed, and now humanity requires a much more militant environmental movement? Or, as you put it so brilliantly in *This Changes Everything*, "the only thing rising faster than our emissions is the output of words pledging to lower them?"[5] How, in the 2020s, do we build opposition movements able to do more than "burn bright and burn out," in your words?[6] Can the momentum of 2019 be regained?

KLEIN: I agree with Andreas in the sense that I was reading some of the reports after COP26, the conference of the parties (the parties to the UN climate convention), and everybody acknowledged it was completely inadequate. But you saw headlines saying, "It Was a Good Start." If you find yourself saying that something is a "good start," and that something is called "COP26"—as in, it has happened twenty-six years in a row—there's something badly amiss, right? We're not at the starting point. We are twenty-six COPs in. We're still patting ourselves on the back for our tiny little gains, even as the impacts are no longer off in the distance but are banging down the doors.

I'm speaking to you from BC, and it's just hard to describe to folks who are not on the West Coast what we've lived through in these past months. We are not located in the most vulnerable climate geography—certainly Pacific islands, the Arctic, parts of Africa are more directly affected—but when it comes to North America, we've been living with these staccato climate events, from the heat dome in June [2021] (the deadliest weather event in Canadian history, six hundred people died in a week, and the estimates are now that ten billion marine creatures also died: these were mussels, clams, and barnacles, and this is the food of the seabirds). Then comes the "atmospheric river." We're learning all these new words—"pineapple express" and "heat dome," and it's just been extraordinary.

We don't need a "good start." We need transformative action. There's no doubt that our movements have failed to produce it. It's not just the COPs that have failed. We've all failed.

Now, I don't know that I agree with Andreas that the missing piece is sabotage, as he's been arguing. I think our movement needs to become broader. I think it needs to become more militant, in the sense of general strikes.

You talked about regaining the momentum of 2019. I think the student youth strikes were incredible, but the youth strikes were never going to be enough. The slogan of the 2014 climate march was "to change everything, it takes everybody." And we've never really had a really broad coalition of social movements, truly engaged. And the missing piece, frankly—more than any other—has been organized labour. Most of the large trade unions have had a much more ambivalent relationship with the kind of transformational climate action we really do need. The hopes of something like a Green New Deal is that the job creation potential and measures like a wage guarantee, a benefits guarantee, a jobs guarantee—that these can be enough to capture the imagination of workers and their representatives so they will fight for it. I don't think it is just going to be a vanguard that's going to win the kind of transformation we need.

MCKAY: Looking at your book for a teenage audience, *How to Change Everything*, I was wondering if that perhaps reflected your sense that it is the young who stand a chance of really transforming the world. *On Fire* has a lot on Greta Thunberg and her gift for unvarnished truth-telling, while also reflecting on the besuited bureaucrats who "clapped and filmed her on their smartphones as if she were a novelty act."[7] Hers was a transnational youth movement in 2019 with perhaps two thousand youth climate strikes in 125 countries, with around 1.6 million young people joining in. And then came the pandemic. And what seemed a movement ready to take on the world really went into reverse.

Does this recent history, and perhaps earlier ones from the 1960s or the '80s, illustrate both the strengths, but also maybe some of the limitations, of a generational emphasis? Do we need something more than a multitude of grassroots movements led by the young? And is it even fair to ask young people to bear this planet-saving burden?

KLEIN: Well, I'll start with the last part of that really important question first. "Is it fair?" It's *not* fair. In championing this extraordinary youth movement, I'm very clear that my generation, generations older than me, those between my generation and the youth strikers—we *all* have to get involved, and we all need to do our parts. One of my minor claims to fame, Ian, is that I sent On Fire to Jane Fonda, when it was still in galleys, and her response was to go get herself arrested every week in Washington. I think the message is very clear: young people are taking extraordinary risks. They are not saying, "We've got this." They're saying, "Show up with us! Do your part!" We all have pieces in this ecosystem. There's no possible replacement for youth energy, but we need intergenerational movements.

One of the most powerful movements I've been a part of in recent years was against the Dakota Access Pipeline. When I was at Standing Rock, what was most striking to me was that it was the most intergenerational movement space I'd ever been in. There really was a role for everybody. I think we have to take that lesson. It really does take everyone.

I think it's too soon to talk about the youth climate movement in the past tense. I have to push back a little bit on that. I think people have had a tough pandemic, as we all have, but I think it's been particularly hard for young people to cope with the isolation and the difficulty of organizing and the weight of the pandemic on top of the climate crisis. There's a lot of grief. But I believe this generation is going to be able to get their fire back. I have a lot of faith in Spring.

One thing I would just say about Greta that I love: there is a new version of Greta that we saw in Glasgow, which is the "blah blah blah" Greta,[8] which is her response to all of those selfies and the way she was paraded around and invited to partake in this weird kind of "tell us how bad we are" ritual, like some sort of political S&M. "Come and tell us how we're failing, and we'll all get our pictures taken with you." And she completely turned the tables on these leaders and refused to play the role of the innocent, pleading with leaders to (please, this time) really listen to her. She just mocks them mercilessly—all of their pledges. And I think her "blah blah blah" speech is the greatest piece of oratory, certainly that I've seen from her, but potentially that I've seen in twenty years. I think it will be studied—it is so brilliant. The way she snuck in on them. At first they thought she was praising them, right? They're kind of clapping as she says, "Build Back Better"—and then she says, "blah blah blah—green economy, blah blah blah . . ." And then she says, "You're not going to save us—we are going to save us." And I think this is a turning point. I think this generation now understands that it isn't going to be the perfect speech to the EU or to the UN that's going to suddenly make these leaders see the light. It's really about building outside power. This story is still being written, I believe.

MCKAY: Your pandemic journalism underlines the message of *The Shock Doctrine*, asking whether all the computer-facilitated discipline we've been subjected to over the past two years will be constrained by democratic oversight—or "will it be rolled out in a state-of-exception frenzy without asking critical questions that will shape our lives for decades to come?" You theorize that the pandemic has been grasped by corporations as a "living laboratory for the permanent and highly profitable no-touch future," which you ironically term "the *screen* new deal." Public schools, universities, hospitals are facing existential questions about their futures. You write, "well before Covid-19, Silicon Valley had an agenda of replacing so many of our personal body experiences by inserting technology in the middle of them."[9] In our years of Covid-19, a principal driver of this transformation has been the state. Does that complicate a narrative that, since *No Logo*, has focused intently on how corporations are transforming our lives? Hasn't the state also revealed itself to be quite capable of its own shock doctrines?

KLEIN: Well, I think there has always been a kind of corporatist collaboration between the state and large multinational corporations. You always need that kind of partnership if you're going to change laws, and what I describe in *The Shock Doctrine* are governments working at the behest of large corporations.

In the piece you're talking about, I was reporting on then New York governor Cuomo collaborating with Google's Eric Schmidt and Michael Bloomberg and Bill Gates to reimagine New York State. Now, thankfully, Cuomo is no longer governor. And organized labour was able to push back on some of the plans they were trying to rush through.

Cuomo was giving speeches at that time, arguing, "Why do we even need classrooms? Why do we even need teachers?" It was similar to what happened after hurricanes that I've reported on, like after Hurricane Katrina when the school system was radically reinvented. It became a laboratory for the charter school system. Same thing happened after Hurricane Maria, where they closed hundreds of schools in Puerto Rico and reversed a law that banned charter schools.

During Covid, we're seeing something quite different. To be honest with you, it's been a little tricky for me. I did write a book about how governments exploit states of emergencies. I do believe we are seeing that. We also are at a time of peak conspiracy theory and misinformation. So, a lot of my ideas are being put into a banana blender. They're being used and abused and being taken places where they really don't belong. They're being used by people who are denying that Covid is real.

I don't like Bill Gates, but I don't like Bill Gates because he has way too much influence over public health. Bill Gates has interfered to protect the patents of drug companies, to keep vaccines that should be available to everyone on earth from being distributed. Bill Gates intervened to say, "No, Pfizer should keep their patents and Moderna should keep their patents." So, he's played a really terrible role. But there are lots of people who are out there claiming Bill Gates is doing all this because he wants to depopulate the earth and the vaccines have tracking devices. It's become part of the tidal wave of misinformation in the context of Covid-19.

It's a new ball game. Conspiracies are always part of disaster ecosystems. After Katrina, you had this kind of disaster opportunism that I call "the Shock Doctrine." It was so convenient for the rich who wanted to clear out the public housing and gentrify New Orleans. You had conspiracy theories that claimed, "Well maybe they blew up the levees to do this on purpose."

I heard the same thing when I was covering the Asian Tsunami. It was so convenient for real estate developers who seized the beaches from the small-boat fishing people. People started saying the whole tsunami was caused by an underground nuclear weapons explosion by the United States, and they did the whole thing so they could have a military occupation. But these things didn't go totally viral in the way the pandemic conspiracies go viral.

Steve Bannon's strategy—which he described to Michael Lewis—is to "flood the zone with shit."[10] The strategy is to make people doubt any kind of fact. So you don't believe anything at all. And if nothing is true, then anything is possible. It creates a very malleable political moment for people to exploit. And what's interesting about the anti-mask and antivax crowd is that, in the US, they've provided incredible cover to the people who want to privatize the school system. So, this same thing that I covered after Katrina, after Maria, is happening in Arizona, in Florida.

Now, the wedge is: "Well, if you don't want your kid to go to school with a mask, you should be able to get a voucher"—which is the same thing they asked for after Katrina, the same thing they asked for after Hurricane Maria. "Parents should be able to get vouchers, so if they don't want their kids to go to schools that are either doing remote learning or requiring vaccines or masks, they should be able to spend that money in private school." So, they're using the pandemic in the same way they use every single disaster—to wage war on public education. Now, they're not just using the pandemic, they're using the misinformation about the pandemic. It's a whole new kind of shock doctrine.

MCKAY: Sounds like it might be a book for you.

KLEIN: I am writing the book [laughter].

MCKAY: One major thrust of left discourse in the pandemic has been that many more such calamities lie in our future, because capitalism has fundamentally disrupted humankind's metabolism with the natural world. So, we think of deforestation, frenzied infrastructure construction, the uprooting of vast peasant populations and their relegation to insalubrious slums, all happening alongside global climate change. Since the 1970s, these have all combined, meaning that we have been living in an Age of Pandemics, as geographer Mike Davis and epidemiologist Rob Wallace have argued. Now, I don't sense this would be a message dramatically out of line with your lifetime of research and writing. Yet, apart from one passage in *On Fire*, this line of inquiry is not really a prominent feature of your work. In *This Changes Everything*, you write that climate change is delivering a "powerful message spoken in the language of fires, floods, droughts, and extinctions."[11] Would you consider it a friendly, or unfriendly, amendment to add "pandemics" to that list of calamities?

KLEIN: Well, I'd hesitate to call the pandemics friendly, but I would certainly agree that they belong on the list. It's an area I have not written about enough. I had a little bit in *The Shock Doctrine* about the disaster of the Tamiflu profiteering that went on under the Bush administration. Donald Rumsfeld, before he became Secretary of Defense, was the CEO of Gilead. He was in the business of producing the key responses to pandemics, and this became one of the examples of disaster profiteering that I documented in *The Shock Doctrine*. And I did add a new forward about Covid to the paperback version of *On Fire*.

And we made a little film, Avi Lewis, my partner, and Molly Crabapple and I, with Alexandria Ocasio-Cortez, a few years ago called *Message from the Future* that told the story, set from the standpoint of a couple of decades into the future, of how we won a Green New Deal. And during the pandemic, we started thinking about doing a sequel to that called *A Message from the Future to the Years of Repair II*.[12] The concept was, what if Covid is a teacher?

MCKAY: Your video seems to agree that we're on the verge of many more pandemics if we don't change the way we live.

KLEIN: There's no doubt of that. What we call for in that video are the real investments that make a society able to weather shocks. You can't put everything on a vaccine mandate. You need to invest in the infrastructure of care (or what we call the infrastructure of care and repair). There have been some great pieces written about this. One, cowritten by Judy Rebick, is about Canada's pandemic response.[13]

In the early days, we did pay people to stay home, but we didn't invest in a community care core. We didn't invest in outdoor education. We didn't make the big infrastructure investments that would have made it possible for people to gather more safely in schools or make our hospitals more resilient. It's just been "the vaccine, the vaccine, the vaccine." This has created an atmosphere that is very ripe for conspiracy theories because people are seeing the huge profits that are being won by a small group of people. It doesn't feel right, so they're looking for explanations. We are going to be seeing more shocks. But that doesn't mean we need to respond in the ways we've been responding. There are ways that we can come together in crisis.

MCKAY: My last question. A dual citizen, born in Montreal, now returned from New Jersey—and welcome home—and resident in British Columbia, you have undoubtedly introduced tens of thousands of young Canadians to progressive environmentalist thought. *On Fire* repeatedly underlines the moral contradictions of our prime minister, who is green-sounding but also pipeline-addicted. And your *Leap Manifesto* caught the eye of Canada's New Democratic Party. Yet, when it comes to *On Fire*, I found the central historical metaphors or analogies—the New Deal and the Marshall Plan—are drawn from the repertoire of US politics of the 1930s and '40s. Now, is there a risk that disregarding national specifics and foregrounding US models inadvertently strengthens some of the colonial relationships of which you are so critical? As someone with rare insights into working on both sides of the border, do you think the next left should work harder to adapt its universal message of human survival to the national contexts in which that message is being articulated?

KLEIN: It's a great question. As a writer, I work with what I have. I'm not inventing this from scratch, and so the decision to call it a "New Deal" was a decision that was made by the Sunrise Movement and the Squad, particularly Alexandria Ocasio-Cortez. It had a lot of traction. The call for a Marshall Plan for Planet Earth actually came from Bolivia, and I was quoting Angelica Navarro, Bolivia's climate and trade negotiator in 2009. As you point out, when we did our own version of this in Canada, we called it "The Leap." We didn't call it a Green New Deal or a Marshall Plan or the Green Industrial Revolution (which is what they call it in the UK). We called it The Leap. And then we got slammed. We were called Maoists.

We weren't modelling it on the Great Leap Forward.[14] But, we were very specific when we had the gathering that led to the writing of the *Leap Manifesto* that we didn't want to appeal to nostalgia. We didn't want to appeal to a Canada that never was because a lot of the left then—the white left in Canada—had sort of fetishized postwar Canada as a moment that we need to return to. It hasn't really reckoned with the exclusions and the violence of that era.

One of the things we are most challenged by, as we organize in the rubble of neoliberalism, is a powerful sense among a lot of people that there's something in human nature that makes it impossible for us to do big things together, that we're just too selfish. That's where I think these drawings on historical precedence are useful, whether it's Canada's own experience during the Second World War or the Civilian Conservation Corps in the US that hired two million young people, planted two billion trees, built eight hundred state parks, and did that in the 1930s. That happened. So, it isn't "human nature" that says we can't do things at that speed and scale again.

QUESTION FROM THE AUDIENCE: How do you feel that neoliberalism has changed or evolved over the past thirty years? What is it today that it wasn't in 1992?

KLEIN: That's such an interesting question. The history of capitalism is a history of enclosure. It's a history of bringing swaths of life that are outside of the market and enclosing them inside the logic of the market—and in the process, transforming them. Once something is within the logic of the market, what it needs to do is completely different. If we think about enclosures of land in the British countryside, it isn't just that a fence was put around previously communal farmland where people who lived around that land used to be able to graze their animals, were able to collect firewood. It's that the role of that land also changed, and it now had to yield crops. So, it's both enclosed and changed.

I would say that the history of neoliberalism is a history of a whole new kind of enclosure that began with enclosing parts of the state that had been kept outside of the reach of the market, like education and health care, and bringing them in.

Where we're at now is so radical because what's being enclosed is us and our relationships. (Enclosing human beings within capital is not new—that's what slavery is. It's turning free human life into a commodity, in the most violent way imaginable.) What we're seeing with surveillance, what Shoshanna Zubov calls "surveillance capitalism"[15] or Nick Couldrey and Ulises A. Mejias called "data colonialism,"[16] is a process of enclosure whereby our friendships, our speech, this conversation are enclosed in a corporate platform (some people are watching it on Google's platform; we're having it on Zoom). The data from our conversations become a raw resource to be extracted, and then the purpose of the conversations changes. The purpose of the conversation for Google is not to facilitate us having a conversation; it's to extract the data to drive more engagement on their platforms so they can sell ads. I think that's the radical edge of what's happening with neoliberalism.

MCKAY: You have that really brilliant analysis of Donald Trump, and his whole family, as a brand.[17] That made me really think that one of the most distinctive things about the changes of neoliberalism since the 1990s has just been that emphasis on branding, taken to be a kind of psychological imperative for each and every one of us. We're supposed to be branding ourselves all the time. It's is, as you say, a radical extension of traditional capitalism.

KLEIN: We are supposed to self-commodify, and do.

QUESTION FROM THE AUDIENCE: What are your thoughts about corporate capitalism creating more emerging diseases and viruses, as long as it continues to destroy nature?

KLEIN: I think that the history of zoonotic diseases would support that claim. There are still debates about the origin of Covid-19, but I think we do know that, as we encroach more and more on wild lands, on the homes of animals, we have more human/animal interfaces, and more opportunities for viruses to jump from animals to humans.

QUESTION FROM THE AUDIENCE: No one is talking about the austerity measures that will surely happen once the pandemic is behind us. What can be done to prepare to fight against them?

KLEIN: Such a great question. I think we're starting to see overloaded hospitals as an excuse for backdoor kinds of privatizations (or partial privatizations) of health care. But I think what you're referring to is the fact that we've seen some huge spending and we're seeing some inflation. These are the conditions under which some of the most brutal austerity measures have been imposed in the history of neoliberalism. So, we must be prepared for that.

This comes back to why we need a broad-based left. It's not just a climate movement. We need a *left*, and we can't all just be in our silos because only a very broad coalition could have the ability to really stage strikes and get the attention of political leaders.

MCKAY: I was wondering about your prognostications for the decade to come. People are just so exhausted—they're so sick of this. Many are bereaved and mourning loved ones. To me, it doesn't strike me as a likely base for an energetic movement of resistance. Do you have a prediction that you'd like to offer?

KLEIN: I think we have a right to a pandemic dividend, and I think we need ambitious movement leaders who demand it and inspire us. And I think we need artists to help revive our spirits after this period of trying to weather these shocks alone. We're in the uncharted territories.

You're a historian, I'm not. While certainly humans have gone through great difficulties before, I think the technology-enabled isolation of Covid is unique: to be two years as separate from one another as possible. So, my hope is that the thrill of being able to be together after such sort of unnatural separation—because we are social beings, we are social animals—will be such that we will be overcome with energy. As depleted as we feel right now, we will be energized by being in each other's company. There's a fantastic role for artists to help give us the soundtrack and the inspiration to alchemize the grief into something energetic.

QUESTION FROM THE AUDIENCE: Do you see fascism creeping into the neoliberal project? A lot of left analysts are talking about imminent fascism and the great debate on the left focuses on the question, is this classical fascism? How does it differ? So, do you see a risk of fascism in our present moment?

KLEIN: I definitely see a risk of eco-fascism. I see a risk of the climate crisis being folded into a narrative around "great replacement" fears and white supremacy, creating an even more toxic cocktail than climate change denial. It's one thing to deny climate change. It's another thing to say, "Okay it's happening, but we need to fortify our countries and our borders and maybe the outsiders should die."

You have a sort of convergence of wellness worlds with the conspiracy and far-right worlds. It's really terrifying because you'll hear things like: "Well, I have a great immune system" and "I take care of myself, so why should I have to sacrifice for all these people who aren't taking care of themselves? Maybe they should die." This is a fascist worldview. Frankly, I see it spreading quickly and in areas that are surprising, like in yoga studios (not all of them). "Conspirituality": a coming together of the wellness world with far-right QAnon worlds. It's a real thing.

QUESTION FROM THE AUDIENCE: How can citizens demand change when the government has been subverted to corporations?

KLEIN: This is not new. Our governments have been doing the bidding of corporations now for a very long time. We have found ways to come together and stand up and out-organize our opponents. We have stopped trade deals before and we have won huge victories for the public good, but there is no substitute for truly broad-based organizing, with a willingness to take action. It isn't just about voicing our opinions. It's actually about interrupting business as usual, withholding labour.

AN INTERVIEW WITH

NOAM CHOMSKY

4 OCTOBER 2021

Throughout his entire academic life, Noam Chomsky has used his knowledge, skills, and stature as a public intellectual to advocate for radical social and economic changes in societies that have failed to live up to the promises and ideals of a socially just society.[1] Professor Chomsky has rightly argued that intellectuals, artists, educators, cultural workers, and others have a responsibility to address grave social problems such as the threat of nuclear war, ecological devastation, and the sharp deterioration of democracy. He is well aware that oppression feeds on mass apathy and manufactured ignorance. In response, his academic work and public interventions have become a model for enriching public life and addressing economic inequality, needless wars, and class and racial injustices. He has worked tirelessly to inspire individuals in social movements to unleash the energy, the insights, and the passion necessary to keep alive the spirit, promises, and ideals of a radical democracy. As a public intellectual and border-crosser, he draws upon a wide variety of disciplinary fields and pushes at the frontiers of the public imagination while reminding us of the need to feel and act upon a passion for a commitment to a free, just, and equal society.

He rightly insists that, in the end, there is no democracy without informed citizens and no justice without a language critical of injustice. He has made clear that we live in dangerous times and that there's an urgent need for more individuals, institutions, and social movements to come together in the belief that the current regimes of tyranny can be resisted, that alternative futures are possible, and that acting on those beliefs through collective resistance will enable social change to happen. Professor Chomsky's work is infused with a vision that merges a sense of moral outrage with the need for civic courage and collective action. His work is more indispensable than ever because the world is more dangerous than ever. I believe that the great playwright Arthur Miller captures the spirit of Noam's work when he wrote, "Writers speak the unspeakable . . . making life possible for those who come after."

CHOMSKY: My talk tonight is entitled: "Rethinking the Civic Imagination and Manufactured Ignorance in The Post-Pandemic World."

You probably know about the Fermi Paradox, posed by the great physicist Enrico Fermi. It's very brief. The paradox is: "Where are they?" His discipline of astrophysics demonstrates that there are a vast number of planets accessible to us with conditions similar enough to earth so that they should be able to support life, over time, intelligent life—maybe even super-intelligent life. So—where are they? With the most diligent search, we cannot find the slightest hint of their existence.

Well, one answer that's been offered, in a kind of morbid jest, is that they're out there, but when they came across humans, they decided to get away from that crazy place as quickly as possible. I could see some justification for that. Another answer in the same vein (but more serious) is that intelligent life in fact developed but proved to be a lethal mutation and quickly destroyed itself. Actually, we know of only one case—humans on earth. We are a new species, only a few hundred thousand years old. That's a blink of an eye in evolutionary time. And we seem to be intent on establishing the thesis.

There have been reasons for such suspicions since August 1945, when we learned that human intelligence had devised the means for self-annihilation. Not quite yet—but it was clear that the day was not far off when technology would reach that point. And it did, a few years later in 1953, when the United States and then the Soviet Union exploded thermonuclear weapons. In acknowledgement of this achievement of human intelligence, the hands of the famous Doomsday Clock—which seeks to encapsulate the world's security situation—were advanced to two minutes to midnight. Midnight is termination. Well, the hands have oscillated since. They did not reach two minutes to midnight again until halfway through the Trump administration. In its final years, the analysts abandoned minutes altogether and shifted to seconds. We're now at one hundred seconds to midnight. Let's take a closer look at what leads to these conclusions.

We are currently facing a confluence of severe crises, something that has never happened before in the brief period of human history. To each of these crises, we know of feasible solutions. In each case, we are rejecting the solutions and racing to the precipice, some of us more rapidly than others.

To be more precise: it is not *we* who are racing to the precipice. Rather, it is those whom Adam Smith called "the masters of mankind."[2] In his day, that was the merchants and manufacturers of England. In our day, it's multinational corporations, financial institutions, other concentrations of private power—and the governments that are, in no small measure, at their service.

On the matter of service to the masters, the evidence is compelling. Illustrative cases feature regularly on the front pages. Right now, for example, as you know, US Congress is debating a major program that, among other things, may be the last chance for the United States to take serious steps to arrest catastrophic global warming. The fate of this measure is largely in the hands of the chairman of the Senate Energy and Natural Resources Committee, who happens to be the champion of Congress in receiving funds from fossil fuel industries. He's now demanding sole jurisdiction in the Senate over the $150 billion clean electricity performance programs. That's Joe Manchin. And he can get what he wants. The Senate is split. The Republicans' half is 100 percent opposed to dealing with the climate crisis. So, the fate of the legislation rests on unity among Democrats. The chief recipient of fossil fuel funding, a Democrat, can ensure that nothing will be done to harm his donors. And he's clear about it. His official position is "innovation but not elimination": no cut-back on fossil fuel use. That's straight from the handbook of the ExxonMobil public relations department. If the denialist party returns to power next year, as well they may, we will be back to racing to the abyss as quickly as possible, picking up from the disastrous Trump years. Well, that may seem like this is an aberration. Just one case.

It's not—and the history is revealing. The Republicans were not always a denialist party. In 2008, when John McCain was running, they were moving towards mild (insufficient but mild) global warming legislation. Their shift to total commitment to cataclysm results directly from fossil fuel funding, specifically the juggernaut deployed by the huge Koch Brothers' energy conglomerate. When it sensed signs that the Republicans were veering towards recognizing that we are destroying the prospects for survival of organized human life on earth and harming short-term profits for the masters, the juggernaut cut the heresy off completely. Decisively. All Republicans turned and haven't changed.

Now that's not an aberration either. There's a good deal of research in mainstream academic political science that has demonstrated a remarkably close correlation between electability and campaign funding—specifically, strategic, business-based campaign funding. And similar scholarship has independently established an immediate corollary of this: namely, a large majority of voters are literally unrepresented. There is no correlation between their views and the votes of their representatives. The representatives are listening to different voices, as they must if they hope to be re-elected.

Well, it's called democracy. Blocking legislation that would harm the fossil fuel industry is not a malady specific to the United States. It's worldwide.

Let's consider what's happening right now, again on the front pages. As we meet, governments of the world are pressuring oil producers to increase production. *Increase* production. They've just been advised in the August 2021 report of the Intergovernmental Panel on Climate Change, by far the most dire yet, that catastrophe is looming unless we begin immediately to reduce fossil fuel use—year by year, effectively phasing it out by mid-century. Petroleum industry journals are euphoric about the discovery of new fields to exploit as demand for oil increases. The business press debates whether the US fracking industry or OPEC is best placed to increase production. You can readily add examples from where you're sitting.

They all know they are racing to catastrophe. We don't have to instruct them. They know it very well. Furthermore, at least if they're minimally literate, they all know there are feasible solutions to the climate crisis that will, furthermore, create a more livable world.

But profit for the rich and political expediency come first. Come first, that is, for the masters and their servants. What about the general population? Well, that's a complex story.

Let's take Joe Manchin of West Virginia, a coal mining state. Not long ago, it was a bastion of working-class militancy. The United Mine Workers, representing the coal miners in West Virginia and elsewhere, recently adopted a program, a transition program, that would shift production towards renewable energy, with better jobs and better lives. All feasible and worked out in detail. But those are *people*, not the masters—their bitter enemy in their relentless class war. Their masters have a different view. Their class war, this one-sided class war, has been continuing with mounting intensity in the past forty years of the neoliberal assault on the population.

That merits a few words. Let's go back to the 1930s. That happens to be my childhood; I remember very well. The world was facing serious crises. There were several ways out. Continental Europe turned to fascism. In the United States, a rising militant working class, with a sympathetic president, turned to social democracy—the New Deal. Later, postwar Europe moved in the same direction. That led to what in Europe is called the *Trente Glorieuses*—the thirty glorious years—and what economists call the "golden age" of capitalism in the United States. The fastest growth rate in history, egalitarian growth rate, for the lowest quintile did as well as the highest quintile. Plenty of flaws—but economically, socially, it was an enormous success.

The business world resisted from the first moment. But, until the 1970s, they were unable to reverse the course. By the late 1970s, under Carter in the United States, the business offensive was making progress. In 1978, the president of the United Auto Workers, Doug Fraser, withdrew from a Carter-initiated management/labour board. He withdrew and condemned the business leaders (I'm quoting him) "for having chosen to wage a one-sided class war in this country. A war against working people, the unemployed, the poor, the minorities, the very young and the very old, and even many in the middle class of our society."[3] And having broken and discarded the fragile unwritten compact previously existing during a period of growth and progress, the New Deal years, under Reagan and Thatcher in the early 1980s, the one-sided class war took off, full steam.

The first acts were to smash unions using illegal methods, like deploying strike breakers, opening the door to the corporate sector and inviting them to follow suit. Such tactics were very effective over the years and severely weakened the unions. They understood (or at least their planners understood) that it was imperative to deprive working people of the main means of defence against what was to come. And for those with eyes open, what was to come was *never* in doubt.

Go back to Reagan's inaugural address. His main principle is "the government is the problem, not the solution," meaning decisions have to be taken out of the hands of government. They don't disappear. They go somewhere else. They go to concentrations of private power. That's a great advantage. The government has a flaw: it's partially responsive to the general population. Concentrated private power is totally unaccountable. So, it's a much better basis for decision-making. This was amplified by the economic guru of the neoliberal assault, Milton Friedman. He came out with his principal articles, giving as his credo, "corporations have no responsibility to the public, only to maximizing profit" (and of course salaries for management.)

So, put that together. Decisions are shifted from the government (partially responsive to the population) to unaccountable private tyrannies (which have no accountability and are responsible only for maximizing their own profit and the salaries of CEOs and management). Doesn't take a genius to figure out what's going to happen. And, in fact, after forty years, even the mainstream institutions are starting to take a look.

So, the super-respectable (quasi-governmental) Rand Corporation recently did a study of what they politely call "the transfer of wealth" from the middle-class and the working-class lower 90 percent of the population to the very top. When you look closely, it's mostly to the top fraction of 1 percent of the population. Their estimate is about fifty trillion dollars in forty years. It's not small change. And that's a vast *underestimate*. They did not take into account the other means of robbing the public that were developed when Reagan and Thatcher opened the spigot and said, "Rob as much as you like."

You can read about the *Pandora Papers*, a huge trove of papers, showing how the ultrarich use various gimmicks (that were illegal prior to Reagan) to stash away huge amounts of money in places where they don't have to pay taxes. It's only a small part of it. The world's largest trillion-dollar corporation has its offices in Ireland, paying very low tax rates. Others play the same game. All of this was illegal prior to Reagan, and the Treasury Department was conscientious in enforcing the laws.

There are many other similar devices: shell companies, changes in rules of corporate governance so CEOs can pick the board that sets their salaries. And guess what happens from that? Of course, that lifts salaries. They have skyrocketed, especially in the United States. That carries all management salaries up with it. So, you get probably seventy or eighty trillion dollars of robbery of the public, putting most of it in the hands of the top fraction of the one percent. In fact, the top 0.1 percent of the US population has increased their wealth from 10 percent to 20 percent of the total. Not quite at that extreme elsewhere—but something like it. A perfectly obvious consequence of the policies that were announced in the 1980s.

Meanwhile, for the general population: stagnation or decline. Up until the late 1970s, the minimum wage and the real wage tracked productivity. That ended with the neoliberal assault. Productivity and growth increased; wages stagnated. Wages for nonsupervisory workers are less in real terms than they were in 1979. Meanwhile services have been cut-back, under the principle that government is the problem. A majority of the population pretty much lives from pay cheque to pay cheque. Can't pay for Covid vaccinations (too much of a co-pay). Cut-back of other services. Precarious existence. Maybe you'll be called to work next week, maybe not. Maybe you'll be called for double-time. That's the result of forty years of sheer highway robbery.

Now the claim is, this has to do with markets. Not quite. What has been created is what economists call "a bailout economy." One of the things done under Reagan was to deregulate, including deregulation of the greatly expanding financial institutions. That immediately leads to crashes. What happens after a crash? The public politely comes and bails you out. And that's a fraction of it.

The government has a tacit insurance policy. It's called "too big to fail." That means that the big guys (the big financial institutions, the big banks, and so on) can get cheap credit. They can take out risky loans, which are profitable. If anything goes wrong, no problem—that's the bailout economy. So, it's markets for the poor and the working class and the middle class. But it's powerful government intervening constantly for the rich. And that's a one-sided class war. Working people and the poor are to suffer the ravages of the market. The masters have to be protected by a powerful state.

Clinton joined in with what are ludicrously called "free trade agreements," which are radically protectionist in a manner that has absolutely no precedent. It's why the prices of drugs go sky-high. Most of the world can't get vaccines. The rich countries (mainly Europe in this case) have to preserve the profits of the masters with a highly interventionist, radically protectionist, global and local system. The poor, the working class and the middle class, are thrown onto the market.

Go across the Atlantic. Thatcher was the same. Her mantra, as you remember, was "there is no society." You survive, somehow, on your own. Unless of course you're among the masters. Then, there's a very rich society. Chambers of commerce. Business roundtables. The American Legislative Exchange Council, corporate funding that imposes business-friendly programs in state legislatures that are easily manipulated and bought off. Trade associations—and more. So, a rich society for the masters. Nothing for the rest. One-sided class war.

Well, the consequences have been profound. That's quite apart from the vast highway robbery of the public. The assault has engendered anger, resentment, conspiracy theories about hidden powers that are causing your malaise, antivax movements. The United States is literally killing hundreds of thousands of people and a lot more. It's also created fertile terrain for demagogues of the Trump variety, who are capable of holding up a banner with one hand saying, "I'm your protector—I love you," while the other hand stabs you in the back. There's been one—one—legislative achievement of the Trump administration: the tax scam of 2017. Sheer robbery. Sharp cut-back of taxes for the rich corporations, imposing, of course, a higher tax burden on everyone else. But that's kind of quiet. You don't talk about that in public. There has also been a sharp attack on democracy. It's an obvious consequence of policies I've described.

Steps towards a kind of protofascism—or all the way, some analysts argue. Well, there are very sober and respected voices sounding the alarm about the possible collapse of American democracy, with dire consequences for the world. Among them are leading commentators of the world's leading business press—the London *Financial Times*—who say that the United States is being driven to autocracy, or worse, by what they call a radical party with a reactionary agenda that ranks alongside the far-right European parties with neofascist origins. I should say that all of this is tragically ironic for people whose lives have been framed by the transition from the 1930s with the US in the lead in social democracy to today, where it's in the lead and moving towards protofascism.

Well, that's a bird's-eye view of where I think we are now. It's not graven in stone. There are plenty of counterforces, with climate the most crucial issue. It's mainly the young. It's a terrible indictment of my generation when Greta Thunberg stands up at an assembly of the masters at Davos and says, "You betrayed us." She was right. The words should be seared into our conscience. It's not too late. But we do not have much time to hear these words.

Well, that's the crisis of global heating, which is actually one aspect of a much broader environmental crisis. Habitat destruction, industrialized agriculture destroying the land and much else (which feeds directly into the Covid crisis, incidentally)—the list goes on.

But let's turn to a different crisis, a comparable one. The one that was initiated seventy-five years ago. The threat of nuclear war is now growing very seriously. It's one of the reasons the Doomsday Clock is moving to seconds, not minutes. There have been slow steps for sixty years towards an arms control regime that would limit the threat of nuclear war. It has been virtually dismantled by this century's radical party with a reactionary agenda, the Republican Party. George W. Bush took time off from invading countries to destroy the ABM treaty; Trump's wrecking ball took care of most of the rest (though Biden was able to rescue the new START treaty hours before it was to expire, accepting finally Russian offers to extend it). The US is, of course, far in the lead in global military power and swamps all potential adversaries combined. It's also well ahead in the mad race to develop even more dangerous weapons and to extend the yearning for global suicide. The US has incomparable security. It's not the way it's perceived in high places—threats everywhere. The gravest perceived threat to the US is China. That deserves some thought.

The China threat is very well-described by the distinguished international diplomat Paul Keating, former prime minister of Australia, right within the reach of the dragon's claws. I'll quote his words: "The threat of China is the fact that, somehow, the rise of 20% of humanity from abject poverty into something approaching a modern state, is illegitimate—but more than that, by its mere presence, it is an affront to the United States. It's not that China presents a threat to the United States, something China has never articulated or delivered—rather its mere presence represents a challenge to United States pre-eminence."[4]

The major point of contention right now is "freedom of navigation" in the South China Sea—or that's the way it's described. It's not accurate. It's accurately described by a leading Australian strategic analyst Clinton Fernandes. As he explains, "the conflict concerns military and intelligence operations in China's exclusive economic zone which extends 200 miles offshore for every country."[5]

The United States holds that military intelligence operations are permissible in these exclusive zones. China holds they're not permissible. India agrees with China's interpretation. Recently, it protested against US military operations in its exclusive zone. These exclusive zones were established by the 1982 Law of the Sea. The United States is the only maritime power not to have ratified the law. It does say that it will not violate it. The law bans the threat or use of force in the exclusive zones. The controversy has nothing to do with freedom of navigation—which is not threatened in the least. It has to do with whether military intelligence operations constitute a threat of force. The United States says no. China and the others say yes. Well, surely this is a clear case where diplomacy is in order, not highly provocative actions like sending in a naval armada in a region of considerable tension with the threat of escalation, possibly without bounds. But it seems to be crucial to establish US pre-eminence everywhere, even off the coast of China, which we are led to believe, unlike the US, faces no threats. Consider the eight hundred military bases the United States has around the world. China has one.

The nature of the China threat is further elaborated by Australia's pre-eminent military correspondent, Brian Toohey. It's worth quoting in detail to help understand world affairs:

> China's nuclear weapons are so inferior that it couldn't be confident of deterring a retaliatory strike from the United States. Take the example of nuclear-powered missile armed submarines. China has four. Each can carry 12 missiles: each with a single warhead. The subs are easy to detect because they're noisy. According to the US Naval Office of Naval Intelligence, each is noisier than a Soviet submarine first launched in 1976. Russian and US subs are now much quieter. China is expected to acquire another four that are a little bit quieter by 2030. However, the missiles on those subs won't have the range to reach the continental United States. They would have to reach suitable locations in the Pacific

Ocean. However, they're effectively bottled up inside the South China Sea. To escape they'd have to pass through a series of US choke points where they could easily be sunk by US hunter killer nuclear submarines. ... In contrast to China, the US has 14 Ohio-class missile armed subs. Each can launch 24 Trident missiles; each containing eight independently targetable warheads, able to reach anywhere on the globe. That means a single US submarine can destroy 192 cities or other targets compared to 12 for the Chinese submarine. The Ohio class is now being replaced by the bigger and more devastating Columbia class.[6]

The US is now sending Australia advanced hunter killer nuclear subs, which Australia will pay for. So, they'll be incorporated in the US naval command. This sale of advanced nuclear subs abrogates an agreement between France and Australia for sale of conventional subs; it's a serious blow to French industry. Washington did not even take the trouble to notify France; it was instructing the European Union on its place in the US global order. Brian Toohey observed further that Australia's submission to the United States does not enhance its security. Quite the contrary. And he further points out that the nuclear subs sale has no discernible strategic purpose. The subs will not even be operational for probably fifteen years, by which time China will surely have expanded its military forces to deal with this new military threat.

The subagreement does serve a purpose, however: to establish more firmly that the United States intends to rule the world, even if that requires escalating the threat of war, possibly terminal nuclear war, in a highly volatile region, and of course is eschewing such specified measures as diplomacy.

Well, these steps to escalate conflict take place against a background that's plain and stark. The United States inherited the mantle of global dominance from Britain and proceeded to substantially extend its reach, becoming far more powerful than Britain ever was. China is a rising power, bound to play a major role in world affairs. The crises we all face—international pandemics, destruction of the environment—know no borders, nor does nuclear war. The US and China will either cooperate in addressing these crises or we are doomed. It's as simple as that. Cooperation is surely achievable just as the other crises we face have solutions that are within reach.

The question we face now is whether we have the will to save ourselves from cataclysm, or whether we will choose to show that higher intelligence really may be a lethal mutation, providing an unhappy answer to Fermi's Paradox.

MCKAY: My questions tonight are all based on your 2021 book *The Precipice: Neoliberalism, the Pandemic and the Urgent Need for Social Change*, brought out with C. J. Polychroniou. In it, you elaborate on the confluence of crises of extraordinary severity, with the fate of the human experiment quite literally at stake.

First of all, among some theorists critical of capitalism, there's been a recovery of a theme developed by Marx, called "the metabolic rift," that speaks to the way capitalism systematically depletes nature of elements necessary for the planet's equilibrium. For such theorists, there aren't *distinct* climate change and pandemic crises—plural—but, rather, one overall multidimensional environmental crisis stemming from the disastrous impact of capitalism upon the natural world. Do you consider this a promising line of inquiry?

CHOMSKY: I hinted that global warming is part of a much broader environmental crisis. That's the metabolic rift. Destruction of habitats, which of course enhances pandemics. Industrialized agriculture, industrialized meat production are not only savage and brutal but exert a huge effect on global warming. And something else I didn't mention: one of the crises that we're facing, not talked about much except in the medical literature, is antibiotic-resistant bacteria. We're coming to a point where going to a hospital is becoming dangerous because there are bacteria mutating that antibiotics can't deal with. Well, the drug companies don't work on that much—it's not really profitable. But cases of antibiotic-resistant bacteria are mounting. And one major reason is industrialized meat production. You cram cows, chickens, under impossible circumstances, in a tight place, diseases are going to spread. Well, you're a good capitalist. You want to maximize profit. So, what you do is pump them full of antibiotics. A huge proportion of the antibiotics that are used, are used basically for that reason. Of course, the antibiotics lead to mutation. Pretty soon, you're getting antibiotic-resistant microorganisms. It's been warned that, in another twenty or thirty years, surgery (and other advanced medical procedures) may be impossible. But you have to make money tomorrow, that's crucial. It doesn't matter what you do to the world's population, to the huge number of species that we're destroying, to animals, to the environment. You have to make profit tomorrow.

So, yes, it's a very profitable line of inquiry. But we have to remember something: time scales. That's critical. The crises we face have to be dealt with today. It's today that the leading democracies are urging the fossil fuel companies to increase production (when the leaders all know certainly that we have to start decreasing production if we hope to survive, but not if you want to improve your electoral prospects or make more profit for the drug companies). That has to be done now.

We can't wait for the capitalist system to be replaced by something more humane, just, concerned with people's needs instead of profit. We can't wait for that. And that's true of the other crises too. All of them have to be dealt with quickly. We're on the verge. They have to be dealt with now. That means working to modify the more destructive aspects of the savage capitalism of the past forty years.

It's not utopian to say we could go back to the kind of capitalism Dwight Eisenhower advocated. It's not super-utopian. In the United States, it's not utopian to say we could rise to the level of the Conservative Party in Germany. That's not a joke. Take a look at Bernie Sanders's programs. One of the editors of the *Financial Times* quipped that, in Germany, he could be running on the Christian Democrat program. It's literally true. Universal health care, free higher education—they're found all over the place. Mexico, Germany, Finland, everywhere you look. But in the United States, that's considered radical. That's part of the extraordinary power of business in the United States. It fought against the New Deal bitterly and shifted the spectrum far to the right. Well, it's not utopian to say we can overcome that. In fact, it's being battled in Congress right now. The Biden programs would move a little bit back towards the kind of more moderate capitalism of earlier years.

Limited social democracy is being fought tooth and nail, 100 percent, by the Republican Party and by the so-called moderate Democrats (who should be called reactionary Democrats, the ones who are awash in corporate funding). They'll probably kill it. That's maybe the last chance to do that.

So, we have to solve the problems within the existing system. Meanwhile, we can be working hard to raise understanding, awareness of the deep flaws in the system that have to be overcome—and also developing institutions that are the seeds of some better society. Worker-managed enterprises, for example, cooperatives that do flourish in Canada (not in the US), localism and so on, all at the same time. But time-scale can't be overlooked.

MCKAY: One distinctive theme I really appreciated in *The Precipice* and in your comments tonight, and I think it sets you apart from a lot of other leftists, is your sympathetic, compassionate treatment of working-class North Americans who are tempted by conspiracy theories and right-wing demagogues. You really are saying that, in a sense, they have some cause to be aggrieved, and they're sort of being lured into a trap by a supremely capable con man. How would you respond to critics who might think you're being too soft on grassroots Trumpians and their reactionary politics?

CHOMSKY: Well, I don't feel that I'm on some high moral pedestal in which I can condemn other people. I'm not living their lives. I didn't have to suffer the precarity of existence, the stagnation of wages, the decline of services that they suffered. I'm privileged. OK, I suffer from the health system. I've had the problem of not being able to get to a hospital because they're overflowing with unvaccinated Covid victims. But that's not like what poor and working people suffer. The last forty years have been a disaster for them and it's the same in England. I think the working-class vote for Brexit, in my view, was suicide. But you can understand it. They want to grasp something. Maybe we can grasp the fact that we can use British currency again; we can feel proud of something. I don't think that's very smart, but you can understand it and I don't feel like condemning.

If you take a look at the Trump voters here in the United States, they've been very carefully studied. The best work is by Tony DiMaggio.[7] Left social scientists have done very detailed work. Turns out that the prime base for the Trump movement is petty bourgeois, relatively affluent small business owners, insurance salespeople, people who own a construction business, rural, Christian, white supremacist, traditional. They feel their country's being taken away from them by minorities. There's even a theory of the "great replacement": the Democrats are trying to get immigrants here so they can undermine the white population. That's one of the wild conspiracy theories that's around.

Well, take a trip through rural America. You can understand it. Jobs are gone, factories are gone, young people are leaving, stores are boarded up, and maybe the bank is boarded up, still some churches—not much future for you. It's declining. It's an elderly, Christian nationalist, traditional, white supremacist population. There was a wonderful notion—it's most largely mythical but there's at least a myth—about a wonderful traditional life where the "coloured people" knew their place, women knew their place, none of this craziness of same-sex marriage, other things that these terrible minorities are doing to us. All being taken away. These are the people who marched on the Capitol—not working people. They're saying, "I'm going to save my country by taking back Congress away from the people destroying the country." Do I approve of it? Of course not. But I think we can understand it, and we could also understand our role in creating it. We tolerated forty years of the neoliberal assault. It has had a devastating effect on its victims. We're in no position to condemn them as "deplorable." They are, but not without reason. So that's the way I feel about it.

Incidentally, it's not basically working class. One of the things Tony DiMaggio showed in his work is that the working class was not won by the Republicans—it was lost by the Democrats. That's where the shift is. Many of the working-class Trump voters voted for Obama. He totally betrayed them—totally. So, what are they supposed to do?

In fact, I could see it in Massachusetts, where I lived at the time. In 2008, Obama was elected with wonderful promises—by 2010, he'd betrayed the working class totally in the way he handled the bailout for the rich (not for the poor, not for the victims). In 2010, there was a by-election for Martha Coakley (who replaced Ted Kennedy, the liberal icon). Even union workers didn't vote for the Democrat. They'd been betrayed, stabbed in the back. "Why should we vote for these guys? They're just the party of rich professionals. They don't care about us." Well, that's the way you lose voters.

MCKAY: I wonder if I could ask a question about what you call the neoliberal assault. Some authorities say it's an all-encompassing logic of rule, others say it's just a specific tradition, a school of economics, the Chicago School; some see it as a particular version of a globalized trade regime, and others see it as an updated version of ruling-class strategies to rob the working class. Would I be right in thinking you essentially incline to that last thrust, which is it's a new variant of a perennial ruling-class scheme to exploit workers? It's very much a class-based attack on the working class? Or would you like to put all these strands of interpretation together with a tilt towards a class-based interpretation?

CHOMSKY: I go along with Doug Fraser it's a one-sided class war. The business classes are basically Marxists, vulgar Marxists. They're fighting a bitter, one-sided class war, using many techniques. None of this has to do with the Chicago School. That's cover. Chicago School doesn't say you should have highly protectionist trade agreements (which you call free trade agreements). Chicago School doesn't say you should bail out the big institutions and give them a government insurance policy so they can be predatory. That's not Chicago School.

The Chicago School had a chance in Chile under perfect experimental conditions—the first 9/11. (This 9/11 in 1973 was much worse than 9/11/2001, but since we were the perpetrators, it's not considered history.) Well, they imposed a vicious, brutal dictatorship and opened the door to huge amount of funds. Investors loved it. The working class was crushed, popular descent was crushed, the Chicago Boys came in. Milton Friedman's students. Friedrich Hayek. All the big shots ran the economy. Perfect conditions. You didn't have any protest: the torture chambers took care of that. They had money pouring in from the wealthy all over the world, the international financial institutions.

Within about five years, they had crashed the economy, totally. The government had to take over more of the economy than it held under Allende (1982). Wags called it the "Chicago road to socialism." But they didn't care. By 1982 they were on to a bigger game. Let's take the whole world. Let's take the whole world and put it under our one-sided class war, masquerading as libertarianism.

So, I think that's a good definition of neoliberalism. Define it by its practices, not its rhetoric—and the practices were perfectly obvious from the beginning.

MCKAY: I really like what you said about Brexit and about American working-class people wanting to believe in their nation, a gut patriotism. In Canada, I think, some of our nationalism derives from taking gleeful pleasure in the troubles of the United States. I really deplore those tendencies and so I really appreciated your pokes at Canada—our so-so Medicare system, the Alberta tar sands and other mega-projects. So, granted that your book is not about Canada, I was wondering, do you think there is a place for progressive nationalism in a future global left? And how do we rid it of this kind of need for *schadenfreude*, watching other nations go through difficult times?

CHOMSKY: I don't remember the exact words, but there was a well-known Canadian diplomat (I think his name might have been John Holmes or something like that), and he once described "the Canadian way." The Canadian way is to stand up for your principles and make sure you violate them. He put it more eloquently.

I've seen the effects of Canadian foreign policy, even in my own experience. I've spent time in southern Colombia, one of the most brutal, vicious parts of the world—horrible atrocities—visiting poor villages where they're desperately trying to preserve their water supplies under the attack of Canadian mining corporations who want to destroy the virgin forest and make profits by killing poor people in Colombia. The scourge of the earth: Canadian mining companies.

You may recall Lester Pearson, the Nobel Prize winner. One of the revelations in the *Pentagon Papers* was that, when Johnson was planning to bomb North Vietnam in 1964, he consulted with the allies. So, he consulted with Canada, with Lester Pearson. Pearson said he didn't think it would be good to use atomic weapons, but iron bombs would be fine. That's the Canadian way. In fact, Canada was serving the United States as basically a US spy.

MCKAY: I really noticed throughout *The Precipice* how many times you make implicit (but also explicit) references to Antonio Gramsci, but I was wondering if you could comment on a theme that Gramsci develops: the Modern Prince. He wants, basically, a cohesive party aiming to build an effective and inclusive state. Libertarian leftists have historically been skeptical of any such state socialist project. Yet the pandemic, to my eye, seemingly shows the need for states with the capacity to plan the economy, institute comprehensive social security, and prevent future pandemics. So, is it time to set aside this libertarian skepticism of the state?

CHOMSKY: Well, I don't know exactly what the libertarian skepticism is. Does it say that, if you don't feel like stopping at a red light, you should drive through it? Especially if there's an old woman pushing a shopping cart there. "I don't want to be inhibited—why should I have the state tell me I have no right to do that?" I haven't heard that from libertarians.

There happen to be vaccine mandates, which have been in place for a long time in schools. You can't send your kids to a school unless they receive a polio vaccine, measles vaccine. So, is a libertarian supposed to say, "I want to send my kid to school and kill those other kids, because I want to be free of state control"? I haven't heard that recently.

In fact, the question is not: Are there general controls? It's who puts them in place. Is it the community—a democratic community that gets together, deliberates, says we want to put these in place because it's for our benefit? Well, that's libertarian socialism. It's not US-style libertarianism, right-wing libertarianism, which says private power does whatever it feels like and the rest of you find a way to survive. It's what was called libertarian socialism—the libertarian wing of the socialist movement—basically anarchism and anarcho-syndicalism. It had nothing to do with what's called libertarianism today.

An interesting measure of the extent to which democracy functions in a society is the attitude towards tax collection. It's a very striking measure. So, if you live in a totalitarian state, when Tax Day comes along, you're furious: they're robbing you. April fifteenth in the United States: "They're robbing us!" Suppose you had a democratic society. Imagine a democratic society, a society where communities get together to decide, here's what we want for next year for ourselves: schools, roads, decent air, water, and so on. Let's figure out how to pay for it. Here's an equitable way to pay for it. Tax Day comes along: it's a day of celebration. It's a day of celebration of the fact that we were able to work together to get what we all want.

It's interesting to place societies on that spectrum. You get an interesting conclusion of the extent to which democracy functions. It's worth thinking about.

So, I don't think the issue is "the horrible state is imposing mandates." We get together, decide we want to protect each other, so we decide we want to protect workers in restaurants. I think they deserve to be protected. So, therefore, we decide that the restaurant should be able to have a vaccine mandate. I want to protect them. It has nothing to do with a powerful state imposing anything else—if it's a democratic society, of course.

MCKAY: My last question. In *The Precipice*, you're asked how one can fight right-wing authoritarianism and, if I can quote you—it's a wonderful quote—you say, "The familiar advice, easy to state, hard to follow, but if there's another way, it's been kept a dark secret: honest, dedicated, courageous, and persistent engagement. . . . Hard work, necessary work, the kind that has succeeded in the past and can again."[8] "Pessimism of the intelligence, optimism of the will" would be how Gramsci would put it. How best can we combat not just right-wing authoritarianism but the ambient despair I'm sensing among some of my students, the sense of many young people that they're just confronting so many interlocking overpowering manifold crises as they inherit the twenty-first-century world. How best can we combat that sense of almost nihilistic, apocalyptic despair?

CHOMSKY: Well, I think several ways. One of them, actually, is history. Take a look at what's been achieved by the dedicated work of completely unknown people. To quote my favourite historian, my old friend Howard Zinn—"the unknown people" do the work that creates the basis for the events that enter history.[9] We'll never know their names. Nobody knows the names of the SNCC workers in 1960 who travelled through Alabama, getting shot at, beaten up, vilified, sometimes killed in order to encourage Black farmers to take their lives in their hands and register to vote. Anybody know their names? I personally happen to know a few of them, but that's by accident. The same is true with everything else. Feminist movement, environmental movement, everything—and a lot succeed.

Just take the United States. Ask what kind of a country it was in the 1960s, before the wave of activism civilized it. The United States had antimiscegenation laws so extreme that the Nazis refused to accept them. It had federally legislated segregated housing. There was, under the New Deal, federal support for public housing, but under the impact of Southern Democrats, it had to be racist. They wouldn't be able to get anything through unless it was segregated. That had a major effect. In the 1950s, in the growth period, an African American man could maybe get a decent job in an auto plant, make a little money, maybe buy a small house. (Property is wealth in the United States.) He couldn't buy a small house. The government said, "No, sorry they're segregated. It's not for you, you don't go there." There were antisodomy laws, of course. By law, women were property, literally. The US still had the laws that were taken over by the founders. Under British common law, women were property owned by the father, handed over to the husband. It wasn't until 1975 that the Supreme Court determined that women were peers with a right to serve on federal juries.

Well, we can go on and on. It was a very different country before the activism of the 1960s. That's why in the general intellectual world, the decade of the '60s is condemned as a time of troubles that disrupted society. It did. It civilized the society in many ways.

The climate strikes a couple of weeks ago—that's young people trying to save the world. Well, one way to support the idea that we should have "optimism of the will" is to look at what's been achieved. A lot young people today don't remember what it was like in the '60s. That's "ancient history."

They should study it—labour history, the whole story. The other major reason, the second major reason, is that there are feasible, workable answers to every crisis that we face. That's important. There's a third reason: you have a choice. You can either give up and make sure that the worst will happen, or you can grasp the opportunities that exist. Maybe it'll make it a better world. It's not a very hard choice.

QUESTION FROM THE AUDIENCE: What kind of organizations, organized by working people, can help to bring about the kind of international cooperation you mentioned? Is there a kind of grassroots democratic globalization that can be contrasted to those that are pursued by the masters of humankind?

CHOMSKY: Well, if you take a look at history, the history of countries like ours, it's overwhelmingly the case that an active militant labour movement was at the forefront of driving progress. That's why Canada has a national health system, for example, and the US doesn't. The labour unions acted differently on the two sides of the border. In the New Deal measures, which brought a measure of social democracy to the United States (which were later imitated in Europe to an extent), labour was at the forefront all the way.

Reagan and Thatcher knew exactly what they were doing when they initiated an attack on the labour movement: no other way to fight a one-sided class war. But then, there's the opposite side of that coin. Rebuild the movement—it can be done. The nineteenth-/early twentieth-century United States happened to have a very violent labour history. There was a vibrant, lively labour movement at that time that was crushed by force (primarily by liberals, incidentally). Woodrow Wilson's Red Scare smashed it. By the 1920s, almost gone. In the 1930s, it arose from the ashes. CIO organizing. (I can remember, it's my family.) In fact, the CIO organizing sit-down strikes put the fear of God into the managing classes. Furthermore, we should remember (it's kind of ancient history) that the labour unions are mostly called "internationals." That can be revived. To some extent, it is being revived. You had longshoremen boycotting trade with South Africa under apartheid when the US government was strongly supporting apartheid (Reagan was the last supporter of the apartheid regime). But the longshoremen were refusing to serve the ships. Internationalism for the labour movement is needed for survival.

The neoliberal globalization programs are designed specifically to pit poor working people in competition with one another. So, you get a race to the bottom. That's Clinton's programs of NAFTA world trade organization and so on. The labour movement can fight against it. The remnants of the labour movement tried to in the 1990s—they weren't strong enough to combat it. But you could have the kind of programs the labour movement put forth: high-growth, high-wage programs for all participants in all countries, labour rights, and so on.

That would be an alternative to the low-growth, low-wage policies of neoliberal globalization. Could be done, so let's help them become strong enough to carry it through.

We can do the same everywhere else. There are labour problems in the universities, plenty of service workers are exploited, adjuncts, graduate students—lots of things that can be done. Everywhere we are, we can organize, work together, build parts of a cooperative society. That's where the common good overrules personal gain. No Ayn Rand.

QUESTION FROM THE AUDIENCE: In an age in which education far exceeds schooling, how can we talk about education as being central to politics? How important is culture as a site of struggle in the twenty-first century?

CHOMSKY: Well, the right wing certainly understands this. They're fighting culture wars all the time. Take the United States. The radical party, the Republican Party—everywhere it has any role in the federal government or the states it is pressing very hard for a deeply reactionary cultural policy. One of their main targets is what's called Critical Race Theory. None of them have a clue what Critical Race Theory is. If they looked into it, they probably wouldn't even understand it. For them, it's a slogan that was set up to mean "the great replacement." "They're trying to destroy the white race, we've got to block them from teaching Critical Race Theory, block them from teaching the history of the vicious oppression of four hundred years of repression of African Americans and the bitter legacy it's left. Can't teach that stuff." Same on everything else. No right to abortion. In fact, let's destroy the public schools.

Mass public education was one of the great contributions of the United States to modern society. That was pretty democratic. It was important. Same on the university level. The great public universities, including MIT where I was, are land-grant universities. They were federally set up to provide education for the general population. There's an ugly side that meant exterminating the native population—but okay, we'll put that in a corner for a moment; you're not supposed to teach that either. Fortunately, where I am, the University of Arizona, they do it. Every large talk begins with an announcement that we're on the territory stolen from the Tohono O'odham Nation, which is in reservations nearby. It's our responsibility not only to acknowledge that but to make up for it by educational programs, cultural programs that enable them to recover somehow from the atrocities we've committed. At least we could do that.

But the Republicans and large number of Democrats want to kill the public education system. For people like Milton Friedman, one of their highest goals was to get rid of public education. In fact, Friedman cooperated with the segregationist movements in the 1970s—white supremacist movements. With the federally-mandated ending to segregation, they could save segregated schooling by putting it under some other rubric—religious education, charter schools, something or other. And Friedman very explicitly cooperated with the racist segregationists as part of the effort to undermine the public education system. The Secretary of Education for Trump, Betsy DeVos, is from a very wealthy family, and the DeVos Foundation is devoted to destroying the public education system and replacing it with right-wing religious education. It's quite open. Defund the schools, defund the state colleges, and so on. So, education is certainly a terrain for popular struggle. We shouldn't give it away to the right wing.

Now, what kind of education? The kind of education that says you don't look at books? The kind of education that says you train for a test? This was ridiculed in the eighteenth century by the Enlightenment, likened to pouring water into a vessel and then the student pours some of it out. We've all had that experience, taking some course that we didn't care about, studying for the exam, getting good marks, and two weeks later forgetting what the course was about. That was institutionalized in the United States under the first Bush and Obama administrations. It's called "teaching to test." The worst imaginable form of education. Get the students to pass a test and then grade the school on the tests. So, if the tests aren't high enough, defund the school and reduce the teachers' salaries.

You have teachers—I've talked to them—who report that a kid comes up after class and says, "You brought up something interesting. I'd like to pursue it. What can I do?" They're supposed just to say, "No, sorry, you have to study for that test to pass the test." This is in Massachusetts, the "liberal state." You've got to pass the test. The teacher doesn't say it, but in the back of her mind is this thought:

"My salary depends on it, school funding depends on it. So don't pursue what you're interested in. Study for the test and then, two weeks later, forget what the course was about." That's teaching to test. That's another way to destroy education.

One thing that's happened, strikingly, is that literacy has sharply declined. There are measures of that. In the United States, there have been studies. The kind of novels that used to be assigned in eighth grade are now assigned to seniors in high school because literacy has declined, reading abilities have declined.

Well, of course, it varies. If you're in a rich community, it's fine. Property taxes pay for decent schools with fairly decent programs. School funding in the United States is based on property taxes. Back in the eighteenth/nineteenth centuries, that didn't matter so much—the populations were mixed. Now it matters enormously, with racially segregated populations.

QUESTION FROM THE AUDIENCE: Is system change the only solution or is transformation of individuals' behaviour also the solution—or is it one or the other? So, do we have to start with the system or can individuals change themselves?

CHOMSKY: Why either/or? You can do both. Look at the major popular movements. Take, say, the Vietnam antiwar movement, which I happened to be very much involved with. We tried to start the movement when John F. Kennedy, one of the major modern criminals, sharply escalated the war in the early 1960s. Nobody cared. Barely reported. There were people around us that said, "Look, it's time to try to organize some opposition to this massive atrocity." We started meeting in a living room with a couple of neighbours, maybe you could get to a church where ten people would show up—long struggle—finally you got to big changes. That's the way *everything* works.

Take the Civil Rights movement. It really took off in 1960, when four Black students (whose names nobody remembers) sat in in a segregated lunch counter in North Carolina. They were immediately arrested and thrown in jail. Could have been the end—except, the next day, a couple of more Black students came, then more. After a while you had some students coming down from the north. Pretty soon you got SNCC [the Student Nonviolent Coordinating Committee] and the Freedom Riders. After a while, you had mass demonstrations, Martin Luther King, you had some institutional changes—nowhere near enough, but some. And that's the way everything works. If we're going to have worker participation or control over enterprises, first it's a matter of consciousness-raising.

You go back to the women's movement. How did it begin in the 1960s? A group of young kids would get together and talk to each other and say, "Look we don't have to live like this; we don't have to be the servants who serve the coffee, we can take part in things." That was a big breakthrough. It wasn't easy to do.

Take the labour movement. You go back to when we had a vibrant labour movement, the late nineteenth/early twentieth centuries. The slogan of the mass labour movement was "Those who work in the mills should own them." The idea that you should be subordinate to a master was considered an intolerable attack on your dignity and rights. (We now call that having a job.)

Well, that consciousness can be revived. I don't think it's much below the surface. It takes a change of attitudes, a change of what Gramsci called hegemonic common sense. Along with that comes institutional changes. They're mutually supportive. You set up a cooperative. That gets people to thinking about how you can work together. In order to set up the cooperative, you have to get people to think, "Yeah, we'd like to cooperate." So, they're mutually reinforcing. I don't think it's one or the other.

NOTES

INTRODUCTION

1. Christian Yates, "All the Coronavirus in the World Could Fit inside a Coke can, with Plenty of Room to Spare," *The Conversation*, 10 February 2021, theconversation.com. The calculations for this estimate rely on ambitious extrapolations from partial evidence. Still, even if the coronavirus would merely fill twenty-four Coke cans, it seems incredible so tiny a contaminant could drive the human world into such a crisis.
2. Deborah Lupton, *COVID Societies: Theorising the Coronavirus Crisis* (London: Routledge, 2022), 86.
3. Salvage Editorial Collective, "The Mask of the Red Death: Dispatch One from a Changing World," *Salvage*, 21 March 2020, salvage.zone.
4. For *Syndemic Magazine*, see syndemic.ca.
5. Richard Horton, "Alarming New Data Shows the UK Was the 'Sick Man' of Europe Even Before Covid," *The Guardian*, 18 October 2020, theguardian.com.
6. Bayla Ostrach, Shir Lerman, and Merrill Singer, eds., *Stigma Syndemics: New Directions in Biosocial Health* (Lanham, MD: Lexington Books, 2017), viii.
7. Mica Jorgenson, "Catastrophic Rhetoric: False Enchantments and 'Unprecedented' Disasters in British Columbia's Punishing 2021"; Matt Sparke and Lucia Vitale, "Covid's Co-Pathognesis," *Syndemic Magazine*, 4 February 2022, syndemic.ca.
8. Ed Dunsworth, "Covid, Class, and Consciousness: Reflections from the Third Year of the Plague"; Nausheen Quayyum, "Global Supply Chains and the Pandemic: Experiences of Readymade Garment Workers in Bangladesh"; and Ranabir Sammadar, "Invisible No More: The Migrant Workers of India," *Syndemic Magazine*, 8 March 2022, syndemic.ca.
9. Jennifer Wallace, "Moving On? Or Masculinist Erasure?"; Heather Howard-Bobiwash, "First Nations, Contagion, and Canada: The Lineages of Pandemic Colonialism"; Paige Castellanos, Carolyn E. Sachs, and Ann R. Tickamyer, "Risking Lives, Averting Hunger, Building Community: The Gendered Dimensions of the Food System in the Pandemic," *Syndemic Magazine*, 25 April 2022, syndemic.ca.
10. Sarah Whitwell, "Structural Barriers to Healthcare, Vaccine Hesitancy, and Racialized Communities"; Angela Mashford-Pringle, "Covid-19, Pandemics and Indigenous People in Canada"; Sandria Green-Stewart, "A Syndemic of Suffering: The Racialized and the Marginalized in Ontario's Long-Term Care Crisis, 2020–2021"; and Brandon Cordeiro, "A Factory for Producing Broken People: Reflections on Covid-19 and the Thunder Bay Jail," *Syndemic Magazine*, 9 May 2022, syndemic.ca.

11   Edward MacDonald, "The Future is Unwritten: Mass Tourism in a Post-Pandemic World"; Ligia Simba-Bolaños, "Yunguilla, Community-Based Tourism, and Covid-19," *Syndemic Magazine*, 7 June 2022, syndemic.ca.

12   Brandon Cordeiro, "The End is the Beginning is the End: Conspiracies and the Right in a Post-Pandemic World"; Zachary Loeb, "Jonah, Cassandra, and the Doomsters: Rereading Lewis Mumford in 2022," *Syndemic Magazine*, 29 June 2022, syndemic.ca.

13   The online "originals" can all be easily located on the *Syndemic* site. In preparing the interviews for publication in the magazine, they were edited for consistency and length; they have undergone a further round of editing for this collection.

14   These include interviews with Gabriel Allahdua (conducted by Ed Dunsworth) on the conditions of migrant farm workers (issue no. 2); Pat Armstrong and André Picard on conditions in homes for the elderly (issue no. 3); Karen Dubinsky and Luc Renaud on tourism (issue no. 5); and Nicholas Christakis on the general historical interpretation of the pandemic (issue no. 6).

15   Naomi Klein, *The Shock Doctrine: The Rise of Disaster Capitalism* (Toronto: Vintage Canada, 2008).

16   Fabian Scheidler, *The End of the Megamachine: A Brief History of a Failing Civilization*, (Winchester, UK: Zero Books, 2020).

17   Ian Angus, *Facing the Anthropocene: Fossil Capitalism and the Crisis of the Earth System* (New York: Monthly Review Books, 2016), 127.

18   Antonio Gramsci, *Subaltern Social Groups: A Critical Edition of Prison Notebook 25*, ed. and trans. Joseph A. Buttigieg and Marcus E. Green (New York: Columbia University Press, 2021), 9, 10, 20, 85–6; Q25§4, §5; Q1§14; Q11§12 (Q for Quaderni or notebook, § for the section referred to). For useful guidance, see Marcus Green, "Rethinking the Subaltern and the Question of Censorship in Gramsci's *Prison Notebooks*," *Postcolonial Studies* 14,4 (2011): 387–404.

19   Dylan Riley, "Lockdown Limbo: March 2020–February 2021," *New Left Review* 127 (January-February 2021): 16–17, newleftreview.org. On this reading, Gramscians appreciate the work of intersectionality theorists but fear they often hypostatize the very categories—race, gender, sexuality—they are committed to interrelating. For a stimulating critique along these lines, see David McNally, "Intersections and Dialectics: Critical Reconstructions in Social Reproduction Theory," in Tithi Bhattacharya, ed., *Social Reproduction Theory: Remapping Class, Recentering Oppression* (London: Pluto Press, 2017), 94–111. For discussions in this volume, see Bhattacharya, Chowkwanyun, and Ryan.

20   Kate Crehan, *Gramsci's Common Sense: Inequality and its Narratives* (Durham, NC: Duke University Press, 2016), 61.

21   Antonio Gramsci, *Selections from the Prison Notebooks*, eds. and trans. Quintin Hoare and Geoffrey Nowell Smith (New York: International Publishers, 1971), 423, Q11, §13. Yet, all attempts to change subaltern common sense require "not the elimination of common sense but the critique and transformation of it." Marcus E. Green and Peter Ives, "Subalternity and Language: Overcoming the Fragmentation of Common Sense," in Peter Ives and Rocco Lacorte, eds.,

     Gramsci, Language, and Translation (Lanham, MD: Lexington Books, 2010), 292.
22   "An Interview with Pat Armstrong" and "An Interview with André Picard," both in *Syndemic Magazine*, 6 April 2022, syndemic.ca.
23   Gramsci, *Selections*, 355; Q10II §54. His close study of Italian history disclosed three "propertied classes" and five "unpropertied" classes, all in motion and all relating to each other.
24   See Mostafa Henaway, "'The Cost of Free Shipping?' Living in the Age of Amazon Capitalism," *Syndemic*, 8 March 2022, syndemic.ca.
25   Cited in Lisa Wade, "Narratives of Outbreak and Survival in English-Language Cinema Prior to COVID-19," *Socius* 8 (21 February 2022): 1–15, doi: 10.1177/23780231221078242.
26   Jie Zhao, Wei Cui, and Bao-ping Tian, "The Potential Intermediate Hosts for SARS-CoV-2," *Frontiers in Microbiology* 11 (2020), doi: 10.3389/fmicb.2020.580137.
27   Harvard psychologist Steven Pinker has repeatedly suggested that pandemics of contagious diseases are on the decline and in 2017 took up a wager from a Cambridge scientist that, by the end of 2020, "bioterror or bioerror" would lead to a million casualties, which Pinker thought unlikely. By September 2020, Covid-19 had claimed at least one million lives. Niall Ferguson, "No More Handshakes: The History of a Pandemic and Its Possible Futures," *Times Literary Supplement*, 30 October 2020, 3quarksdaily.com.

NANCY FRASER

1   Antonio Gramsci, *Selections from the Prison Notebooks*, ed. and trans. Quintin Hoare and Geoffrey Nowell Smith (New York: International Publishers, 1971), 276, Q3§34. For an excellent contextualizing discussion, see Gilbert Achcar, "Morbid Symptoms: What Did Gramsci Really Mean," *Notebooks: The Journal for Studies on Power* 1 (2021), 379–87, brill.com.
2   "Virus Lays Bare the Frailty of the Social Contract," *Financial Times*, 3 April 2020, ft.com. For commentary, see Rutger Bregman, "The Neoliberal Era Is Ending. What Comes Next?" *The Correspondent*, 14 May 2020, thecorrespondent.com.
3   Nancy Fraser and Rahel Jaeggi, *Capitalism: A Conversation in Critical Theory*, ed. Brian Milstein (Oxford: Polity, 2018): 222.
4   Cited in George Eaton, "Is the Neoliberal Era Finally Over?" *New Statesman*, 16 June 2021, newstatesman.com.
5   Fraser and Jaeggi, *Capitalism*, 200.
6   Cinzia Arruzza, Tithi Bhattacharya, and Nancy Fraser, *Feminism for the 99%: A Manifesto* (London: Verso, 2019).
7   Fraser and Jaeggi, *Capitalism*, 208–9.
8   Antonio Gramsci: "Our motto is still alive and to the point: Pessimism of the intellect, optimism of the will," *L'Ordine Nuovo*, 4 March 1921; the publication's motto was borrowed from French writer Romain Rolland. For discussion, see Francesca Antonini, "Pessimism of the Intellect, Optimism of the Will:

Gramsci's Political Thought in the Last Miscellaneous Notebooks," *Rethinking Marxism* 31,1 (2019), 42–57, doi: 10.1080/08935696.2019.1577616.

MIKE DAVIS

1. Mike Davis, *The Monster at Our Door: The Global Threat of Avian Flu*, rev ed. (New York: Henry Holt and Company, 2006), 63.
2. Rob Wallace, *Big Farms, Big Flu: Dispatches on Influenza, Agribusiness, and the Nature of Science*. (New York: Monthly Review Press, 2016).
3. Justin S. Brashares, Peter Arcese, Moses K. Sam, Peter B. Coppolillo, A. R. E. Sinclair, and Andrew Balmford, "Bushmeat Hunting, Wildlife Declines, and Fish Supply in West Africa," *Science* 306 (12 November 2004), 1180–82, doi: 10.1126/science.1102425.
4. Chuang [闯], *Social Contagion: And Other Material on Microbiological Class War in China* (Chicago: Charles Kerr, 2020), chuangcn.org.
5. Mike Davis, *The Monster Enters: COVID-19, Avian Flu and the Plagues of Capitalism* (New York: OR Books, 2020), 1.

MACK PENNER

1. Johanna Bockman, *Markets in the Name of Socialism: The Left-Wing Origins of Neoliberalism* (Stanford, CA: Stanford University Press, 2011).
2. Quinn Slobodian, *Globalists: The End of Empire and the Birth of Neoliberalism* (Cambridge, MA: Harvard University Press, 2018).
3. Amy Offner, *Sorting Out the Mixed Economy: The Rise and Fall of Welfare and Developmental States in the Americas* (Princeton, NJ: Princeton University Press, 2019).
4. Wendy Brown, *Undoing the Demos: Neoliberalism's Stealth Revolution* (New York: Zone Books, 2015).
5. Daniel Rodgers, "The Uses and Abuses of 'Neoliberalism,'" *Dissent* (Winter 2018), dissentmagazine.org.
6. Damien Cahill and Maritjn Konings, "Neoliberalism: A Useful Concept?" *The Bullet*, 1 December 2017, socialistproject.ca
7. For a libertarian assessment of Spencer and Hayek, see Scott Boykin, "Spencer and Hayek's Liberal Evolutionism, and Why It Should Omit the Nation-State," *The Journal of Libertarian Studies* 24,2 (2020), 385–422, mises.org.
8. Michele Filippini, *Using Gramsci: A New Approach*, trans. Patrick J. Barr (London: Pluto Press, 2017), 8.
9. Donald Sassoon, *Morbid Symptoms: Anatomy of a World in Crisis* (London: Verso, 2021), 205.
10. Jamie Peck and Nik Theodore, "Still Neoliberalism?" *The South Atlantic Quarterly* 118,2 (April 2019), 260, dukeupress.edu.
11. Offner, *Sorting Out*, 289.
12. Offner, *Sorting Out*, 284.
13. Greta Krippner, *Capitalizing on Crisis: The Political Origins of the Rise of Finance* (Cambridge, MA: Harvard University Press, 2011), *passim*.

14 Grégoire Chamayou, *The Ungovernable Society: A Genealogy of Authoritarian Liberalism*, trans. Andrew Brown (Cambridge, UK: Polity Press, 2021), 136.
15 Adam Tooze, *Crashed: How a Decade of Financial Crises Changed the World* (New York: Viking, 2018).
16 Perry Anderson, "Situationism à L'envers?" *New Left Review* 119 (Sept-Oct 2019): 74.
17 Lars Lih, "The Pre-war Roots of the Comintern," in *Cataclysm 1914*, ed. Alex Anievas (Leiden: Brill, 2014).
18 Quinn Slobodian, *Globalists: The End of Empire and the Birth of Neoliberalism* (Cambridge, MA: Harvard University Press, 2018), 2.
19 Cited in Peck and Theodore, "Still Neoliberalism?" 251.
20 See David Harvey, *A Brief History of Neoliberalism* (Oxford, UK: Oxford University Press, 2005), 120–51.
21 Lisa Adkins, Melinda Cooper, and Martijn Konings, *The Asset Economy: Property Ownership and the New Logic of Inequality* (Cambridge, UK: Polity, 2020), *passim*.
22 See Evgeny Morozov, "Critique of Techno-Feudal Reason," *New Left Review* 133/134 (Jan-Apr 2022): 89–126.
23 Ian McKay, "The Liberal Order Framework: A Prospectus for a Reconnaissance of Canadian History," *The Canadian Historical Review* 81,4 (December 2000), 623.
24 "46% of Canadians Sympathize with Trucker Convoy, but Many Disagree with Their Tactics: Poll," *Global News*, 11 February 2022, globalnews.ca.
25 See Wendy Brown, *In the Ruins of Neoliberalism: The Rise of Antidemocratic Politics in the West* (New York: Columbia University Press, 2019).
26 See Andreas Malm, *Fossil Capital: The Rise of Steam Power and the Roots of Global Warming* (New York: Verso, 2016).
27 Andreas Malm, *Corona, Climate, Chronic Emergency: War Communism in the Twenty-First Century* (New York: Verso, 2020), *passim*.
28 Aaron Benanav, *Automation and the Future of Work* (London: Verso, 2020), *passim*.
29 See Andreas Malm, *How to Blow up a Pipeline: Learning to Fight in a World on Fire* (New York: Verso, 2021).
30 Thea Riofrancos, "A Burning Planet: Should the Climate Movement Embrace Sabotage?" *The Nation*, 25 July 2022, thenation.com.

ANDREAS MALM

1 Andreas Malm and the Zetkin Collective, *White Skin, Black Fuel: On the Danger of Fossil Fascism* (London: Verso Books, 2021).
2 Andreas Malm, *Corona, Climate, Chronic Emergency: War Communism in the Twenty-First Century* (New York: Verso, 2020), 100.
3 Malm, *Corona*, 26.
4 Luiz Inácio Lula da Silva, president of Brazil, 2003–10, 2022–.
5 Michael Ryan of the WHO, as cited in "Coronavirus Outbreak: WHO Official Says Countries Must Rely On Speed, Not Perfection in Response," *Global News*, 13 March 2020, globalnews.ca.

MERRILL SINGER

1. Richard Horton, "Alarming New Data Shows the UK Was the 'Sick Man' of Europe Even Before Covid," *The Guardian*, 18 October 2020, theguardian.com.
2. See Paul Farmer, *AIDS and Accusation: Haiti and the Geography of Blame*, second edition (Berkeley: University of California Press, 2006); *To Repair the World: Paul Farmer Speaks to the Next Generation* (Berkeley: University of California Press, 2013); *Fevers, Feuds, and Diamonds: Ebola and the Ravages of History* (New York: Farrar, Straus and Giroux, 2020).
3. Merrill Singer and Rebecca Allen, *Social Justice and Medical Practice: Life History of a Physician of Social Medicine* (New York: Routledge, 2018).
4. Merrill Singer, *Introduction to Syndemics: A Critical Systems Approach to Public and Community Health* (San Francisco: Jossey-Bass, 2009), 226.
5. Merrill Singer, Nicola Bulled, and Bayla Ostrach, "Whither Syndemics? Trends in Syndemics Research, a Review, 2015–2019," *Global Public Health* 15,7 (2020), 943.
6. Bayla Ostrach, Shir Lerman, and Merrill Singer, eds., *Stigma Syndemics: New Directions in Biosocial Health* (Lanham, MD: Lexington Books, 2017), viii.
7. See William W. Dressler, *Stress and Adaptation in the Context of Culture: Depression in a Southern Black Community* (Albany: State University of New York Press, 1991); "Social Inequality and Health: A Commentary," *Medical Anthropology Quarterly* 24 (January 2010), 549–54.
8. See D. Ann Herring with Merrill Singer, Judith Littleton, and Melanie Rock, "Syndemics in Global Health," in *A Companion to Medical Anthropology*, eds. Merrill Singer and Pamela I. Erickson, (Chichester, UK: Wiley-Blackwell, 2011), 159–80.
9. Merrill Singer, *Anthropology of Infectious Diseases* (London: Routledge, 2016), 191.
10. Emily Mendenhall, *Unmasked: COVID, Community, and the Case of Okoboji* (Nashville: Vanderbilt University Press, 2022).
11. Alfred W. Crosby, *America's Forgotten Pandemic: The Influenza of 1918* (Cambridge: Cambridge University Press, 2003).
12. Merrill Singer, *Anthropology*, 222.
13. Merrill Singer, *Climate Change and Social Inequality: The Health and Social Costs of Global Warming* (London: Routledge, 2019).
14. See, for example, Merrill Singer and Hans Baer, eds., *Killer Commodities: Public Health and the Corporate Production of Harm* (Lanham, MD: Altamira Press, 2009).
15. Merrill Singer, *Introduction*, 133.
16. Singer, *Introduction*, 132–34.
17. For discussion of this insight from Virchow, see J. R. A. with Siân Anis, "Virchow Misquoted, Part-Quoted, and the Real McCoy," *Journal of Epidemiology and Community Health* 60,8 (2006), 671.
18. For Fauci's relationship with Larry Kramer, who cofounded the Gay Men's Health Crisis in 1982 and the AIDS Coalition to Unleash Power (ACT UP) in 1987, see Chris Riotta, "From HIV to Covid-19: Fauci on His 'Complicated

Relationship' with Activist Larry Kramer," *NBC News*, 2 October 2020, nbcnews. com.
19   "'I Want You to Panic': 16-Year-Old Issues Climate Warning at Davos—video," *The Guardian*, 25 January 2019, theguardian.com.
20   Singer, Bulled, and Ostrach, "Whither Syndemics?" 943–55.

NORA LORETTO

1   sandyandnora.com.
2   Cited in Athina Khalid, "Mismanaged Crisis: Nora Loreto's *Spin Doctors*," *Montreal Review of Books*, 2 March 2022, mtlreviewofbooks.ca.
3   Cited in John Dugdale, "The Wicked Wit and Enigma of Dorothy Parker—50 Years On," *The Guardian*, 16 June 2017, theguardian.com.
4   Nora Loreto, *Spin Doctors: How Media and Politicians Misdiagnosed the Covid-19 Pandemic* (Halifax: Fernwood, 2021), 130.
5   Margaret Thatcher famously declared in an interview with *Woman's Own* in 1987: "I think we have gone through a period when too many children and people have been given to understand 'I have a problem, it is the Government's job to cope with it!' or 'I have a problem, I will go and get a grant to cope with it!' 'I am homeless, the Government must house me!' and so they are casting their problems on society and who is society? There is no such thing! There are individual men and women and there are families and no government can do anything except through people and people look to themselves first." newlearningonline.com.
6   For commentary from Vancouver-based disability activist Gabrielle Peters, see cbc.ca.
7   CERB is the Canadian Emergency Response Benefit, which offered financial aid to both employed and self-employed Canadians (under certain conditions) directly affected by Covid-19.
8   See Susanna Trnka and Sharyn Graham Davies, "Blowing Bubbles: COVID-19, New Zealand's Bubble Metaphor, and the Limits of Households as Sites of Responsibility and Care," in *COVID-19: Volume I: Global Pandemic, Societal Responses, Ideological Solutions*, ed., J. Michael Ryan (London: Routledge, 2021), 167–83.
9   *The Breach* (breachmedia.ca), *Briarpatch Magazine* (briarpatchmagazine.com), *Canadian Dimension* (canadiandimension.com), *Rabble* (rabble.ca).
10   *Passage Magazine* (readpassage.com); *The Maple* (readthemaple.com).
11   *The Rover* (rover.substack.com/about).
12   Sandy Hudson and Nora Loreto, *Sandy & Nora*, podcast, sandyandnora.com.
13   Loreto, *Spin Doctors*, 335.

TITHI BHATTACHARYA

1   Tithi Bhattacharya, ed., *Social Reproduction Theory: Remapping Class, Recentering Oppression* (London: Pluto Press, 2017).
2   Cinzia Arruzza, Tithi Bhattacharya, and Nancy Fraser, *Feminism for the 99%: A Manifesto* (London: Verso, 2019).

3   Tithi Bhattacharya in conversation with Sarah Jaffe, "Social Reproduction and the Pandemic," *Dissent Magazine*, 2 April 2020, dissentmagazine.org.
4   Arruzza, Bhattacharya, and Fraser, *Feminism*, 68.
5   Bhattacharya, *Social Reproduction Theory*, 3.
6   "Hindutva" is a term subject to various interpretations, all of which can be related to the idea of a universal, essential Hindu identity, sharply distinguished from others, in particular those related to Islam.
7   A public procession in a chariot, often with particular reference to annual commemorations in East Indian states.
8   A conspiracy theory maintaining that Muslim men target Hindu women in order to transform India into an Islamic state.
9   See Susan Ferguson, *Women and Work: Feminism, Labour, and Social Reproduction* (Toronto: Between the Lines, 2019).
10 David McNally, "Intersections and Dialectics: Critical Reconstructions in Social Reproduction Theory," in *Social Reproduction Theory*, ed., Bhattacharya, 94–111.
11 Bhattacharya and Jaffe, "Social Reproduction."

CHANDRIMA CHAKRABORTY

1   Chandrima Chakraborty, Amber Dean, and Angela Failler, eds., *Remembering Air India: The Art of Public Mourning* (Edmonton: University of Alberta Press, 2017).
2   Iyko Day, "The Yellow Plague and Romantic Anticapitalism," *Monthly Review*, 1 July 2020, monthlyreview.org.
3   A small number of Chinese artisans and carpenters had arrived in British Columbia earlier, in the late eighteenth century. See John Price, "Relocating Yuquot: The Indigenous Pacific and Transpacific Migrations," *BC Studies* 204 (Winter 2019/2020), 21–44.
4   27-year-old Vincent Chin, a Chinese American draftsman, was killed outside a club in Highland Park, Michigan, by three white men who evidently assumed he was of Japanese descent and in some way responsible for the success of the Japanese auto industry at the expense of the American.
5   Chandrima Chakraborty, "Contagious Minorities: Chinese Canadians during the COVID-19 Pandemic," *Journal of Canadian Studies* 56,3 (November 2022), doi: 10.3138/jcs-2022-0017.
6   Chakraborty, "Contagious Minorities."
7   Audre Lorde, "The Uses of Anger: Women Responding to Racism," *BlackPast*, 12 August 2012, blackpast.org.
8   "COVID-19: Ethno-Racial Identity and Income," *City of Toronto, Covid-19: Pandemic Data*, toronto.ca.

MERLIN CHOWKWANYUN

1   Merlin Chowkwanyun, *All Health Politics Is Local: Community Battles for Medical Care and Environmental Health* (Chapel Hill: University of North Carolina Press, 2022).

2   Merlin Chowkwanyun and Adolph L. Reed, Jr., "Racial Health Disparities and Covid-19—Caution and Context," *New England Journal of Medicine* 383,3 (16 July 2020): 201–3, doi: 10.1056/nejmp2012910.
3   Merlin Chowkwanyun, "The Strange Disappearance of History from Racial Disparities Research," *Du Bois Review* 8,1 (2011): 254.
4   Chowkwanyun, "Strange Disappearance," 259.
5   Adolph Reed, Jr., and Merlin Chowkwanyun, "Race, Class, Crisis: The Discourse of Racial Disparity and Its Analytical Discontents," *Socialist Register* (2012): 150, socialistregister.com.
6   Joanna Wuest, "The Racial Disparity Politics of Biomedical Research: Disaggregating Categories into New Essentialisms," *Nonsite*, 29 December 2019, nonsite.org.
7   Charles Tilly, *Durable Inequality* (Berkeley: University of California Press, 1998).
8   Reed and Chowkwanyun, "Race," 152, 166–7.
9   Loïc Wacquant, "From Slavery to Incarceration: Rethinking the 'Race Question' in the US," *New Left Review* 13 (January-February 2002), 41–60; "Resolving the Trouble with 'Race,'" *New Left Review* 133/134 (January-April 2022), 67–88.
10 Chowkwanyun and Reed, Jr., "Racial Health Disparities," 202.
11 theatlantic.com.
12 Karen E. Fields and Barbara J. Fields, *Racecraft: The Soul of Inequality in American Life* (New York: Verso, 2014).
13 Mara Loveman, "Is 'Race' Essential?" *American Sociological Review* 64,6 (December 1999): 891–98.
14 Adolph Reed, Jr., *Class Notes, Posing as Politics, and Other Thoughts on the American Scene* (New York: New Press, 2000), xiv.
15 As in, for example, Anne Case and Angus Deaton, *Deaths of Despair and the Future of Capitalism* (Princeton, NJ: Princeton University Press, 2020).
16 Landon R. Y. Storrs, *The Second Red Scare and the Unmaking of the New Deal Left* (Princeton, NJ: Princeton University Press, 2012).
17 For an overview, see David Spiegelhalter and Anthony Masters, *Covid by Numbers: Making Sense of the Pandemic with Data* (London: Pelican Books, 2021).
18 See Richard Evans, *Eric Hobsbawm: A Life in History* (Oxford: Oxford University Press, 2019).
19 On 22 December 2008, a dike at the Kingston Fossil Plant in Roane County, Tennessee, managed by the Tennessee Valley Authority, failed, releasing 4.2 billion cubic metres of coal fly ash slurry into nearby waters, in one of the largest industrial spills in American history.
20 Jon Zelner, Nina B. Masters, Ramya Naraharisetti, Sanyu A. Mohola, Merlin Chowkwanyun, and Ryan Malosh, "There Are No Equal Opportunity Infectors: Epidemiological Modelers Must Rethink Our Approach to Inequality in Infection Risk," *PLOS Computational Biology*, 9 February 2022, plos.org.
21 Howard Markel, "History Won't Help Us Now: We Have No Historical Precedent for This Moment," *The Atlantic*, 19 August 2021; theatlantic.com.

SANJAY NEPAL

1. Sanjay Nepal, "Residents' Attitudes to Tourism in Central British Columbia, Canada," *Tourism Geographies* 10, 1 (2008): 42–65.
2. See Sanjay Nepal and T. B. Jamal, "Resort-Induced Changes in Small Mountain Communities in British Columbia, Canada," *Mountain Research and Development* 31,2 (2011): 89–101.
3. Sanjay Nepal, Jarkko Saarinen, and Erin McLean-Purdon, "Introduction: Political Ecology and Tourism—Concepts and Constructs," in *Political Ecology and Tourism*, eds., Sanjay Nepal and Jarkko Saarinen, (Milton Park and New York: Routledge, 2016), 10.
4. Sanjay Nepal, Yang Mu, and Po-Hsin Lai, "The Beyul: Perspectives on Landscape Characteristics and Tourism Development in Khumbu (Everest), Nepal," in *Religious Tourism and the Environment* eds., K. A. Shinde and D. H. Olsen, (CAB ebooks, 2020), cabi.org.
5. David Harvey, "Anti-Capitalist Politics in the Time of COVID-19," *Jacobin Magazine*, March 2020, jacobinmag.com.
6. Sanjay Nepal, "Adventure Travel and Tourism after Covid-19—Business as Usual or Opportunity to Reset?" *Tourism Geographies* 22,3 (2020): 646–50, doi: 10.1080/14616688.2020.1760926.
7. Nepal, "Adventure."
8. United Nations World Tourism Organization, *Framework Convention on Tourism Ethics* (Madrid: UNTWO, 2020), doi: 10.18111/9789284421671. Article 10 addresses the "right to tourism."
9. For discussion, see Jamie D'Souza, Jackie Dawson, and Mark Groulx, "Last Chance Tourism: A Decade Review of a Case Study on Churchill, Manitoba's Polar Bear Viewing Industry," *Journal of Sustainable Tourism* 29 (8 April 2021), doi: 10.1080/09669582.2021.1910828.
10. Rabindra Nepal and Sanjay Kumar Nepal, "Managing Overtourism through Economic Taxation: Policy Lessons from Five Countries," *Tourism Geographies* 23,5–6 (2021), 1107, lib.mcmaster.ca.
11. Mary Jane Grant, "A Travel Writer Unlocks the Secrets of Her Best-Loved Trips: Mindful Travel," *Globe and Mail*, 23 June 2020, theglobeandmail.com.
12. Elaine Glusac, "Move Over, Sustainable Travel. Regenerative Tourism Has Arrived," *New York Times*, 27 August 2020, nytimes.com.

J. MICHAEL RYAN

1. J. Michael Ryan and Serena Nanda, *COVID-19: Social Inequalities and Human Possibilities* (New York: Routledge, 2022), 166.
2. Ryan and Nanda, *COVID-19*, 21.
3. George Ritzer, *The McDonaldization of Society* (Los Angeles: Sage and Pine Forge Press, 2011).
4. Ryan and Nanda, *COVID-19*, xxvii.
5. Ryan and Nanda, *COVID-19*, 25.
6. Ryan and Nanda, *COVID-19*, 124.

LAURA SPINNEY

1. Laura Spinney, "Coronavirus Is Evolving. Whether It Gets Deadlier or Not May Depend On Us," *The Guardian*, 19 November 2020, theguardian.com.
2. Devi Sridhar, "Continual Lockdowns Are Not the Answer to Bringing Covid Under Control," *The Guardian*, 10 October 2020; theguardian.com.
3. Richard Horton, "Coronavirus is the Greatest Global Science Policy Failure in a Generation," *The Guardian*, 9 April 2020, theguardian.com.
4. As Zeynep Tufecki remarked to journalist Ed Yong, "We can't even deal with a starter pandemic?" Ed Yong, "How the Pandemic Defeated America," *The Atlantic*, September 2020, theatlantic.com.
5. See Laura Spinney, "Has Covid Changed the Price of a Life?" *The Guardian*, 14 February 2021, theguardian.com.
6. Laura Spinney, "We Need to Mark the Countless Lives Covid Has Claimed. But How To Do It?" *The Guardian*, 18 March 2021, theguardian.com.
7. See Laura Spinney, "'Humans Weren't Always Here. We Could Disappear': Meet the Collapsologists," *The Guardian*, 11 October 2020, theguardian.com.
8. Stephen Buranyi, "Ignore the Pessimism: Covid Vaccines Are Quietly Prevailing," *The Guardian*, 12 April 2021, theguardian.com.

NAOMI KLEIN

1. Naomi Klein, *This Changes Everything: Capitalism vs. the Climate* (New York: Simon and Schuster, 2014), 21.
2. Pope Francis in conversation with Austen Ivereigh, *Let Us Dream: The Path to a Better Future* (New York: Simon and Schuster, 2020), offers a distillation of his thought.
3. Nigel Lawson, *An Appeal to Reason: A Cool Look at Global Warming* (London: Duckworth Overlook, 2008). See also Will Potter, *Green Is the New Red: An Insider's Account of a Social Movement Under Siege* (San Francisco: City Lights Publishers, 2011).
4. Naomi Klein, *On Fire: The Burning Case for a Green New Deal* (London: Penguin Random House UK, 2020), 169.
5. Klein, *This Changes Everything*, 11.
6. Klein, *This Changes Everything*, 9.
7. Klein, *On Fire*, 12.
8. See "Greta Thunberg's 'blah blah blah' speech, Milan, 2021," Carbon Independent org., carbonindependent.org.
9. Naomi Klein, "How Big Tech Plans to Profit from the Pandemic," *The Guardian*, 13 May 2020, theguardian.com.
10. Michael Lewis, "Has Anyone Seen the President?" *Bloomberg*, 9 February 2018, bloomberg.com.
11. Klein, *This Changes Everything*, 25.
12. For the film, an excerpt from which was shown during the interview, see The Leap and The Intercept, *Message from the Future II: The Years of Repair* (2020), youtube.com.

13 Judy Rebick and Corvin Rusell, "The Left Is Nowhere on COVID. And That's a Big Problem," Rabble.ca, 4 February 2022, rabble.ca.
14 In the Great Leap Forward in China (1958–1962), the communist regime attempted a rapid process of industrialization based on steel-making, the chaotic implementation of which led to millions of deaths in rural areas.
15 Shoshana Zuboff, *The Age of Surveillance Capitalism: The Fight for a Human Future at the New Frontier of Power* (New York: PublicAffairs, 2020).
16 Nick Couldry and Ulises A. Mejias, *The Costs of Connection: How Data Is Colonizing Human Life and Appropriating It for Capitalism* (Stanford: Stanford University Press, 2019).
17 Naomi Klein, "How to Jam the Trump Brand," *The Intercept*, 12 April 2017, theintercept.com.

NOAM CHOMSKY

1 Dr. Henry Giroux offered the introduction for Noam Chomsky's talk.
2 Adam Smith, *An Inquiry into the Nature and Causes of the Wealth of Nations* (1776), book 3, chap.4, available at Project Gutenberg, gutenberg.org.
3 "Doug Fraser's Resignation Letter from the Labor-Management Group," 17 July 1978, historyisaweapon.com. Fraser was the president of the United Autoworkers Union. "I believe leaders of the business community, with few exceptions, have chosen to wage a one-sided class war today in this country—a war against working people, the unemployed, the poor, the minorities, the very young and the very old, and even many in the middle class of our society."
4 "Former Australian PM Critiques AUKUS Deal, 'Quad,'" *China Daily*, 4 October 2021, chinadaily.com.
5 For a fuller exposition, see Clinton Fernandes, *Sub-imperial Power: Australia in the International Arena* (Melbourne: University of Melbourne Press, 2022).
6 Brian Toohey, "Australia's Nuclear Submarine Deal Won't Make Us Any Safer," *Pearls and Irritations*, 29 September 2021, johnmenadue.com.
7 See Anthony DiMaggio, "Election 2020: A Democratic Mandate or a Vote Against Trump?" *CounterPunch*, 24 November 2020, counterpunch.org. His views are more fully expounded in *Rebellion in America: Citizen Uprisings, the News Media, and the Politics of Plutocracy* (New York: Routledge, 2020) and *Unequal America: Class Conflict, the News Media, and Ideology in the Era of Record Inequality* (New York: Routledge, 2021).
8 Noam Chomsky with C.J. Polychroniou, *The Precipice: Neoliberalism, the Pandemic, and the Urgent Need for Social Change* (Chicago: Haymarket Books, 2021), 73.
9 See Noam Chomsky, "Remembering Howard Zinn," *Resist Newsletter*, March/April 2010, chomsky.info.

INDEX

1918–20 influenza global pandemic. *See* Great Influenza Epidemic
2008 financial crisis, 65–6, 192, 248

ableism, 130
academics, 75, 83–4, 116–17, 227–8
accumulation, 16, 18–19
activism and scholarship, 83–4, 116–17
Adkins, Lisa, 68
Advani, Lal Krishna, 152
affordable housing, 56
Africa, 40, 115, 283
African Americans, 107, 162, 166–7, 185–6, 282, 284. *See also* civil rights; segregation
AIDS. *See* HIV/AIDS
Air India Tragedy, 166, 167–8
air travel/trade, 46. *See also* tourism
Alberta, 74, 81
alien life, 264
All Health Politics is Local (Chowkwanyun), 173
Allende, Salvador, 44, 278
Alliance for Progress, 49
Alma Ata Declaration, 44
Alzheimer's disease, 107
Amazon (corporation), 8, 45
Amazon (forest), 95
American Federal Reserve, 65–6
anarchism, 32–4, 93–4, 280
Anderson, Perry, 66, 189
anger, 91–2, 96–7, 165
Angus, Ian, 5
animals. *See* bats; factory farms; zoonotic diseases
Antarctica, 1
antibiotic-resistant bacteria, 274–5
antiracism, 157
antivax movement, 233
apartheid, 283

Aronowitz, Robert, 174
Asia, 111. *See also* China
Asian Canadians/Americans, 161–3, 166. *See also* Chinese Canadians/Americans
Asian Tsunami, 254–5
austerity, 260
Australia, 90
automation, 4, 78, 79
Automation and the Future of Work (Benanav), 78
Avian Flu in 2003, 41

bacteria, 274–5
Baer, Hans, 104, 113
bailout economy, 269, 277
Baker, Michael, 238–9
banks, 269
Bannon, Steve, 255
Barcelona, 206
bats, 1, 9, 20, 41–2, 85–6, 216–17
Benanav, Aaron, 78, 79–80
Benjamin, Walter, 75–6
Bharatiyia Janata Party (BJP), 153
Bhattacharya, Tithi, 145–59; about, 145. *See also Feminism for the 99%*
Biden, Joe, 149–50, 241, 271, 275
Big Farms, Big Flu (Wallace), 40
Big Pharma, 44, 45
biomedical model, 104–5, 111–12
biosocial model, 104–5, 108
Black Lives Matter, 22–3, 37, 53, 157–8
Bloomberg, Michael, 254
Bolsheviks, 88
Bolsonaro, Jair, 61, 95
branding, 259
Brazil, 61, 94–5
Brexit, 276
Britain, 47, 276

British Columbia, 99–100, 197, 198, 250–1
Brown, Wendy, 70, 75
bubbles, 131–2, 142
Bulled, Nicola, 118–19
Bush, George W., 271
bush meat, 40

Cahill, Damien, 61
Calgary School, 59
Canada, 99–100, 111, 123–6, 154–5, 165. *See also various provinces*
Canada Emergency Response Benefit (CERB), 128, 131, 136, 295n7
Capital (Marx), 32
Capital attack (2021), 43
capitalism: overview, 28; and care work, 17, 21–2; China vs. US, 217; contradictions, 16, 17–18, 19; Covid-19 pandemic as perfect storm, 15, 23; and ecology, 17, 20, 22 (*See also* climate change); effects of, 215; and enclosures, 258–9; and expropriation, 18; and fossil fuels, 78; "golden age," 267; and governance, 19; and hegemony, 19; and imperialism, 18; impulses of, 147–8; laissez-faire capitalism, 26; logical capitalism, 46; and neoliberalism, 62, 63–5 (*See also* neoliberalism); New Deal capitalism, 26, 267; as primed for crisis, 19, 24; priorities of, 150; and public power, 18–19, 20–1; and racism, 22; relation to noneconomic conditions, 17, 19; and robo-automatic Marxism, 189; and sacrificial zones, 249; social democratic, 26, 28–9; vs. socialism, 49; surveillance capitalism, 259. *See also* neoliberalism
Capitalism: A Conversation in Critical Theory (Fraser), 15, 24, 27, 34
care work, 17, 21–2. *See also* health care
caregivers. *See* essential workers
Carter, Jimmy, 267
case-fatality rate (CFR), 10

categorical inequality, 179
cell phones, 69
Chakraborty, Chandrima, 161–72; about, 161
Chamayou, Grégoire, 65
cheap goods, 68–9
cheap labour, 96
Chicago School, 278
Chile, 44, 278
Chin, Vincent, 296n4
China: blaming, 219; as challenging US, 271–3; emissions, 96; Great Leap Forward, 300n14; lockdowns, 88, 239; and neoliberalism, 68; popular organizing, 51; and SARS, 111, 240; US military and Covid, 164; and WHO, 42
Chinese Canadians/Americans, 161–4, 296n3
Chomsky, Noam, 263–87; about, 263
Chowkwanyun, Merlin, 173–94; about, 173
Christianity, 51
Churchill, Winston, 168
CIO, 283
civil rights, 162, 281–2, 286
class: alliances, 8; analysis of, 190; as ascriptive category, 189; and Covid-19 pandemic deaths, 191; defined, 188; discussions of, 47; and earthquakes, 86–7; essential workers, 23; in India, 48; and Indian migration, 154; and intersectionality, 188; and migration, 154; and race intersection, 166–7, 177; and racialized people, 23; as relational, 8; SES approach to, 188. *See also* essential workers; subalterns; working class
class war, 266–7, 269, 270, 278, 300n3
climate change: and academia, 83; and anger, 91–2, 96–7; bats and bridging species, 20; in BC, 250–1; climate strikes, 282; commitment to fighting, 250–1; COP26, 250; vs. Covid quarantines, 88; vs. Covid-19 pandemic,

302 / CRISIS AND CONTAGION

88–9, 91; and Democratic Party, 265; deniers, 250, 265; and global effort, 80; and Global North, 91, 92–3; and Global South, 89, 93; goals, 80; and gradualism, 98–9; and historians, 87–8; and infectious diseases, 113; and intergenerational movements, 252; and Republican Party, 46, 265–6; and Senate Energy and Natural Resources Committee, 265; and tourism, 208; and unions, 251; and white supremacy, 261; and working class, 92; as youth movement, 93, 100
Climate Change and Social Inequality (Singer), 112–13
Clinton, Bill, 269
Clinton, Hillary, 31
coal, 96
Coal Ash disaster, 193
Cold War, 11, 49. *See also* New Cold War
collapsology, 244–5
collectivity, 70
Colombia, 279
colonialism, 47, 60, 259
"Color of Coronavirus" project, 166–7
commemoration, 139–40, 167–9, 232, 243–4
commensalism, 109–10
commodification, 216
commodities, 17, 216, 259
common sense, 6–7, 287, 290n21
community, 127, 140, 142
comorbidities, 106, 107, 114–15, 128–30
complacency, 237. *See also* passivity
conservation, 204–5
conspiracy theories, 164, 254–5, 261, 276, 277, 296n8
conspirituality, 261
consumption, 3, 69
Contagion (film), 9
contradictions, 16, 17–18, 19
control trials, 114
Cooper, Melinda, 68
COP26, 250

Copenhagen, 149
Corona, Climate, Chronic Emergency (Malm), 78, 79, 86, 88–9
coronavirus. *See* Covid-19 pandemic; Covid-19 pandemic deaths; Covid-19 virus
corporate livestock, 5, 39–41, 274
corporations, 45, 268–9
Couldrey, Nick, 259
Coutts border crossing, 74
"Covid Racial Data Tracker," 184
"Covid Tracking Project," 184
Covid-19 pandemic: overview, 1; allowing spread of, 54; as anticipated/predicted, 41–2, 55; avoiding, 90; vs. climate change, 88–9, 91; commemorating, 139–40, 168–9, 232, 243, 244; as contemporary history, 138; as finished, 109, 110, 231–3; Global South vs. North reactions, 89; as group of syndemics, 106; historical accounts, 8–9, 191–2; as one-off, 8–9, 10; and other diseases, 106, 107, 115, 129–30; social factors involved, 106, 107; and social movements, 90–1; as teacher, 256
Covid-19 pandemic deaths: and class, 191; and comorbidities, 129–30; and gender, 130; institutionalized seniors, 55; Latinos, 46; and lockdowns, 237–8; and media reporting, 138; and milestones of deaths, 139, 191, 232–3; as multifaceted, 169; number of, 80; and Pinker's ideas, 291n27; as preventable, 46; and Republican Party, 46; and variants, 110
COVID-19: Social Inequalities and Human Possibilities (Ryan), 217–18
Covid-19 virus, 1, 20, 109–10, 164, 289n1
creative destruction, 69
Crehan, Kate, 6
crisis, 19, 24–6, 27
critical materialist interpretation, 10
critical medical anthropology, 104, 117
Critical Race Theory, 37, 284

critical utopian energy, 193–4
Cuba, 42
Cuomo, Andrew, 253–4
customs, 185–6

dads, 130
Dakota Access Pipeline, 252
data colonialism, 259
data sets, 173, 174, 183–4, 242
Davis, Mike, 39–57, 76; about, 39
Day, Iyko, 161
deaths from Covid. *See* Covid-19 pandemic deaths
debt, 35–6
Deep State, 77
deforestation, 5, 20, 89, 94–5
deglobalization, 70–1
democracy, 280–1
Democratic Party, 45–6, 265, 275
Denmark, 139
deregulation, 269
despair, 281
developmental crisis, 26
DeVos, Betsy, 285
digital content, 243–4
DiMaggio, Tony, 276–7
disability activists, 128
disasters, 86–7, 97
diversity, 165
Doomsday Clock, 264, 271
Durable Inequality (Tilly), 179

earthquakes, 86–7
Ebola, 42
ecological Marxism, 85
ecology, 17, 20, 22, 29, 86–7, 274. *See also* climate change; metabolic rift thesis
ecopolitics, 37
ecosyndemics, 112–13
education, 51, 165, 170–1, 284–6. *See also* schools
electoral politics, 76
elimination of Covid, 238–9
elite dominance, 76–7
enclosures, 258–9

Engels, Frederick, 46–7
entrepreneurs, 68, 69
environmental crisis, 274. *See also* climate change
Environmental Protection Agency, 29
epidemiologists, 192, 193
epochal crisis, 26
essential workers: overview, 22; Chinese Canadians as, 163–4; and class and race intersection, 167; defined, 23; as disrespected, 191; in health care, 50, 53; vs. investment banking, 145; protecting, 281
European Union, 42
evolution of viruses, 48, 108, 109, 110, 236
exclusive zones, 272
expert knowledge, 73–4

factory farms, 5, 39–41, 274
farm workers, 46
Farmer, Paul, 104–5
fascism, 11, 88, 152–3, 261, 270
fatalism, 194, 245
Fauci, Anthony, 109, 117
fear, 127, 132–3
feminism, 30–1, 157–8
Feminism for the 99% (Arruzza, Fraser, and Bhattacharya), 31, 145, 146–7
feminist strike, 146
Ferguson, Sue, 154, 155–6, 157–8
Fermi Paradox, 264
Fernandes, Clinton, 272
fictional commodities, 216
Fields, Barbara and Karen, 177, 186
financial institutions, 269
First World War, 11, 26, 47, 235, 243
On Fire (Klein), 251, 257
Flanagan, Tom, 67
Floyd, George, 92, 159
flu. *See* Great Influenza Epidemic; influenza
Fonda, Jane, 252
food, 115–16
forgetfulness, 192. *See also* memory

Forgotten Pandemic, The (study), 111
Fossil Capital (Malm), 78
fossil fuels, 5, 87–8, 96, 265–6, 297n19
Foster, John Bellamy, 84–5
France, 245, 273
Francis (pope), 49, 247
Fraser, Doug, 267, 300n3
Fraser, Nancy, 15–37; about, 15
free trade agreements, 269
Freedom Convoy, 73, 74, 75, 81, 127
French fries, 209
Friedman, Milton, 268, 285

Gates, Bill, 254
gay men, 11, 104, 130
GDP, 68
gender, 129–30
general crisis, 25–6, 27
gentrification, 57
George, Henry, 56
Germany, 275
global interconnectedness, 224
Global North, 7–8, 36, 89, 91, 92–3, 99
global public health, 46
Global South: and climate change, 89, 93; and Covid-19 pandemic, 99; feminism for the 99%, 31; migration, 4, 14, 87, 162; and pandemics, 9–10; tourism (*See* tourism); and vaccines, 7–8
global warming. *See* climate change
globalization, 70–2, 218, 283
gradualism, 98–9
Gramsci, Antonio: and common sense, 6; and intersectionality, 290n19; Modern Prince theme, 98, 279–80; organic crisis, 24; on pessimism/optimism, 36–7; pillars of hegemony, 28; on working class, 8
Great Influenza Epidemic: accessing knowledge of, 111–12; authorities reactions to, 111; and big picture, 243; commemorating, 140, 243; commensalism, 109; Covid following pattern of, 111; as Covid-19 pandemic reference point, 9, 194, 236–7; humans shaping, 236; in India, 47; as "Spanish Flu," 241; tone of presentation, 111–12; virus and bacterium, 109; and vulnerabilities, 236
Green New Deal, 248, 251, 256
Greenspan, Alan, 66
grief, 141–2
growth imperative, 249–50

Harper, Stephen, 59
Harvey, David, 199–200
Hayek, F. A., 61, 66
health care: antibiotic-resistant bacteria, 274–5; care work, 17, 21–2; countries missing, 43; data sets, 176, 183–4; as eroded, 21, 43; global public health, 46; and historians, 173–4; investing in, 256–7; mental hospitals, 56; national vs. local, 173; outcomes, 176; privatization, 260; public health education, 50; and racial disparities, 173–4; research funding, 174–6; sexual health, 131; social medicine, 43–4; workers, 50, 53–4
hegemony, 19, 28, 30, 31, 69–70
Herring, Ann, 103, 109, 111–12, 119
Hinduism, 151–2, 153, 296n6, 296n8
Hispanic Health Council, 103–4, 115–16, 117
Hitler, Adolf, 152
HIV/AIDS: commonalities, 108; deaths from, 9, 112; in Hartford, 104; and inequality, 223–4; as "supply driven," 42; syndemic patterns, 114–15
Hobbes, Thomas, 51
Hobsbawm, Eric, 192
homelessness, 52, 55–6
homophobia, 222
hope, 53, 117–18, 171
Horton, Richard, 1–2, 106, 237
"How Not to Skip Class" (Bhattacharya), 149
How to Blow up a Pipeline (Malm), 79
Hurricane Katrina, 254, 255

INDEX / 305

Hurricane Maria, 254, 255
hyperindividualism. *See* individualism

identitarians, 187
immigration, 97, 162, 165, 166. *See also* migration
immunological humanities, 48
imperialism, 18
inconvenient truth, 250
India, 47–8, 115, 151–4, 170
Indigenous Peoples, 48, 284–5
individualism, 62, 70, 125, 140–1, 220–1
inequality: 0.1% of population, 269; 1% of population, 268; categorical inequality, 179; class divisions, 6; diseases reflecting, 105, 107; as element in Covid-19 pandemic, 1–2; and emissions, 92, 93; in Global North, 8, 36; and Great Influenza Epidemic, 111, 238; and HIV/AIDS, 223–4; and medicine, 223; and neoliberalism, 68; and vaccines, 7–8, 220; and workplace, 186. *See also* syndemics
influenza, 10, 39, 41, 237. *See also* Great Influenza Epidemic
innovations, 69
insurance companies, 45
interconnectedness, 224
interdependence, 169
Intergovernmental Panel on Climate Change, 266
International Women's Day, 146
internationalism, 49, 100–1, 283
Internet, 140, 142–3, 243–4, 253. *See also* social media
intersectional feminism, 157–8
intersectionality, 156–7, 166–7, 177, 187–9, 290n19
Introduction to Syndemics (Singer), 115, 118
investigative journalism, 137–8
Islamophobia, 152–3
isolation, 127, 141, 260

January sixth riot, 46

jobs, 52

Kaplan, E. Ann, 91
Kathmandu, 196, 199–203, 205–6
Keating, Paul, 271
Kennedy, John F., 286
Kenney, Jason, 74
Klein, Naomi, 247–61; about, 247
Koch Brothers, 265–6
Konings, Martijn, 61, 68
Krippner, Greta, 64

lab leak theory, 164
laissez-faire capitalism, 26
land, 56–7
Late Victorian Holocausts (Davis), 47
Latinos, 46, 167. *See also* Hispanic Health Council
Lawson, Nigel, 247, 249–50
lean-in feminism, 146
Leap Manifesto, 257–8
leftists: overview of Covid response, 72–3; academics, 75; and Alberta border blockade, 74; and anarcho-libertarian politics, 93–4; and community, 127; hope for Covid-19 pandemic, 11; left melancholia, 76; media of, 136–7; and neoliberalism as term, 62; and populism, 72–3, 77; rethinking strategies, 11–12; and social media, 100–1; and visions of alternatives, 74–6; and working class, 34; and Zionist pressure, 159
Lehman Brothers, 66
LGBTQ+, 130, 131, 222
liberal feminism, 30–1
liberalism, 11, 67, 73, 123–4
libertarian socialism, 280
libertarians, 280
Lippmann Colloquium, 67
lockdowns/quarantines: and borders, 218; bubbles, 131–2, 142; in China, 88, 239; vs. climate crisis, 88; of countries by neoliberalism, 48–9; and deaths, 237–8; fatigue from, 142; in India, 153;

and loneliness, 141; as patchwork, 226, 239; schools, 132–4; as term, 227; timing of, 225–6, 239
Locke, John, 67
logical capitalism, 46
long-term-care facilities (LTC), 54–5, 137–8
loneliness, 141
Lorde, Audre, 165
Loreto, Nora, 123–43; about, 123
"Love jihad" campaign, 154, 296n8
Loveman, Mara, 187
Lula, 95

Macpherson, C. B., 27
malaria, 223
Malm, Andreas, 78–80, 83–101, 250; about, 83–4
malnourishment, 115
Malthus, Thomas Robert, 244, 245
Manchin, Joe, 265, 266–7
Markel, Howard, 194
Marxism, 32, 79, 85, 155–6, 189
masking, 110, 225, 226, 255
materialist analysis, 155–6
McCain, John, 265
McCarthyism, 190
McNally, David, 156, 157
meat production, 274
media, 123–6, 129–30, 136–8, 165
media consolidation, 124
medical trials, 114
medicine as social science, 116
Mejias, Ulises A., 259
memory, 230, 232–3, 236–7, 242–3. See also commemoration
Mendenhall, Emily, 106, 110
mental hospitals, 56
Message from the Future (film), 256
metabolic rift thesis: vs. conventional theories, 9; defined, 39, 84–5, 274; history of, 5; and O'Connor, 40; and Singer, 113
metaphors, 231
migrant workers, 162, 167

migration, 4, 87, 154, 162. *See also* immigration
military bases, 272
Mill, John Stuart, 66
Miller, Arthur, 263
mining, 279
Ministry for the Future, The (Robinson, Kim Stanley), 93
mitigation/suppression, 239
model minority stereotype, 161, 164–5
model-builders, 192, 193
"Modern Prince" (Gramsci), 98, 280
Modi, Narendra, 151, 152–3, 159
money, 35–6
Monster at Our Door, The (Davis), 39–40, 52
Monster Enters, The (Davis), 39
Mont Pelerin Society, 67
Montevideo, 244
Moore, Jason, 85
Morrison, Scott, 90
Mount Everest, 199–203. *See also* Nepal
Mucormycosis, 115
Muslims, 152–3, 296n8
mutual aid, 143

nation terminologies, 217–18
National Institutes of Health (NIH), 175–6
National Union of Nurses, 50
nationalism, 71–2, 168, 170, 218–19, 279
nationalization, 94
Native Americans, 48
neoliberalism: and capitalism, 62, 63–5 (*See also* capitalism); Covid-19 pandemic as most negative aspect of, 70–1; death of, 27–8, 45, 81–2; Deep State, 77; defined, 278–9; and entrepreneurs, 69; and feminism, 30–1; and hegemony, 69–70; history of, 26, 60, 61–2, 63–6, 258–9; in India, 152–4; and individualism, 62, 70, 220–1; and inequality, 68; interpreted, 278; and Klein's writing, 248–9; and liberalism, 67; literature influencing

Canadians, 60; and lockdowns, 48–9; logic of rule, 7; market rule, 67; Penner studying, 59–60; progressive, 31; and race intersection, 179–80; as repackaged, 27; and right wing, 75–6; vs. social democratic capitalism, 28–9; and social medicine, 44–5; and social reproduction, 147; strengths of, 67–8; as term, 61–3; and tourism, 206; as unoriginal, 66; and wages, 269
Nepal, 199–202, 205–6, 209
Nepal, Sanjay, 195–209; about, 195
New Cold War, 11, 163–4, 241, 271–2
New Deal, 267, 275, 282, 283
New Deal capitalism, 26, 267
New Zealand, 131
No Is Not Enough (Klein), 247, 248
No Logo (Klein), 249
"normal," 74, 82, 171–2
nostalgia, 258
nuclear war, 52, 264, 271, 272
nursing homes, 54–5, 137–8

Obama, Barack, 277
obesity, 115
Ocasio-Cortez, Alexandria, 257
Occupational Health and Safety Administration (OSHA), 54
Occupy Wall Street, 33
O'Connor, Jim, 40
Offner, Amy, 59–60, 63
oil industry, 266
Old Gods, New Enigmas (Davis), 50
Old Order Is Dying and the New Cannot Be Born, The (Fraser), 15
Ontario, 135
Ostrach, Bayla, 118–19
outcomes, 176

Pale Rider (Spinney), 235, 243
Palestinians, 159
pandemics: and animals (*See* zoonotic diseases); as continuing, 10, 20, 43, 112, 231–2, 256–7; downplaying, 8–9; humans shaping, 236; number per century, 239; and passivity, 235
panic, 117, 237
passivity, 90, 235, 241
Pearson, Lester, 279
Penner, Mack, 59–82; about, 59
physical distancing, 225
Pinker, Steven, 291n27
podcasts, 137
Polanyi, Karl, 216
polio, 112
political autonomy, 6
Polychroniou, C. J., 274
popular self-help, 51
populism, 28, 72–5, 76–7
postmodernism, 87
potable water, 48
poverty: and Alzheimers, 107; diseases of, 114; as element in Covid-19 pandemic, 1–2; and food, 115; and protein consumption, 40; as reduced, 68
Precipice, The (Chomsky and Polychroniou), 274, 279–80, 281
pretrauma, 91
prisons, 56
privatization, 255, 260
production, 3, 16
professionalization, 228
profit: and antibiotic-resistant bacteria, 274–5; and climate change, 5, 20; corporations' responsibility, 268; and deforestation, 20; in disasters, 45; and fossil fuels, 78; neoliberalism megamachine, 4; vs. people, 147, 148; sacrifice for, 150–1; and senior citizens, 6–7
Progress of This Storm, The (Malm), 85
progressive neoliberalism, 31
protectionism, 28
protein consumption, 40
protests as episodic, 159
public power, 18–19, 20–1
Puerto Rico, 254

quantitative easing (QE), 66
quarantines. *See* lockdowns/quarantines
Quebec, 133, 134–5

race, 166–7, 177–80, 181–9
"Race, Class, Crisis" (Chowkwanyun and Reed), 176, 183, 185
Race for Profit (Taylor), 35
race-baiting, 164–5
Racecraft (Fields and Fields), 186
racialized people, 18, 23, 161, 165, 175. *See also* essential workers; *various groups*
racism: anti-Asian, 163–5, 166, 296n4; and aphoristic statements, 178; and capitalism, 22; Chin murder, 163, 296n4; and global environmental load, 22; neologisms of, 180–2; NIH funding, 176; opportunistic racists, 35; and real estate, 35; structural, 22, 35, 176, 180–1. *See also* antiracism; Black Lives Matter; white supremacy
Rand, Ayn, 67
Rashtriya Swayamsevak Sangh (RRS), 152–3
Ratha Yatra, 152
Reagan, Ronald, 267–8, 269, 283
realm of necessity/freedom, 79
recovery period, 194
red scare, 190, 283
Reed, Adolph, 176, 183, 185, 187
Republican Party, 46, 265–6, 275, 284
responsibility, 47, 51, 125, 263, 268
revolutionary change, 143
right wing: and Alberta border blockade, 74; combatting, 281; and conspiracy theories, 261, 276, 277; and Critical Race Theory, 37, 284; and neoliberalism, 75–6; and "normality," 74, 82, 171–2; and populism (*See* populism); and skepticism, 73–4
Roberts, Michael, 65
Rodgers, Daniel, 60
Rumsfeld, Donald, 256

Ryan, J. Michael, 213–34; about, 213

sabotage, 79, 80
Sanders, Bernie, 49, 50, 76, 275
SARS, 240
Scandinavia, 148–9. *See also various countries*
Scheidler, Fabian, 4
Schmidt, Eric, 253–4
schools, 132–5, 150, 228, 254–5, 284–6. *See also* education
science, 229–30
screen new deal, 253
Second Red Scare, The (Storrs), 190
Second World War, 5
sectoral crisis, 25–6
segregation, 149, 282, 285, 286
Senate Energy and Natural Resources Committee, 265
senior citizens, 6–7, 54–5, 137–8
sex workers, 131
sexual health, 131
Sherpas, 200–1, 205, 209
Shock Doctrine, The (Klein), 247, 248, 253–4, 256
Simon, Roger, 170–1
Singer, Merrill, 2, 103–19; about, 103
Sinophobia, 162–3
skepticism, 74
slavery, 18, 284
Slobodian, Quinn, 65
smart phones, 69
Smith, Adam, 265
SNCC (Student Nonviolent Coordinating Committee), 281–2, 286–7
social democracy, 267, 275
social democratic capitalism, 26, 28–9
social media, 100–1, 178
social medicine, 43–4. *See also* health care
social murder, 46–7
Social Reproduction (Bhattacharya), 149

social reproduction theory, 147–8, 154–5, 157–8
social vs. physical distancing, 225
socialism, 49. *See also* Marxism
socioeconomic status (SES) approach, 188
solidarity, 49, 165–6
Sorting Out the Mixed Economy (Offner), 59–60, 63
South Africa, 283
"Spanish Flu." *See* Great Influenza Epidemic
Spencer, Herbert, 61, 66
Spin Doctors (Loreto), 123, 128–9, 135, 138–9, 143.
Spinney, Laura, 235–46; about, 235
Squad, the, 31
Sridhar, Devi, 236
Standing Rock, 252
stereotypes, 161–3
stigmatization, 184
stimulus, 35–6
Storrs, Landon R. Y., 190
"Strange Disappearance of History from Racial Health Disparities Research" (Chowkwanyun), 173
structural racism, 22, 35, 176, 181
subalterns: and class and race intersection, 166–7; as heroes, 11; killed by Covid-19, 22; and political autonomy, 6; uniting, 11. *See also various groups*
submarines, 272–3
Superfund, 29
supersyndemics, 113
surveillance capitalism, 259
Sweden, 90, 96–7
Syndemic Magazine, 1–3
syndemics: overview, 214–15; defined, 105–6; and disease treatment, 108; ecosyndemics, 112–13; and ethnography, 119; evolution of, 118–19; growth of, 119; local, 106; and social factors, 106, 107; supersyndemics, 113; as term, 1–2, 105–6

Tam, Theresa, 164–5
taxes, 268, 270, 280–1
teaching to test, 285–6
techno-feudalism, 69
technology, 4, 78, 79, 253–4, 264. *See also* Internet; social media
Tennessee, 193, 297n19
testing and tracing, 226, 240
Thatcher, Margaret, 267, 268, 270, 283, 295n5
Third World urbanization, 39
This Changes Everything (Klein), 247, 248–9, 250
Thunberg, Greta, 117–18, 251, 252–3, 271
ticks, 113
Tilly, Charles, 179, 187
Toohey, Brian, 272–3
Tooze, Adam, 27–8, 66
Toronto, 167
Toronto Star (newspaper), 137–8
tourism: overview, 196–7, 198–9; as business, 196; and climate change, 208; as human right, 203–4; and masks, 225; Nepal, 199–203, 205–6, 209; S. Nepal overview, 195–6; and poverty, 204–5; prohibited, 203–4; resistance to, 206; spreading viruses, 208; Valemount, BC, 197–8
ToxicDocs, 173
transnational history, 182
transnational organizations, 94–5
transphobia, 222
trauma, 91, 140, 141
Trente Glorieuses, 267
Trotsky, Leon, 57
Trump, Donald: 2016 elections, 31; as brand, 259; China and Covid, 164; and Doomsday Clock, 264; and feminism, 146; handling of Covid pandemic, 230; and OSHA, 54; supporters as racists, 35; tax scam, 270; and Virology Institute, 41
Trump voters, 35, 276–7
two-earner family, 29

unions: overview, 287; Canada vs. US, 283–4; and climate change, 92, 251; and protection, 150; and public social care system, 148; United Mine Workers, 266–7; voting Republican, 277
United Auto Workers, 267
United Mine Workers, 266–7
United Nations, 48, 62
United Nations World Tourism Organization (UNWTO), 204
United States national public health system, 183
universal basic income, 150
universal health care, 43–4
"Uses of Anger" (Lorde), 165
utopia, 79–80

vaccines: antivax movement, 233; cost of, 269–70; and Covid predictions, 43; and evolution of viruses, 236; as focus, 256–7; and Global North/South, 7–8; and India, 47; and inequality, 7–8, 220; nationalism of, 170; political resistance to, 110; and profit, 45
Valemount, BC, 197–8
variants, 110
Venice, 206
Vietnam, 50, 111
Vietnam War, 286
Virchow, Rudolf, 43, 116
Virology Institute, 41
Vitamin D, 185

wages, 269
Wallace, Rob, 40
war as metaphor, 240–1
West Africa, 40
Western Front, 236
wet markets, 41. *See also* factory farms
White Skin, Black Fuel (Malm and Zetkin Collective), 83, 88

white supremacy, 261, 276–7, 284, 285. *See also* racism
Wiesner, Ben, 86
wildlife trading, 86
Wilson, Woodrow, 283
women: and care work, 17, 21–2; in India, 47–8; and Marxist theory, 32; rights of, 282; women's movement, 287. *See also* feminism
Woods, Bretton, 28, 29
work, 36, 78–9, 96, 150–1
working class: beyond workplace, 8; and climate change, 92; and conspiracy theories, 276; and historical agency, 50; and inequality in Global North, 36; leftists condescending to, 34; and Obama, 277; as topic, 227–8; United Mine Workers, 266–7. *See also* unions
workplaces, 186
World Health Organization (WHO), 42, 44, 241
Wuest, Joanna, 177
Wuhan, China, 51, 164, 239

yellow peril stereotype, 161
York University, 154–5
young people, 7, 53, 251–3, 282

Zelner, Jon, 193
Zetkin Collective, 83, 88
Zinn, Howard, 281
zoonotic diseases: overview, 259; animals meeting, 9; and capitalist development, 41, 216–17; case-fatality rate, 10–11; and deforestation, 85–6; and factory farms, 5; and passivity, 90
Zubov, Shoshanna, 259